369 0240061

Fundamentals of
Revision Knee Arthroplasty
Diagnosis, Evaluation, and Treatment

Fundamentals of
Revision Knee Arthroplasty
Diagnosis, Evaluation, and Treatment

EDITED BY

David J. Jacofsky, MD
Chairman
The CORE Institute
Center for Orthopedic Research and Education
Phoenix, Arizona

Anthony K. Hedley, MD, FRCS
Arizona Institute for Bone & Joint Disorders
Phoenix, Arizona

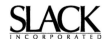

SLACK
INCORPORATED

www.Healio.com/books

ISBN: 978-1-55642-974-3

Copyright © 2013 by SLACK Incorporated

The procedures and practices described in this publication should be implemented in a manner consistent with the professional standards set for the circumstances that apply in each specific situation. Every effort has been made to confirm the accuracy of the information presented and to correctly relate generally accepted practices. The authors, editors, and publisher cannot accept responsibility for errors or exclusions or for the outcome of the material presented herein. There is no expressed or implied warranty of this book or information imparted by it. Care has been taken to ensure that drug selection and dosages are in accordance with currently accepted/recommended practice. Off-label uses of drugs may be discussed. Due to continuing research, changes in government policy and regulations, and various effects of drug reactions and interactions, it is recommended that the reader carefully review all materials and literature provided for each drug, especially those that are new or not frequently used. Some drugs or devices in this publication have clearance for use in a restricted research setting by the Food and Drug and Administration or FDA. Each professional should determine the FDA status of any drug or device prior to use in their practice.

Any review or mention of specific companies or products is not intended as an endorsement by the author or publisher.

SLACK Incorporated uses a review process to evaluate submitted material. Prior to publication, educators or clinicians provide important feedback on the content that we publish. We welcome feedback on this work.

Published by: SLACK Incorporated
6900 Grove Road
Thorofare, NJ 08086 USA
Telephone: 856-848-1000
Fax: 856-848-6091
www.Healio.com/books

Contact SLACK Incorporated for more information about other books in this field or about the availability of our books from distributors outside the United States.

Library of Congress Cataloging-in-Publication Data

Jacofsky, David J.
Fundamentals of revision knee arthroplasty : diagnosis, evaluation, and treatment / [edited by] David J. Jacofsky and Anthony K. Hedley. -- 1st ed.
    p. ; cm.
 Includes bibliographical references and index.
 ISBN 978-1-55642-974-3 (hbk. : alk. paper)
 I. Jacofsky, David J. II. Hedley, Anthony K.
  [DNLM: 1. Arthroplasty, Replacement, Knee--methods. 2. Knee Joint--surgery. 3. Knee Prosthesis. 4. Periprosthetic Fractures--surgery. 5. Reoperation--methods. WE 870]

 617.5'820592--dc23

2012031399

Printed in the United States of America.

Last digit is print number: 10 9 8 7 6 5 4 3 2 1

DEDICATION

To my mentors... you know who you are.
David J. Jacofsky, MD

To my fellows, past and present.
Anthony K. Hedley, MD, FRCS

CONTENTS

ABOUT THE EDITORS

David J. Jacofsky, MD was born in Long Island, New York and is an international authority on adult reconstruction of the hip and knee. He received his residency training at the Mayo Clinic in Rochester, Minnesota and did his fellowship training at Johns Hopkins University in Baltimore, Maryland, during which time he was awarded the Mayo Scholar's Award and the Joe Janes' Humanitarian Award. Dr. Jacofsky started his career as an attending at the Mayo Clinic and subsequently moved to Phoenix, Arizona where he founded The Center for Orthopedic Research and Education (CORE) Institute. Dr. Jacofsky has published over 40 articles and 20 book chapters and has lectured around the world. He has a keen interest in health care reform, cost containment, improved outcomes, and the changing demographics of arthroplasty. Dr. Jacofsky is an avid martial artist and enjoys weight-lifting and running.

Anthony K. Hedley, MD, FRCS is a fellow of the Royal College of Surgeons of Edinburgh and an acclaimed orthopedic surgeon, author, researcher, and educator specializing in joint reconstruction.

After graduating from medical school in South Africa, Dr. Hedley completed his general and orthopedic residency training at Natalspruit Hospital in Johannesburg. He then sat for the exams and was named a Fellow of The Royal College of Surgeons of Edinburgh. Dr. Hedley returned to South Africa to complete an orthopedic residency at Johannesburg General Hospital. After, having registered as a Specialist Orthopedic Surgeon with the South African boards, he traveled to London and did a brief sojourn with the late, world-famous teacher and author Alan Apley at St. Thomas Hospital. Dr. Hedley came to the University of California, Los Angeles (UCLA) in 1977 to start a fellowship in Orthopedic Bioengineering with Dr. Harlan Amstutz of the Division of Orthopedic Surgery at UCLA. This was followed by 4 years in the Junior Professor ranks as an Assistant Professor.

Dr. Hedley left UCLA at the end of 1982 and moved to Phoenix, Arizona to join a private practice partnership. He served as the Chairman of the Department of Orthopedics at St. Luke's Hospital from 1987 to 2005. He became an inventor with Howmedica in 1982. He is currently an inventor and consultant with Stryker Orthopaedics and is involved in several clinical research projects.

Dr. Hedley is well known in the arthroplasty world for his various contributions both from the podium and in referee journals. He has headed a joint replacement fellowship since 1983 and continues to do so. From this, he is now associated with 45 fellows who have gone out into the community to continue their work as hip or knee arthroplasty surgeons.

CONTRIBUTING AUTHORS

Christopher L. Anderson, MD (Chapter 12)
Fellow
Adult Joint Reconstruction
Department of Orthopedics
RUSH University Medical Center
Chicago, Illinois

Wael K. Barsoum, MD (Chapter 7)
Department of Orthopaedic Surgery
Department of Surgical Operations
Cleveland Clinic
Cleveland, Ohio

Michael R. Bloomfield, MD (Chapter 7)
Department of Orthopaedic Surgery
Cleveland Clinic
Cleveland, Ohio

John J. Bottros, MD (Chapter 7)
Department of Orthopaedic Surgery
Cleveland Clinic
Cleveland, Ohio

Mark D. Campbell, MD (Chapter 10)
The Center for Orthopedic Research and
    Education
Phoenix, Arizona

Robert M. Cercek, MD (Chapter 4)
The Center for Orthopedic Research and
    Education
Sun City West, Arizona

Henry D. Clarke, MD (Chapter 14)
Associate Professor of Orthopedic Surgery
Mayo Clinic College of Medicine
Phoenix, Arizona

Dermot Collopy, MBBS, FRACS (Chapter 9)
Department of Orthopaedic Surgery
Royal Perth Hospital
Chairman, Western Orthopaedic Clinic
Perth, Western Australia

Craig J. Della Valle, MD (Chapter 5)
Associate Professor of Orthopedic Surgery
Director, Adult Reconstructive Fellowship
RUSH University Medical Center
Chicago, Illinois

Douglas A. Dennis, MD (Chapter 1)
Colorado Joint Replacement
Adjunct Professor of Biomedical Engineering
University of Tennessee
Knoxville, Tennessee
Adjunct Professor of Bioengineering
University of Denver
Director, Rocky Mountain Musculoskeletal
    Research Laboratory
Denver, Colorado

Ian M. Gradisar, MD (Chapter 2)
Clinical Instructor Orthopedic Surgery
Northeast Ohio Medical University
Summa Health System
Crystal Clinic Orthopaedic Center
Akron, Ohio

Curtis W. Hartman, MD (Chapter 5)
Assistant Professor
University of Nebraska Medical Center
Department of Orthopaedic Surgery and
    Rehabilitation
Omaha, Nebraska

Kirby D. Hitt, MD (Chapter 8)
Head of Adult Reconstruction & Joint
    Replacement Surgery
Scott & White Memorial Hospital
Assistant Professor
Texas A&M University
College Station, Texas

Aaron J. Johnson, MD (Chapter 11)
Rubin Institute for Advanced Orthopedics
Center for Joint Preservation and
    Reconstruction
Sinai Hospital of Baltimore
Baltimore, Maryland

Vamsi K. Kancherla, MD (Chapter 3)
St. Luke's University Health Network
Department of Orthopedics
Bethlehem, Pennsylvania

Harpal S. Khanuja, MD (Chapter 11)
Rubin Institute for Advanced Orthopedics
Center for Joint Preservation and
    Reconstruction
Sinai Hospital of Baltimore
Baltimore, Maryland

Raymond H. Kim, MD (Chapter 1)
Colorado Joint Replacement
Adjunct Associate Professor of Bioengineering
Department of Mechanical and Materials
    Engineering
University of Denver
Denver, Colorado

Viktor E. Krebs, MD (Chapter 2)
Director, Center for Adult Reconstructive
    Surgery & General Orthopaedics
Cleveland Clinic
Cleveland, Ohio

Steven M. Kurtz, PhD (Chapter 13)
Exponent Inc
Philadelphia, Pennsylvania

Michael T. Manley, FRSA, PhD (Chapter 13)
Homer Stryker Center for Orthopaedic
    Education and Research
Mahwah, New Jersey
Visiting Professor
Department of Biomechanics
University of Bath
Bath, United Kingdom

David A. McQueen, MD (Chapter 12)
Clinical Professor of Surgery (Orthopedics)
University of Kansas School of Medicine–
    Wichita
Medical Director
Orthopedic Research Institute
Wichita, Kansas

R. Michael Meneghini, MD (Chapter 6)
Director of Joint Replacement, IU Health
    Saxony Hospital
Director, IU Lower Extremity Adult
    Reconstruction Fellowship
Assistant Professor of Clinical Orthopaedic
    Surgery
Indiana University School of Medicine
Indianapolis, Indiana

Michael A. Mont, MD (Chapter 11)
Rubin Institute for Advanced Orthopedics
Center for Joint Preservation and
    Reconstruction
Sinai Hospital of Baltimore
Baltimore, Maryland

Trevor G. Murray, MD (Chapter 7)
Department of Orthopaedic Surgery
Cleveland Clinic
Cleveland, Ohio

Qais Naziri, MD (Chapter 11)
Rubin Institute for Advanced Orthopedics
Center for Joint Preservation and
    Reconstruction
Sinai Hospital of Baltimore
Baltimore, Maryland

Kevin L. Ong, PhD (Chapter 13)
Senior Managing Engineer
Exponent Inc
Philadelphia, Pennsylvania

Adam J. Schwartz, MD (Chapter 14)
Assistant Professor of Orthopedic Surgery
Mayo Clinic College of Medicine
Phoenix, Arizona

Scott M. Sporer, MD, MS (Chapter 3)
Associate Professor Orthopaedic Surgery
RUSH University Medical Center
Chicago, Illinois

Bryan D. Springer, MD (Chapter 1)
Fellowship Director
OrthoCarolina Hip and Knee Center
Charlotte, North Carolina

Joseph F. Styron, MD, PhD (Chapter 7)
Department of Orthopaedic Surgery
Cleveland Clinic
Cleveland, Ohio

Creighton C. Tubb, MD (Chapter 2)
Adjunct Assistant Professor of Surgery
Uniformed Services University of
    the Health Sciences
Bethesda, Maryland
Orthopaedic Surgery Service
Madigan Healthcare System
Tacoma, Washington

INTRODUCTION

This book is designed for surgeons who are not necessarily in the academic field, but who are encountering revisions more commonly in their practice and are capable of managing simpler revision cases. Unlike most texts in the revision arena, this text does not focus on the most difficult and challenging of cases to be tackled by experienced and high-volume revision surgeons. Rather, it is intended to guide the surgeon in the evaluation of the painful total joint replacement, review the basic tenants and principles of revision arthroplasty, and help the surgeon determine whether a given case is one he or she is competent and capable of managing, or whether it might best be managed via referral to a tertiary orthopedic center. As the number of these cases exponentially increases, this book is designed to serve as a concise resource to turn to for guidance.

This book is aimed at the orthopedic surgeon's formative years, namely residency, fellowship, and the early years of practice. The chapters have been contributed by well-known orthopedic surgeons who have expertise in the field of knee arthroplasty; their expertise is brought to the forefront with their contributions.

Evaluation of the Painful Total Knee Arthroplasty

Raymond H. Kim, MD; Bryan D. Springer, MD; and Douglas A. Dennis, MD

While total knee arthroplasty (TKA) has been a successful procedure with excellent survivorship and functional outcomes,[1-3] it is not without complications. A common patient complaint is that of a painful TKA. In the differential diagnosis, one must consider the variety of intra-articular and extra-articular causes of pain in a TKA. Evaluation of a patient with a painful TKA includes a meticulous gathering of the patient's history, a thorough physical exam, laboratory tests, possible arthrocentesis, and imaging studies. This chapter will discuss the evaluation process of the painful TKA.

DIFFERENTIAL DIAGNOSIS

The etiology of a painful TKA can be divided into intra-articular and extra-articular causes. Common intra-articular causes include infection, prosthetic loosening, instability, component failure, patellofemoral disorders, and periprosthetic osteolysis. Less common intra-articular causes include periprosthetic fracture, particulate-induced synovitis, patellar crepitus (Figure 1-1) or clunk syndrome, patellar ischemia, patellar nonresurfacing, soft tissue impingement syndrome, fabellar impingement, popliteus tendon dysfunction, component overhang, heterotopic ossification (Figure 1-2), recurrent hemarthrosis, and intramedullary stem pain. Extra-articular causes include hip pathology (arthritis, avascular necrosis, or fracture), lumbar spine pathology (degenerative disc disease or nerve root impingement), vascular disease (insufficiency, aneurysm, or thrombosis), tendinitis, bursitis, cutaneous neuromas, reflex sympathetic dystrophy, and psychological illness. A history and physical—in conjunction with appropriate laboratory and imaging testing—is then used to narrow down the differential diagnosis list.

HISTORY

Evaluation of a patient with a painful TKA begins with a meticulous gathering of the patient's history. The history begins with the initial reason for the index arthroplasty procedure.

Jacofsky DJ, Hedley AK, eds.
Fundamentals of Revision Knee Arthroplasty:
Diagnosis, Evaluation, and Treatment (pp 1-10).
© 2013 SLACK Incorporated.

Figure 1-1. Arthroscopic view of hypertrophic synovium causing patellar crepitus.

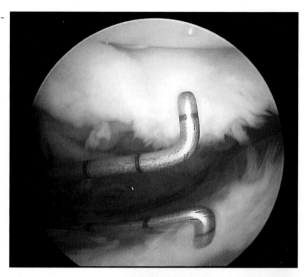

Figure 1-2. Heterotopic ossification visible on lateral radiograph.

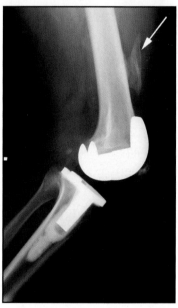

If preoperative radiographs are available, they should be reviewed to confirm the presence of end-stage arthritic changes within the knee joint. Preoperative radiographs demonstrating minimal degenerative changes should alert the surgeon to scrutinize the hip and spine even more carefully to assess for referred pain.

The characteristics of the pain should also be obtained with regard to the exact location, localization versus radiation, onset and duration of pain, the quality of the pain (sharp, aching, or burning), intensity, exacerbating activities, and ameliorating factors. Weightbearing pain must be distinguished from pain at rest. Pain with weightbearing is commonly due to prosthetic loosening or instability, while pain at rest should lead to suspicion for infection.

The chronology of events regarding the pain is also significant. If the patient was initially doing well after the TKA and then subsequently developed pain months later, diagnoses such as hematogenous seeding of infection, component loosening, or late instability should be considered. If pain relief was never obtained since the initial surgery, infection, instability, component malalignment, or nonarticular etiology must be considered. Additionally, one must consider initial misdiagnosis prior to the index procedure.

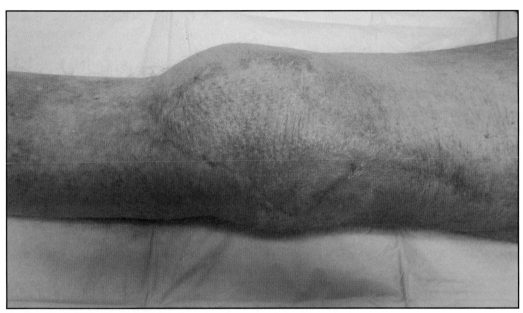

Figure 1-3. Assessment of surgical scars.

Infection should always be suspected and must be ruled out prior to moving onto other items on the differential diagnosis list. Pertinent risk factors such as history of infection prior to TKA,[4] medical conditions leading to host compromise (rheumatoid arthritis,[5] corticosteroid use,[6] diabetes,[7] malnutrition,[8] obesity,[9] or psoriatic arthritis[10]), wound healing problems or drainage after TKA, fevers, chills, or pain at rest should be investigated. Recent invasive procedures such as dental work and gastrointestinal or urogenital procedures without antibiotic prophylaxis should also be noted. Concomitant active infections should also be recognized and include pneumonia, urinary tract infections, dental abscesses, lower extremity skin ulcerations, cardiac valve vegetations, or any other condition that can lead to bacteremia.

Finally, operative records should be reviewed to determine the type of implant and the level of constraint utilized in the initial procedure, as well as any potential complications that may have occurred intraoperatively.

PHYSICAL EXAMINATION

The physical examination should be utilized by the surgeon to sequentially rule out extra-articular etiologies in the differential diagnosis list. Thus, physical examination begins with examination of the extra-articular aspects of the patient and ends with an examination of the knee itself. Starting with the general appearance of the patient, the surgeon may determine the severity and intensity of the knee pain. Acute distress may be due to an acutely septic joint or a periprosthetic fracture. Gait analysis should be performed to assess antalgia, spinal posture, hip contractures, Trendelenburg gait, and limb alignment. Thorough examination of the lumbar spine and ipsilateral hip are imperative in order to rule out radicular pain or referred hip pain. The examination of the spine includes a neurologic evaluation that pays particular attention to any motor or sensory deficits. Vascular examination is also critical not only to rule out possible claudicatory sources of pain, but to also document baseline pulses for postoperative reference.

Examination of the knee begins with the skin. Previous scars should be noted, which often paint the story of the patient's past surgical history (Figure 1-3). Old scars from arthroscopic portals, open meniscectomies, ligament reconstructions, tibial tubercle procedures, or fracture fixation may provide information that the patient may have failed to disclose either due to complex procedures not thoroughly explained to the patient, or procedures in the remote past that he or she simply could not remember. Erythema and warmth of the skin should warn the surgeon of acute inflammation and possible infection. Effusion within the knee may be assessed by ballottement of the patella, which indicates synovial irritability within the knee joint or hemarthrosis. Tenderness around the knee should be correlated with the patient's perception of whether that particular pain is consistent with his or her symptoms. The patient's knee may then be brought through both active and passive range of motion. Patellar crepitus or clunk may be clinically present with active extension of the knee but absent with passive extension. Range of motion should be documented with both active and passive flexion and extension. Extensor mechanism compromise will be apparent when there is a discrepancy between passive extension and active extension with an extension lag. Hyperextension should invoke suspicion of extensor mechanism weakness and may have resulted as a compensatory mechanism. Stability of the knee should be assessed with both varus and valgus stressing in full extension to determine collateral ligament competency. Anteroposterior stability can be assessed with the knee at 90 degrees of flexion with the patient relaxing his or her hamstrings and quadriceps. Evaluation of flexion instability may also be performed with the patient sitting with his or her knee suspended over the edge of the examination table in order to eliminate the weight of the thigh, artificially inducing a false sense of flexion stability. With the leg dependent, a gap may be balloted between the upper surface of the tibial component and the posterior condyles of the femur by pulling and pushing sharply up and down on the ankle with a stabilizing hand on the thigh. A large flexion gap may be appreciated. The effusion found with instability is often large, but the capsule and skin are soft and essentially pliable, unlike infection and inflammatory effusions. Patellar tracking should also be assessed as the knee is brought through a range of motion in order to assess maltracking or patellar tilt.

After reviewing radiographic imaging, repeating the physical examination may be warranted in order to correlate radiographic findings with the clinical findings in the physical exam.

Laboratory Tests

Laboratory analysis is utilized to distinguish septic and aseptic causes of knee pain. Hematologic evaluation should include obtaining a complete blood count with differential, erythrocyte sedimentation rate (ESR), and C-reactive protein (CRP). Although an elevated white blood cell (WBC) count is indicative of active infection, a normal count does not exclude infection.[10] After an uncomplicated TKA, the ESR is typically elevated for 3 to 6 months postoperatively.[11] Barrack et al studied the use of a preoperative ESR and observed that an ESR of greater than 30 mm/hour demonstrated a sensitivity of 80%, specificity of 62.5%, a positive predictive value of 47.1%, and a negative predictive value of 88.2% for the diagnosis of a septic TKA.[12] CRP is another acute phase reactant which peaks in 2 to 3 days after an uncomplicated TKA. An elevated CRP in conjunction with an elevated ESR has been found to be 96% sensitive and 95% specific in diagnosing infection.[13]

Arthrocentesis

Aspiration of a painful TKA is a valuable tool for evaluation of a septic joint. Barrack et al reviewed 69 revision TKA cases and found a sensitivity of 65.4%, a 96.1% specificity, an accuracy of 85.7%, a 89.5% positive predictive value, and a 84.5% negative predictive value when utilizing knee aspiration for diagnosing infection.[12] Mason et al observed a high likelihood of infection (98% sensitivity, 95% specificity) if the knee aspirate possessed greater than $2500/10^{-3}$ cm^3 WBC in conjunction with a polymorphonucleocyte (PMN) percentage of greater than 60%.[14] Similarly,

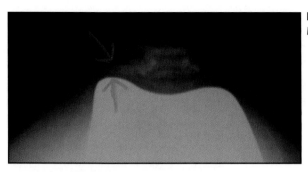

Figure 1-4. Facet impingement seen on Merchant view.

a study by Trampuz and Hanssen et al found that a WBC count of greater than 1700 or a PMN differential of greater than 65% is 97% sensitive and 98% specific for a prosthetic knee infection.[15]

RADIOGRAPHIC ANALYSIS

Radiographic evaluation includes standard anteroposterior, lateral, and Merchant views.[16] The lateral view is useful for evaluating femoral component size, sagittal alignment and component positioning, tibial slope, the presence of posterior femoral osteophytes, heterotopic ossification, component loosening, level of the joint line, and patellar baja. The Merchant view allows assessment of facet impingement (Figure 1-4) and patellar tracking. Full-length radiographs of the entire lower extremity may be indicated to evaluate extra-articular pathology such as malunion, tumor, or stress fractures that would not be visible on standard knee radiographs. Views of the hip and pelvis are also warranted when suspecting hip pathology with referred pain to the knee. As mentioned previously, preoperative radiographs prior to the initial TKA should also be reviewed, if available, to ensure substantial degenerative change was present to confirm that the knee was the true source of pain. Comparative films from previous years are also valuable to assess for progressive radiolucent lines at the fixation interface, component migration, and osteolysis. Varus or valgus stress radiographs may also be used to evaluate collateral ligamentous instability. Use of fluoroscopically guided radiographs has been described by Fehring and McAvoy to assess for component loosening.[17] Fluoroscopy is utilized to ensure that the x-ray beam is perfectly tangential to the fixation interface in order to determine the status of component fixation.

OTHER DIAGNOSTIC STUDIES

Additional types of imaging studies are available for evaluating the painful TKA. The role of nuclear medicine scans (including technetium-99m HDT, gallium citrate, indium[111]-labeled WBC scan, and the sulfur colloid bone marrow scan) have not been clearly outlined. Nuclear scans demonstrate high sensitivity with variable specificity and commonly display increased uptake for many months following an uncomplicated TKA.[18] Rand and Brown[19] reviewed 38 indium[111] scans in 18 infected and 20 noninfected cases of TKA and observed a sensitivity of 83%, a specificity of 85%, and a diagnostic accuracy of 84%. False-positive results were occasionally observed in cases of rheumatoid arthritis or those with massive osteolysis. A nuclear scan may perhaps be most useful in ruling out component loosening or infection if the scan is negative.

Computed tomography (CT) scans can be utilized for evaluation of component malrotation (Figure 1-5).[20,21] Thin axial cuts through the knee will allow assessment of femoral component rotation relative to the transepicondylar axis. Tibial component rotation can also be gauged with reference to the tibial tubercle. It is also useful in evaluating the size of osteolytic lesions.

Figure 1-5. CT scan utilized to assess component malrotation.

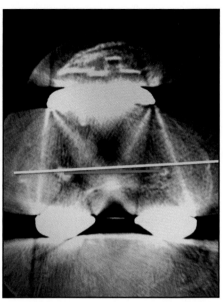

Use of magnetic resonance imaging (MRI) has been described in evaluation of the painful TKA. Sofka et al[22] performed MRI evaluations with metal subtraction software in 46 cases of problematic TKA. MRI scans were found to be of diagnostic value in 20 of the 46 cases (43.5%), providing various diagnoses including osteolysis, synovitis, bursitis, ligamentous or tendinous injury, fat pad scarring, pigmented villonodular synovitis, and intramuscular hematoma.

UNIQUE INTRA-ARTICULAR CAUSES OF PAINFUL TOTAL KNEE ARTHROPLASTY

Once the surgeon has taken a complete history, performed a thorough physical exam, and ordered the appropriate tests, the differential diagnosis list may be reassessed. Priority should be given to initially rule out extra-articular causes of knee pain prior to focusing on intra-articular etiology of pain. Once extra-articular causes have been eliminated, attention should be paid to the most common causes of TKA failure. Sharkey et al described the most common causes of failure of TKA, which include polyethylene wear, loosening, instability, infection, arthrofibrosis, and malalignment.[23] If the common modes of failure have also been ruled out, other less recognized sources of pain in a TKA may be pursued.

Particulate-induced synovitis may present months to years after TKA with a chronic knee effusion. In severe cases of polyethylene wear through the full thickness of the tibial insert or patellar button of a metal-backed patellar component, metal-on-metal crepitus may be observed. Confirmatory diagnosis is facilitated with use of aspiration with fluid analysis using polarized light microscopy or through direct visualization with arthroscopic evaluation.

Intra-articular irritation may be a source of pain in TKA. Overhang of the femoral or tibial components beyond the osseous periphery may cause painful irritation of the collateral ligaments or joint capsule. This is most commonly observed at the medial aspect of the tibia due to the close proximity of the medial collateral ligament. Slight lateral tibial component overhang is often well tolerated since the lateral collateral ligament is slightly offset from the periphery of the tibia due to its insertion onto the fibular head. Intra-articular soft tissue pain can also result from impingement of either the patellar fat pad[24] or posterior impingement due to fabellar enlargement.[25] Intra-articular soft tissue irritation can also occur from retained distal femoral osteophytes,[26] extruded bone cement, or intra-articular fibrous bands.[27] Barnes and Scott[28] described popliteus tendon dysfunction resulting in lateral pain and snapping. In this condition, the popliteus tendon typically subluxes over either a retained lateral femoral osteophyte or overhanging lateral edge of the femoral component. Heterotopic ossification may occasionally be seen postoperatively on a lateral radiograph and is usually unassociated with pain unless the osseous mass is large in size.[29]

Painful recurrent hemarthroses have been reported by numerous authors[30-33] and are usually due to synovial impingement or entrapment and may also be present in the rare case of pigmented villonodular synovitis. Cutaneous neuromas have also been described as an infrequent cause of pain following TKA. Dellon et al[34] followed 70 patients with painful cutaneous neuromas following TKA. These may occur along the infrapatellar branch of the saphenous nerve at the distal pole of the TKA incision. Successful relief of pain was obtained in 86% of patients with denervation procedures. "End-of-stem" pain in either the femur or tibia has been reported as a source of pain in TKA in cases in which diaphyseal-engaging stems have been utilized.[35]

Patellar sources of pain in TKA have also been described. Irritation of the uncovered periphery of the lateral patellar facet following patellar resurfacing in TKA can occur. This may be associated with use of an inset patella positioned medially, which then leaves a portion of the lateral facet uncovered by the patellar component. This may result in chronic lateral patellar pain, well-localized tenderness along the lateral border of the patella, and may demonstrate increased isotope uptake about the patella on bone scan. Anterior knee pain secondary to patellar ischemia has also been reported and documented with bone scintigraphy.[36] Similarly, anterior knee pain can occur in cases of TKA in which the patella is not resurfaced. While resurfacing the patella versus leaving the patella nonresurfaced in primary TKA remains controversial, evidence continues to emerge that nonresurfaced patellae deteriorate with time, resulting in anterior knee pain rates as high as 29%.[37] In addition, the incidence of residual patellofemoral pain after secondary resurfacing is substantially higher than when patellofemoral resurfacing is done primarily.[38] Lastly, prospective, randomized studies favor patellar resurfacing and report reoperation rates to convert nonresurfaced to resurfaced patellae exceeding those for complications after patellar resurfacing.[39,40]

Another cause of pain in TKA is patellar crepitus or clunk syndrome, which occurs secondary to the development of peripatellar fibrosynovial hyperplasia at the junction of the superior pole of the patella and the distal quadriceps tendon. During deep knee flexion, the fibrosynovial hyperplasia may become entrapped within the intercondylar box of a posterior-stabilized femoral component and cause painless or painful crepitation or clunk. The incidence of this condition has been reported up to 14%.[41-45] In some cases, patellar crepitus is painful and debilitating enough to warrant surgical treatment with either arthroscopic or open débridement of the synovial hyperplasia.[41,44,45] A recent analysis compared a group of 60 TKA subjects who developed patellar crepitus symptomatic enough to merit surgical intervention to a matched group of control subjects who did not experience postoperative patellar crepitus.[46] The mean time to presentation of patellar crepitus was 10.9 months. The incidence of patellar crepitus correlated with a greater number of previous knee surgeries, decreased patellar component size, a decreased composite patellar thickness, shorter preoperative and postoperative patellar tendon length, and placement of the femoral component in a flexed posture.

Metal hypersensitivity has been implicated as a cause of pain in TKA. A recent report of a patient with a painful and stiff TKA revised to a ceramic femoral component and a titanium tibial component achieved pain relief and improved motion.[47] A study performed by Granchi et al revealed a 4-fold likelihood of component loosening confirmed with radiographs and bone scan in patients who had a preoperative medical history of delayed-type hypersensitivity to metal.[48] Benzoyl peroxide, a component in bone cement, has also been reported as a rare allergen that may cause pain, swelling, inflammatory skin reactions, and implant loosening.[49] Although the presence of dermal sensitivity in patients with failed total joint arthroplasty is substantially higher than that in the general population, there is currently no universally accepted test for determining metal hypersensitivity.[50]

SUMMARY

Multiple articular and nonarticular causes can lead to a painful TKA. A systematic approach should be utilized to determine the etiology of pain through obtaining a thorough history, conducting a physical examination, laboratory testing, and radiographic evaluation. Proceeding to revise a TKA without determining a clear source of pain will frequently lead to inferior results.[51] For these patients, periodic repeat evaluations or even referral to a high-volume revision total joint surgeon may be necessary to determine the etiology of pain.

REFERENCES

1. Colizza WA, Insall JN, Scuderi GR. The posterior stabilized total knee prosthesis: assessment of polyethylene damage and osteolysis after a ten-year-minimum follow-up. *J Bone Joint Surg Am*. 1995;77:1713.
2. Dennis DA, Clayton ML, O'Donnell S, Mack RP, Stringer EA. Posterior cruciate condylar total knee arthroplasty. Average 11-year follow-up evaluation. *Clin Orthop Relat Res*. 1992;281:168-176.
3. Ranawat CS, Luessenhop CP, Rodriguez JS. The press-fit condylar modular total knee system: four to six year results with a posterior-cruciate-substituting design. *J Bone Joint Surg Am*. 1997;79:342.
4. Jerry GJ, Rand JA, Ilstrup D. Old sepsis prior to total knee arthroplasty. *Clin Orthop Relat Res*. 1988;236:135-140.
5. Green JP. Steroid therapy and wound healing in surgical patients. *Br J Surg*. 1965;52:523-525.
6. England SP, Stern SH, Insall JN, Windsor RE. Total knee arthroplasty in diabetes mellitus. *Clin Orthop Relat Res*. 1990;260:130-134.
7. Dickaut SC, DeLee JC, Page CP. Nutritional status: importance in predicting wound-healing after amputation. *J Bone Joint Surg*. 1984;66A:71-75.
8. Wilson MG, Kelley K, Thornhill TS. Infection as a complication of total knee arthroplasty: risk factors and treatment in sixty-seven cases. *J Bone Joint Surg*. 1990;72A:878-883.
9. Stern SH, Insall JN, Windsor RE, Inglis AE, Dines DM. Total knee arthroplasty in patients with psoriasis. *Clin Orthop Relat Res*. 1989;248:108-110; discussion 111.
10. Della Valle CJ, Sporer SM, Jacobs JJ, Berger RA, Rosenberg AG, Paprosky WG. Preoperative testing for sepsis before revision total knee arthroplasty. *J Arthroplasty*. 2007;22(6 suppl 2):90-93.
11. Evans BG, Cuckler JM. Evaluation of the painful total hip arthroplasty. *Orthop Clin North Am*. 1992;23:303.
12. Barrack RL, Jennings RW, Wolfe MW, Bertot AJ. The Coventry Award. The value of preoperative aspiration before total knee revision. *Clin Orthop Relat Res*. 1997;345:8-16.
13. Sanzen L, Carlsson AS. The diagnostic value of C-reactive protein in infected total hip arthroplasties. *J Bone Joint Surg*. 1989;71B:638-641.
14. Mason JB, Fehring TK, Odum SM, Griffin WL, Nussman DS. The value of white blood cell counts before revision total knee arthroplasty. *J Arthroplasty*. 2003;18(8):1038-1043.
15. Trampuz A, Hanssen AD, Osmon DR, Mandrekar J, Steckelberg JM, Patel R. Synovial fluid leukocyte count and differential diagnosis of infection. *Am J Med*. 2004;117(8):556-562.
16. Merchant AC, Mercer RL, Jacobsen RH, Cool CR. Roentgenographic analysis of patellofemoral congruence. *J Bone Joint Surg Am*. 1974;56(7):1391-1396.
17. Fehring TK, McAvoy G. Fluoroscopic evaluation of the painful total knee arthroplasty. *Clin Orthop Relat Res*. 1996;331:226-233.
18. Oswald SG, Van Nostrand D, Savory CG, Anderson JH, Callaghan JJ. The acetabulum: a prospective study of three-phase bone and indium white blood cell scintigraphy following porous coated hip arthroplasty. *J Nucl Med*. 1990;31:274-280.
19. Rand JA, Brown ML. The value of indium 111 leukocyte scanning in the evaluation of painful or infected total knee arthroplasties. *Clin Orthop Relat Res*. 1990;259:179-182.
20. Boldt JG, Stiehl JB, Hodler J, Zanetti M, Munzinger U. Femoral component rotation and arthrofibrosis following mobile-bearing total knee arthroplasty. *Int Orthop*. 2006;30(5):420-425.
21. Berger RA, Crossett LS, Jacobs JJ, Rubash HE. Malrotation causing patellofemoral complications after total knee arthroplasty. *Clin Orthop Relat Res*. 1998;356:144-153.
22. Sofka CM, Potter HG, Figgie M, Laskin R. Magnetic resonance imaging of total knee arthroplasty. *Clin Orthop Relat Res*. 2003;406:129-135.

23. Sharkey PF, Hozack WJ, Rothman RH, Shastri S, Jacoby SM. Insall Award paper. Why are total knee arthroplasties failing today? *Clin Orthop Relat Res.* 2002;404:7-13.

24. Dye SF, Vaupel GL, Dye CC. Conscious neurosensory mapping of the internal structures of the human knee without intra-articular anesthesia. *Am J Sports Med.* 1998;26(6):773-777.

25. Larson JE, Becker DA. Fabellar impingement in total knee arthroplasty. A case report. *J Arthroplasty.* 1993;8(1):95-97.

26. Dennis DA, Channer M. Retained distal femoral osteophyte: an infrequent cause of postoperative pain following total knee arthroplasty. *J Arthroplasty.* 1992;7:193-195.

27. Lintner DM, Bocell JR, Tullos HS. Arthroscopic treatment of intraarticular fibrous bands after total knee arthroplasty. A followup note. *Clin Orthop Relat Res.* 1993;309:230-233.

28. Barnes CL, Scott RD. Popliteus tendon dysfunction following total knee arthroplasty. *J Arthroplasty.* 1995;10(4):543-545.

29. Barrack RL, Brumfield CS, Rorabeck CH, Cleland D, Myers L. Heterotopic ossification after revision total knee arthroplasty. *Clin Orthop Relat Res.* 2002;404:208-213.

30. Ballard WT, Clark CR, Callaghan JJ. Recurrent spontaneous hemarthrosis nine years after a total knee arthroplasty. A presentation with pigmented villonodular synovitis. *J Bone Joint Surg Am.* 1993;75(5):764-767.

31. Kindsfater K, Scott R. Recurrent hemarthrosis after total knee arthroplasty. *J Arthroplasty.* 1995;10(suppl):S52-S55.

32. Worland RL, Jessup DE. Recurrent hemarthrosis after total knee arthroplasty. *J Arthroplasty.* 1996;11(8):977-978.

33. Cunningham RB, Mariani EM. Spontaneous hemarthrosis 6 years after total knee arthroplasty. *J Arthroplasty.* 2001;16(1):133-135.

34. Dellon AL, Mont MA, Mullick T, Hungerford DS. Partial denervation for persistent neuroma pain around the knee. *Clin Orthop Relat Res.* 1996;329:216-222.

35. Barrack RL, Stanley T, Burt M. Hopkins S. The effect of stem design on end-of-stem pain in revision total knee arthroplasty. *J Arthroplasty.* 2004;(7 suppl 2):119-124.

36. Gelfer Y, Pinkas L, Horne T, Halperin N, Alk D, Robinson D. Symptomatic transient patellar ischemia following total knee replacement as detected by scintigraphy. A prospective, randomized, double-blind study comparing the mid-vastus to the medial para-patellar approach. *Knee.* 2003;10(4):341-345.

37. Picetti GD 3rd, McGann WA, Welch RB. The patellofemoral joint after total knee arthroplasty without patellar resurfacing. *J Bone Joint Surg Am.* 1990;72(9):1379-1382.

38. Boyd AD Jr, Ewald FC, Thomas WH, Poss R, Sledge CB. Long-term complications after total knee arthroplasty with or without resurfacing of the patella. *J Bone Joint Surg Am.* 1993;75(5):674-681.

39. Barrack RL, Bertot AJ, Wolfe MW, Waldman DA, Milicic M, Myers L. Patellar resurfacing in total knee arthroplasty. A prospective, randomized, double-blind study with five to seven years of follow-up. *J Bone Joint Surg Am.* 2001;83-A(9):1376-1381.

40. Nizard RS, Biau D, Porcher R, et al. A meta-analysis of patellar replacement in total knee arthroplasty. *Clin Orthop Relat Res.* 2005;(432):196-203.

41. Beight JA, Yao B, Horzack WJ, Hearn SL, Booth RE. The patellar "clunk" syndrome after posterior stabilized total knee arthroplasty. *Clin Orthop Relat Res.* 1994;299:139-142.

42. Clarke HD, Fuchs R, Scuderi GR, Mills EL, Scott WN, Insall JN. The influence of femoral component design in the elimination of patellar clunk in posterior-stabilized total knee arthroplasty. *J Arthroplasty.* 2006;21:167-171.

43. Fukunaga K, Kobayashi A, Minoda Y, Iwaki H, Hashimoto Y, Takaoka K. The incidence of the patellar clunk syndrome in a recently designed mobile-bearing posterior stabilized total knee replacement. *J Bone Joint Surg Br.* 2009;91-B:463-468.

44. Lonner JH, Jasko JG, Bezwada HP, Nazarian DG. Incidence of patellar clunk with a modern posterior-stabilized knee design. *Am J Orthop.* 2007;36:550-553.

45. Ranawat AS, Ranawat CS, Slamin JE, Dennis DA. Patellar crepitation in the P.F.C. Sigma total knee system. *Orthopedics.* 2006;29(suppl):S68-S70.

46. Dennis DA, Kim RH, Johnson DR, Springer BD, Fehring TK, Sharma A. The John Insall Award: control-matched evaluation of painful patellar crepitus after total knee arthroplasty. *Clin Orthop Relat Res.* 2011;469:10-17.

47. Bergschmidt P, Bader R, Mittelmeier W. Metal hypersensitivity in total knee arthroplasty: revision surgery using a ceramic femoral component—a case report. *Knee.* 2012;19(2):144-147.

48. Granchi D, Cenni E, Tigani D, Trisolino G, Baldini N, Giunti A. Sensitivity to implant materials in patients with total knee arthroplasties. *Biomaterials.* 2008;29:1494-1500.

49. Bircher A, Friederich NF, Seelig W, Scherer K. Allergic complications from orthopaedic joint implants: the role of delayed hypersensitivity to benzoyl peroxide in bone cement. *Contact Dermatitis.* 2012;66(1):20-26.

50. Hallab N, Merritt K, Jacobs JJ. Metal sensitivity in patients with orthopaedic implants. *J Bone Joint Surg Am.* 2001;83A:428-436.

51. Mont MA, Serna FK, Krackow KA, Hungerford DS. Exploration of radiographically normal total knee replacement for unexplained pain. *Clin Orthop Relat Res.* 1996;331:216-220.

Modes of Failure in Total Knee Arthroplasty

Viktor E. Krebs, MD; Creighton C. Tubb, MD; and Ian M. Gradisar, MD

A knee replacement that has failed or is functioning at a level below the expectations of the patient is a difficult situation to address. The evaluation process must be individualized, and all potential causes for the failure or dissatisfaction must be considered. Knee replacement failure is usually multifactorial, and the evaluating surgeon must define the most likely cause while considering all other potentially contributing issues. The evaluation involves a complete history and exam followed by radiographic and often laboratory evaluations. A systematic approach is useful, but a diagnosis can remain elusive even in the hands of an experienced joint replacement surgeon. Defining the patient's expectations and physical demands is as critical as gaining a thorough understanding of the patient's medical, surgical, and social history. It is then important to appreciate what the patient perceives as the problem; in many situations, this will guide your focus. For example, patients may describe the knee as stiff, painful, or unstable. Though this does not seal the diagnosis, the patient's perspective provides meaningful clues as to what needs to be addressed. Putting a time frame on when the patient began to have problems with the knee further focuses the problem solving. Some cases will have been problematic from the time of the index arthroplasty, which is concerning for indolent infection or component malposition. Other knees may have functioned well for a period of time before becoming problematic, as in the case of aseptic loosening from polyethylene wear. Simply performing a thorough initial history allows the surgeon to develop a context for this particular problematic knee. Addressing why the knee failed requires further investigation; a thorough musculoskeletal and neurovascular exam is warranted. Review of the operative record provides critical information on implants used and technical variables. Investigation of perioperative complications—such as persistent wound drainage or unexpected returns to the operating room—and postoperative rehabilitation protocols provides further useful data. The surgeon can build a differential diagnosis for the etiology of the failed knee arthroplasty by answering who, what, when, and why. The final step to fully define the problem requires an understanding of how knee replacements fail. That is the focus of this chapter.

There are numerous mechanisms by which a knee replacement can fail, and several are usually involved in any given case. The failure modes will always overlap to varying degrees, and it is this complex interaction that will make a definitive diagnosis for the failure difficult. To avoid confusion and the focus on a single cause, it is important to categorize the various modes of failure

Jacofsky DJ, Hedley AK, eds.
*Fundamentals of Revision Knee Arthroplasty:
Diagnosis, Evaluation, and Treatment* (pp 11-30).
© 2013 SLACK Incorporated.

Table 2-1. Modes of Failure in Total Knee Arthroplasty

- Technical factors
  - Instability
  - Stiffness
  - Extensor mechanism complications
  - Component loosening
- Implant-related factors
- Traumatic complications
- Infection
- Dysfunction resulting from disease of the spine or other joints

and then determine the predominating mode. Vince et al[1] describe and utilize a worksheet that lists 9 categories useful when evaluating a failed total knee replacement. Deviating slightly from that model, the modes of failure can be broken down into 5 major categories: technical factors, implant-related factors, traumatic complications, infection, and dysfunction resulting from disease in the spine or other joints (Table 2-1). The technical factors are subcategorized as knee instability, knee stiffness, extensor mechanism complications, and component loosening. When disease in other parts of the musculoskeletal system affects the function of a knee replacement, it is not truly a failure of the arthroplasty. If the knee never functioned well, there may have been an initial patient selection misjudgment; however, if it functioned well and then became problematic, it is commonly due to progression of contiguous joint disease.

Several authors have studied the prevalence of the various failure modes. Fehring et al[2] found in their referral practice that the majority of failures occurring within 5 years of the index procedure were related to infection and tibiofemoral instability. Failure patterns, however, may differ in other areas or practice scenarios and may change with time. Sharkey et al[3] retrospectively evaluated revision knee arthroplasties at their institution during a later time frame. This study included both early and late failures. In order of prevalence, they found polyethylene wear, aseptic loosening, instability, and infection to be the top offenders for failure.[3] The most recent epidemiologic study of revision knee arthroplasty in the United States found infection to be the root cause of 25.2% of the revisions performed. Mechanical loosening accounted for 16.1% of revisions.[4] Ultimately, the surgeon considering revision of a failed knee replacement must consider all the possible modes of failure in each case. The remainder of this chapter will look at each aforementioned category in greater detail.

INSTABILITY

Arthroplasty surgeons can most directly control technical factors that lead to knee failure. Of these, instability of the tibiofemoral articulation is quite debilitating—according to the study by Fehring et al,[2] it accounts for 27% of the early knee failures requiring revision arthroplasty. Knee instability after arthroplasty is subcategorized as sagittal plane, coronal plane, global, or hyperextension.[5] A careful knee examination makes the diagnosis. When these symptoms present early, technical factors during the index procedure are most assuredly the cause. However, instability symptoms can occur later after years of good function. When late instability occurs, polyethylene wear, component loosening, and traumatic ligament injury should be considered.

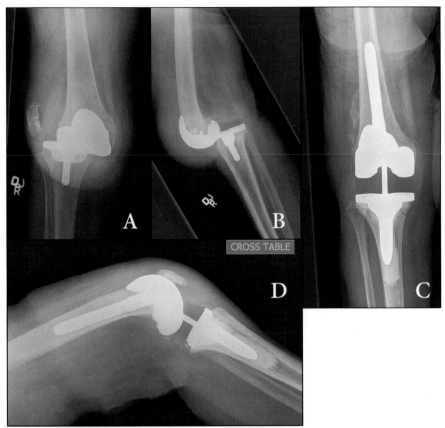

Figure 2-1. (A) Anteroposterior radiograph of the right knee of an 87-year-old female with dislocation of a posterior-stabilized total knee prosthesis. (B) Lateral view. (C) Anteroposterior view of the same patient after revision knee arthroplasty for instability. (D) Lateral view after revision. (Reprinted with permission of Robert Molloy, MD.)

Sagittal plane instability is typically the result of a flexion gap that is greater than the extension gap or a deficient posterior cruciate ligament in posterior cruciate-retaining implant designs. Techniques utilized to ensure adequate gap balancing are essential in preventing this complication, regardless of the implant design.[6] Patients with sagittal plane instability often complain of pain in or around the knee, recurrent effusions, and difficulty with descending stairs. Factors to consider in evaluating patients with flexion instability are the degree of posterior tibial slope, the size of the femoral implant, and the competency of the other stabilizing structures of the knee. Sierra and Berry[7] reviewed some of the technical differences in handling the flexion gap with posterior cruciate-retaining and substituting knee replacements. It is worth noting that resection of the posterior cruciate ligament opens the flexion space and has a significant impact on the release of other soft tissue restraints in the knee.[8] Patients presenting with anterior to posterior instability after an index posterior cruciate-retaining knee replacement typically require revision surgery to a posterior stabilized implant or deep dish insert. Obviously, careful gap balancing is required. Converting to a posterior stabilized design in these cases has been reported to be the most predictable solution.[9] Flexion instability can still occur in the posterior stabilized designs and must be scrutinized at the time of surgery. In severe flexion gap mismatch cases, knee dislocation can occur, especially when there is concomitant laxity of the lateral ligaments, particularly the posterolateral corner. This is not a common complication with current knee designs.[10] If dislocation does occur and is recurrent, revision surgery is indicated and usually requires a varus-valgus constrained or hinged implant design (Figure 2-1). A loose flexion gap can still result in patient dissatisfaction with a posterior

Figure 2-2. Clinical photograph of a knee at revision surgery demonstrating laxity of the medial structures.

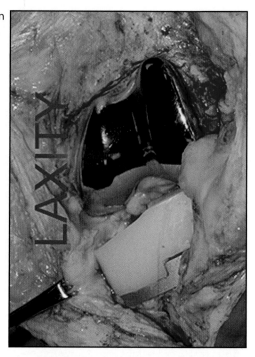

Figure 2-3. Radiograph of the right knee of a 53-year-old female complaining of persistent knee pain and giving way symptoms. Note the asymmetry of her extension gap. (Reprinted with permission of Mark I. Froimson, MD.)

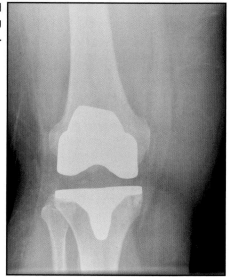

stabilized knee replacement without having frank knee dislocation. In these cases, revision surgery to address the cause of the flexion gap mismatch can lead to successful outcomes.[11]

Coronal plane instability leads to abnormal varus and valgus mobility and is often noted in extension. If this is purely a symmetric imbalance in extension, the likely cause is overresection of the distal femur at the index procedure. The solution is revision surgery with distal femoral augments to correct the elevated joint line in extension.[10] Asymmetric coronal plane instability results from ligament disruption or poor soft tissue balancing (Figure 2-2). The diagnosis relies on demonstrating abnormal varus or valgus laxity. Radiographs may show widening on the side of incompetent ligaments or asymmetry related to poor correction of a preoperative deformity (Figure 2-3). An incompetent collateral ligament will not heal by conservative measures. Revision surgery to a constrained implant is indicated, and reconstruction of the damaged ligament should also be undertaken, as noted by McAuley et al.[9] If there is such gross instability or lack of adequate tissue for reconstruction of the ligaments, a rotating hinged prosthesis affords the revision surgeon the ability to provide the patient with a functional knee joint. Another common cause for coronal plane asymmetry is poor initial soft tissue balancing despite intact collateral ligaments.[10] If not overly severe, these cases may not present until the abnormal forces on the bearing surface generate sufficient wear to compromise the function of the implant. When these cases do present and are symptomatic, revision arthroplasty is indicated and involves appropriate soft tissue balancing to result in equal, rectangular gaps. Soft tissue release techniques vary by surgeon preference but should be well thought out preoperatively. Bottros et al[6] reviewed the various releases for both varus and valgus knee deformities. If the knee components are well aligned and stable, soft tissue releases followed by appropriate insert exchanges may be successful. However, careful selection and scrutiny is required. Good functional results and patient satisfaction have been reported with revision of components for coronal plane instability as long as care is taken to address the underlying cause.[12]

Global instability is essentially a problem in both the coronal and sagittal planes. It is extremely debilitating. If this is caused by pure undersizing of the polyethylene liner in the face of balanced and rectangular gaps, logic would suggest placing a thicker insert would be beneficial. This logic should be approached cautiously to ensure all other factors are considered and the knee is truly stable and balanced after the exchange. The experience at the Anderson Orthopaedic Research Institute demonstrates that highly constrained or hinged prostheses provided the most optimal results for cases of global instability.[9] The underlying causes for instability must also be addressed if the implant is expected to have a reasonable chance for long-term survival.[5]

Hyperextension or genu recurvatum is an especially difficult form of instability that has significant consequences on gait and patient function. Risk factors for this debilitating complication are preoperative recurvatum, neuromuscular disorders, rheumatoid arthritis, quadriceps weakness, and poor surgical technique.[10] Results for managing this complication are often dissatisfying, and some even argue for fusion rather than revision in some of these cases.[5,10] An extension stop placed in a rotating hinge prosthesis provides a solution, but the longevity of this is not reported; Vince et al[5] argue that this has a poor long-term survivorship.

STIFFNESS

The opposite extreme from instability is knee stiffness. A knee replacement with poor motion has functional consequences that prevent the patient from realizing the full benefit of arthroplasty. The true incidence of this complication is unknown, as there is disagreement on what constitutes a stiff knee. Patients require approximately 83 degrees of knee flexion for stair climbing, 93 degrees for rising from a chair, greater than 106 degrees for shoe tying, and 117 degrees for lifting an object from the floor.[13] These requirements may fall short of individual patient demands but provide a basis for discussing requirements of activities of daily living. Ritter et al[14] found that Knee Society scores in patient status following a posterior cruciate-retaining knee replacement were best when the patient gained 128 to 132 degrees of postoperative motion, excluding those with a knee flexion contracture or recurvatum. With regard to knee extension, a flexion contracture decreases the working arc of the quadriceps muscles, making ambulating less efficient and resulting in early fatigue. Poor Knee Society pain and functional scores have been documented with postoperative knee flexion contractures of greater than 5 degrees.[15] Kim et al[16] defined stiffness after total knee arthroplasty (TKA) as a flexion contracture greater than or equal to 15 degrees or less than 75 degrees of knee flexion. Others have broadened the definition placing higher expectations on postoperative knee motion.[17,18] Certainly, each patient's expectations and definition of an acceptable outcome is different. Understanding this, it is worthwhile as surgeons to have a working definition of what constitutes a postoperative stiff knee. Generally, there should be no more than a 5 degrees flexion contracture, and the knee should bend beyond 90 degrees. Despite inconsistent definitions, the incidence of a stiff total knee replacement is probably between 1% and 4%.[16,17] It is worth exploring what causes a knee to be stiff after surgery and why there is a relatively high incidence of this complication. The problem is multifactorial and involves technical, rehabilitative, and patient-related factors. A common technical factor is poor gap symmetry affecting either flexion or extension. This may be due to inappropriate component sizing, poor soft tissue balancing, component malposition, an overstuffed patellofemoral articulation, residual osteophytes, or a combination of these. Another technical variable is a tibial component that is too thick due to underresection of the tibia or a polyethylene component that is inappropriately sized for the gaps. The result is a limitation in both flexion and extension. Other technical variables, although debated, include the position of the knee at the time of arthrotomy closure[19] and/or the surgical approach utilized.[20-22] Pain management after knee replacement can also be critical in the early period in order to regain knee motion. Lavernia et al[23] found using a small-incision surgical technique combined with patient education and a multimodal pain management protocol resulted in a 47% decrease in the number of patients requiring postoperative manipulation under anesthesia to regain motion.

Aside from the technical factors that impact knee motion, certain patient characteristics are worth noting as well. One of the more predictive patient-related factors for poor postoperative knee motion is limited preoperative knee motion.[14-17] In addition to those patients with a preoperative flexion contracture, males and patients with advanced age seem to be at risk for a postoperative flexion contracture that interferes with function.[15] Gandhi et al[17] reviewed 1216 primary total knee replacements and cited poor preoperative motion, preoperative patella baja, increased medical comorbidities, increased surgical difficulty, less intraoperative flexion, and intraoperative complications as risk factors for limited postoperative motion. Finally, postoperative physical therapy and rehabilitation play important roles in returning patients to an acceptable level of function. The patient's ability and willingness to comply is certainly important. Rehabilitative protocols vary widely but should be considered in the evaluation of the stiff knee to determine if particular protocols or programs contributed to the lack of motion.

The etiology of the stiffness does provide some insight into management decisions. Several modalities have been used with varying degrees of success. Well-timed manipulation under anesthesia may be of benefit in the face of appropriately placed and sized components. Other options include arthroscopic releases and lysis of adhesions, open arthrolysis with or without polyethylene exchange, or revision arthroplasty. For the most part, these techniques have a role in treatment and have some success at improving motion, but often with only moderate improvement in outcomes.[16,24-27] Having keen insight into the contributing factors for postoperative knee stiffness may provide some benefit to successful management of this mode of failure.

EXTENSOR MECHANISM COMPLICATIONS

Complications related to the extensor mechanism encompass a myriad of challenges for the revision surgeon. The most obvious source of failure related to the extensor mechanism is its discontinuity. Any complication that results in an incompetent extensor mechanism severely affects the function of the knee. Patellar fractures, which will be discussed later, can be dissatisfying to manage. Patellar tendon ruptures can occur intraoperatively or postoperatively and tend to result in poorer outcomes. The incidence of this complication is quite low. A retrospective study from the Mayo Clinic showed the incidence to be 0.17%[28]; the North American Knee Arthroplasty Revision study group reported a 0.48% need for revision due to extensor mechanism disruption.[29] Risk factors for this complication include patients with poor preoperative knee motion, multiple previous knee surgeries, or associated medical comorbidities, such as rheumatoid arthritis, chronic renal insufficiency, or diabetes mellitus.[30] Management of the disrupted patellar tendon in knee arthroplasty patients involves direct repair typically with either autograft (semitendinosus

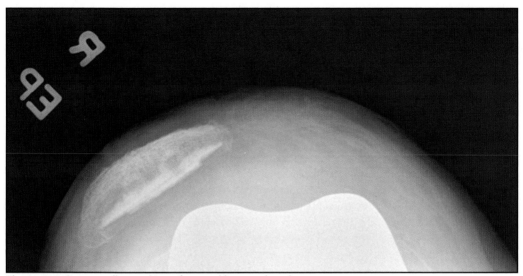

Figure 2-4. Poor patellar tracking after total knee arthroplasty.

tendon) or allograft tissue augmentation or reconstruction.[31,32] Though the numbers studied by Schoderbek et al[29] were low, their results supported the perception that functional outcomes were worse in patients with extensor mechanism disruption compared to other patients undergoing knee revision. Quadriceps tendon ruptures occur less frequently but likely are associated with similar risk factors.[30] Complete quadriceps tendon ruptures that compromise the extensor mechanism should be repaired and augmented with autograft or allograft tissue if needed to bolster support to the local tissue.

Poor patellar tracking may not be quite as debilitating as the ruptured extensor mechanism, yet it is a common cause of failure after knee arthroplasty (Figure 2-4). The exact incidence is not well defined, but is likely decreasing as surgeons are more cognizant of the impacts of proper implant alignment and positioning on patellar tracking.[33] Poor patellar tracking seems more apt to occur following a traditional medial parapatellar approach when compared to some version of a quadriceps-sparing arthrotomy.[34,35] Additionally, patient factors, such as an excessively valgus knee or preoperative history of lateral patellar subluxation, increase the risk for this complication. Reconstructive surgeons must be aware of these risk factors, but understanding the role of component position and how that impacts patellar tracking is paramount. Essentially, any scenario that increases the lateral pull of the quadriceps mechanism or increases the lateral retinacular tension will negatively impact patellar tracking. Plain radiographs to include long-length films provide a means for assessing axial alignment. A neutral mechanical alignment is the goal in knee arthroplasty; valgus alignment greater than 10 degrees increases the risk for patellar maltracking.[33] Berger et al[36] described a technique for measuring femoral and tibial component rotation on computed tomography (CT) scans. Their study showed that with increasing combined tibial and femoral internal rotation in patients with appropriate axial alignment there were more severe problems with patellar tracking. Likewise, excessive medialization of the femoral or tibial components will predispose to lateral subluxation of the patella.[37] Position of the patellar component when resurfaced also plays a significant role in that a central or lateralized button will increase the lateral retinacular tension and lead to increased tracking problems.[38,39] An "overstuffed" patellofemoral articulation from either an inappropriately sized femoral component or underresected patellar resurfacing will result not only in maltracking but often poor knee flexion as well.[37] The solution to patellar tracking problems is directed at the cause. A thorough preoperative radiographic evaluation to include a CT scan where appropriate is helpful. Often, component revision is indicated to improve patellofemoral tracking.

Other symptoms related to the patellofemoral articulation may result in patient dissatisfaction. The debate on patellar resurfacing is ongoing.[40,41] Good results have been reported for nonresurfacing in patients with noninflammatory arthritis that spares the patella.[42,43] For those who have persistent anterior knee pain after knee replacement without patellar resurfacing, secondary resurfacing can be considered. Care should be taken to ensure no other conditions are causing these symptoms, as the results for this approach are often unsatisfactory.[43,44] Additional factors that affect the patellofemoral articulation include significant deviations from the original joint line in primary and revision knee arthroplasty.[45,46] Cases of excessive patella baja or patella alta may require revision to restore the anatomic joint line, as these cases likely affect gap balancing overall and not just the patellofemoral articulation.[6] Patellar clunk syndrome may be an additional extensor mechanism-related cause of poor knee function. This is associated with posterior stabilized knee designs of which many have made modifications to decrease the incidence of this complication. Unlike the previously mentioned patellofemoral complications, patellar clunk syndrome may respond well to conservative management. If not, arthroscopic débridement may be useful.[47,48]

COMPONENT LOOSENING

Component loosening is either a problem of initial fixation or late loosening—typically as a result of osteolysis—and remains a common cause of failure, as demonstrated in the studies by Sharkey et al[3] and Bozic et al.[4] Cementing total knee components provide immediate stable fixation and has proven clinical success when proper cement techniques have been utilized. Interest exists for uncemented TKA especially in the young, active population in need of a knee replacement. The sought-after goal is to outperform current cemented designs by creating a more biologic fixation of the implants. To date, uncemented TKA has not been proven to be superior to cemented TKA. A recent meta-analysis supported cemented TKA as the current standard based on the available literature, which includes randomized and observational studies. The investigators admit that the few randomized, controlled trials available failed to find a significant difference between the techniques with respect to survivability and knee function, but offer caution as these studies had low numbers with short follow-up periods.[49] Regardless of the technique used at the index procedure, the revision surgeon should carefully evaluate the radiographs for extensive radiolucent lines developing in the early postoperative period, suggesting failed fixation for patients presenting with activity-related pain or a sense of instability.

The once-stable, well-fixed total knee implant can go on to loosen. The cause of this can be multifactorial and likely related to component positioning and gap balancing. Early reports found that there was a significant correlation with implant failure and axial limb alignment.[50] With changes in implant design and the advent of computer technologies, questions regarding the importance of limb alignment as it relates to implant survivability arise. Yet, Fang et al[51] recently reviewed a large series of primary knee replacements and found a statistically higher failure rate in knees that did not have a postoperative tibiofemoral angle between 2.4 and 7.2 degrees of valgus when followed for an average of 6.6 years. Osteolysis as a result of the generation of wear particles plays a pivotal role. A great deal of research has gone into understanding the process of bone resorption that occurs as a result of the immune system's response to wear debris. Polyethylene wear in TKA is different than that found in total hip arthroplasty.[52] Not only does component alignment affect wear, implant features such as the degree of constraint between the bearing and the femoral condyles, tibial base plate locking mechanisms in modular designs, and whether the bearing is fixed or free to rotate will impact how polyethylene wears. Moreover, polyethylene manufacturing and sterilization processes can alter wear characteristics.[52,53] Finally, most surgeons believe that wear is a function of use and is accelerated by high activity levels.[54]

Manufacturing and sterilization processes are beyond most surgeons' control; likewise, patient activity levels are difficult to directly influence. However, surgeons should recognize factors, such

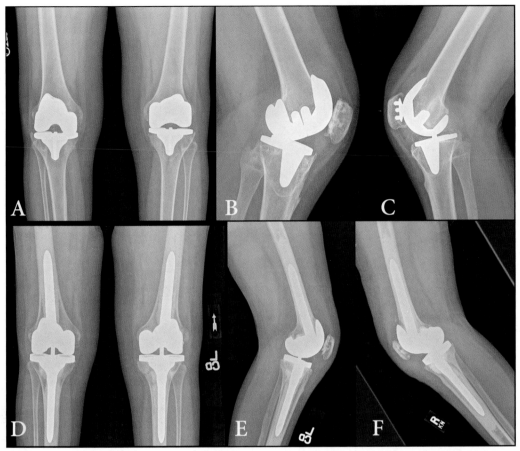

Figure 2-5. (A) Anteroposterior and (B, C) lateral radiographs of progressively painful bilateral knee replacements 15 years after the index arthroplasty. Note the osteolysis about the implants. (D) Anteroposterior and (E, F) lateral views following revision surgery to stemmed implants for both knees resulting in resolution of symptoms.

as component and limb malalignment or gap asymmetry, and consider how these can be corrected in the case of revision surgery for component loosening or progressive osteolysis. Routine radiographs are the mainstay for follow-up of a TKA. When components appear well fixed but osteolysis is present, the frequency of radiographic follow-up should increase to every 6 to 12 months as long as the patient is asymptomatic.[53] If symptoms develop or the osteolysis progresses, surgical intervention is warranted (Figure 2-5). CT scans can be very instructive in not only looking at component alignment but also in evaluating the degree of bone loss that will be faced in the revision scenario. Well-aligned and stable implants may respond well to polyethylene liner exchange, provided the components are modular.[55] Single-component or full-knee revision is the solution for component or limb malalignment resulting in implant loosening or osteolysis.

IMPLANT FAILURE

The preceding modes of failure relate closely to technical factors. Implant failure in the presence of appropriate surgical technique constitutes another mode of failure of which the revision surgeon must be aware. In many cases this may be quite obvious, whereas others may be more subtle and can make revision surgery a challenge (Figure 2-6). The key is knowing the implants used and

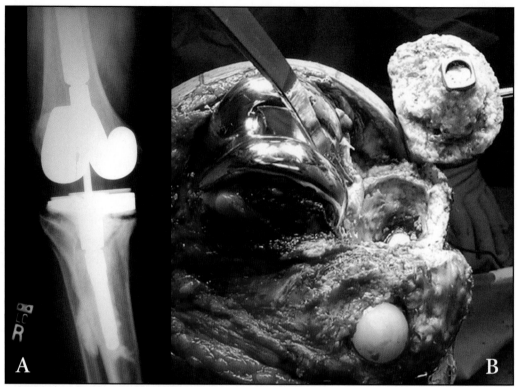

Figure 2-6. (A) Radiograph showing broken tibial stem. (B) Intraoperative image of the same broken stem making extraction more difficult. Recognizing this preoperatively allows for proper planning for the revision surgery.

having an honest and open relationship with industry representatives. Historically, arthroplasty implants and techniques have continued to evolve in a positive manner, but not without some setbacks along the way. Certain design features and manufacturing or sterilizing techniques were complicated by early failure. The most obvious example is the evolution of sterilization techniques for polyethylene. Gamma irradiation of polyethylene in air produced free radicals that would oxidize. As these components sat on the shelf, the oxidative process led to mechanical inferiority of the product. Large areas of delamination would occur, resulting in early wear-related failures. Recognition of this has led to a decrease in the failure rates associated with wear by developing improved sterilization and packaging techniques.[56] As another example, Bal et al[57] reported on a 12% failure rate of the tibial post in 564 posterior-stabilized total knee replacements performed by one surgeon using a single-implant design. Though retrospective analyses such as these do not control for other variables, the trend is worth noting. Large joint registries and databases will likely have the most to offer in the early identification of these failures so that arthroplasty surgeons can be appropriately alerted and industry engineers can make rapid adjustments. The value of learning which components were utilized in each particular case cannot be emphasized enough. Armed with this information, the revision surgeon can work with implant industry colleagues to identify these particular cases and develop useful solutions.

PERIPROSTHETIC FRACTURE

Often, external factors such as trauma play a role. Periprosthetic fractures of the distal femur, proximal tibia, or patella can compromise the results of a knee replacement. The incidence of this

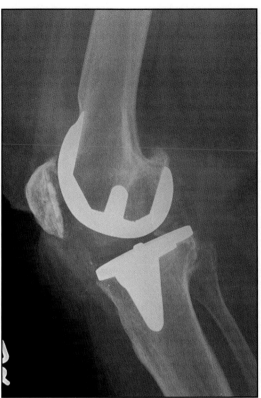

Figure 2-7. Anterior notching after knee replacement.

complication is not well defined but may be as high as 2.3%, as was noted during a review of a large number of cases from the Mayo Clinic total joint registry which included femoral, tibial, and patellar fractures.[58] These fractures can be classified as occurring intraoperatively or postoperatively, as was done in the Mayo Clinic study. For the purposes of this review, intraoperative fractures will not be addressed under the assumption that this is noted and addressed at the time of the index arthroplasty and not typically a cause for failure. Specific classifications do exist for femoral, tibial, and patellar periprosthetic fractures, which are reviewed in an article by Parvizi et al.[59] Postoperative periprosthetic fractures are typically quite evident on radiographs. The challenge is not in diagnosis but in determining the status of the knee implants. Asking the patient how the knee replacement functioned prior to the incident that resulted in his or her fracture can help elucidate other more subtle modes of failure, if present. Likewise, a review of previous radiographs, especially if recent, is helpful in evaluating the prosthesis. The presence of anterior cortical notching of the femur decreases bending strength by 18% and torsional strength by 39.2%, as shown in a cadaveric study.[60] This is an frequently discussed risk factor for subsequent periprosthetic distal femur fracture (Figure 2-7). Others have argued against this theoretical risk.[61] Most critically, radiographs can help determine if there were signs of loosening, excessive wear, or suggestions of malalignment.

If the knee components are stable and the patient had a well-functioning knee, the surgeon merely faces a fracture that requires stabilization. The goals are fracture union and restored functionality for the patient. Various techniques have been utilized for fracture fixation ranging from nonoperative care to external or internal fixation. Internal fixation methods vary but account for the most popular means for handling these fractures. The methods have included traditional plating techniques using fixed angled devices, to the more biologically friendly indirect reduction maneuvers followed by an intramedullary nail or a locking plate construct.[59] A recent systematic review of the literature found that intramedullary nails resulted in a significantly higher union

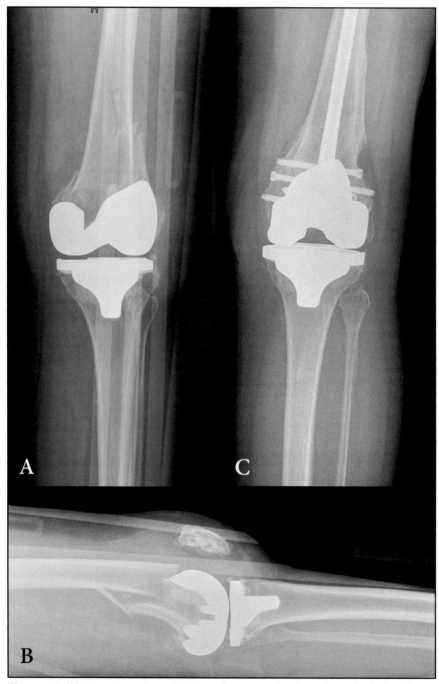

Figure 2-8. (A) Anteroposterior and (B) lateral radiographs of a periprosthetic distal femur fracture. (C) Complete union of the same fracture after fixation with an intramedullary nail.

rate and decreased reoperation rate compared to nonoperative treatment or conventional plating of periprosthetic distal femur fractures (Figure 2-8).[62] But, the investigators do note that observational studies without control groups compose the available literature on the topic.[62] For periprosthetic distal femoral fractures, the newer plating techniques offer some theoretical benefits and can be utilized on most implant designs, unlike intramedullary nails, which require an access point through the center of the distal femur. Data suggest that locked plates may also have improved union rates compared to nonoperative treatment or traditional plating techniques, but this correlation has yet to be definitively proven.[62] Periprosthetic tibial fractures occur less frequently with an incidence of 0.4% in the Mayo Clinic registry study.[58] Moreover, with modern tibial implant designs, this problem may occur less frequently than previously reported.[59] Optimal management is dependent upon the status of the implants as well as limb alignment and fracture stability. Treatment options include nonoperative management, fracture fixation with plating devices, or revision arthroplasty.[59]

The case of loose components or a previously poorly functioning knee associated with a periprosthetic fracture has the same ultimate goal of returning the patient to an acceptable degree of function. The path to achieve this goal will likely require revision arthroplasty with or without fracture fixation depending on the fracture pattern. The particular circumstances will determine if this is a staged process or accomplished in one operative setting. These cases can certainly become quite complex and require a wide range of available techniques and implants, whether that be fracture fixation and conversion to revision implants using stemmed components or, in some circumstances, the use of distal femoral or proximal tibial replacing hinged prostheses.

Patella fractures also can occur intraoperatively or postoperatively. Large series suggest that postoperative patella fractures occur in less than 1% of primary cases in which the patella is resurfaced, though other reports have shown a higher incidence.[63] Risk factors for this complication include technical factors such as patellar resurfacing, overresection of the patella, a single-peg implant design, patellar maltracking, and possibly the combination of a lateral release and medial parapatellar approach, as this diminishes patellar blood supply. The latter complication is debated as to its relevance to a clinically significant increase in the risk for patellar fracture.[63] Though periprosthetic patella fractures may occur following direct trauma, they typically are more insidious in nature and often found on routine radiographs or in the evaluation of persistent anterior knee pain.[64] The management decision process involves determining if the implant is loose and if the extensor mechanism is intact. Nonoperative management is indicated when the patellar component is well fixed and the extensor mechanism is intact. If the component is loose, management should consist of ensuring the extensor mechanism is repaired then consideration for revision of the patellar component, but only if adequate bone stock remains to do so. An incompetent extensor mechanism should be repaired. Results in the surgical management of these cases are often disappointing, as noted in recent reviews of the literature on this topic (Figure 2-9).[63,64]

INFECTION

Periprosthetic knee infection is one of the more common modes of failure arthroplasty surgeons will face. Because of its implications toward further revision, it is a source of failure that must always be considered and systematically ruled out. Infection probably occurs in approximately 1% of primary knee replacements, but the increasing number of knee replacements being performed ensures a solid presence for this difficult complication. Moreover, the burden to the health care system from periprosthetic knee infections is notable.[65] Finnish registry data recently noted a 0.90% incidence of revision for infection in 40,135 primary knee replacements performed in Finland during the study time period.[66] Kurtz et al[67] recently studied the United States Medicare population and found a 1.55% incidence of the diagnosis of periprosthetic knee infection within 2 years of the index primary knee arthroplasty, with this incidence increasing to 2.01% when carried out to 10 years postoperatively. The challenge for orthopedic surgeons has always been the ability to readily diagnose the problem; however, it is incumbent upon the surgeon to do so when evaluating any failed TKA.

The classification for periprosthetic joint infections is well known.[68-70] An early postoperative infection develops within 4 weeks of the index procedure, whereas a late chronic infection develops later than 4 weeks after the procedure and typically arises insidiously. An acute onset of symptoms

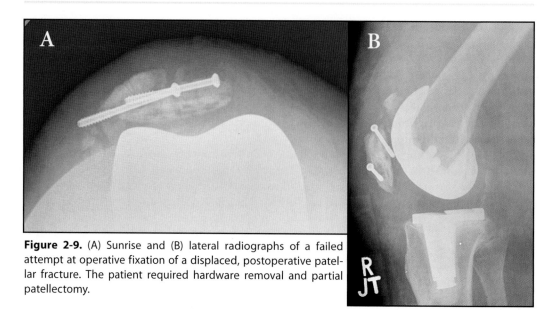

Figure 2-9. (A) Sunrise and (B) lateral radiographs of a failed attempt at operative fixation of a displaced, postoperative patellar fracture. The patient required hardware removal and partial patellectomy.

following a suspected bacteremic event is referred to as an acute hematogenous infection. Finally, a positive intraoperative culture at the time of revision makes for the fourth category. Typically, this is characterized by the same organism grown from at least 2 specimens when infection was not suspected. Segawa et al[69] found this clinical classification system useful in guiding treatment. Certainly, it provides a means for effective communication and for thinking about these cases.

Patients who present with a swollen knee that is warm, erythematous, and associated with pain or systemic symptoms such as fever make the diagnosis fairly certain. Likewise, persistent wound drainage following knee replacement is a worrisome finding that necessitates early intervention.[71,72] But, more often than not, the presentation is more subtle. In these cases, diagnosis can be difficult. All patients who present with a painful or poorly functioning knee replacement must be evaluated for underlying periprosthetic joint infection. Numerous surgical factors and patient-related factors can influence the risk of infection. Kurtz et al[67] found that increased operative time significantly increased the risk for postoperative infection. Likewise, bilateral knee replacements done at the same operative setting may increase the risk.[73] Obviously, poor sterile technique or careless soft tissue management are risk factors that are in the surgeon's control. Patients with notable medical comorbidities have an increased risk for infection.[67] Specifically, rheumatoid arthritis, diabetes mellitus, obesity, renal failure, smoking, immunosuppressive therapy, male gender, and previous knee surgery have been associated with a higher risk of periprosthetic knee infection.[66,73,74] Many patients carry these risk factors, so they are only helpful in understanding the problem of periprosthetic knee infections and do not necessarily make the diagnosis any more clear. Appropriate radiographs of the knee are a part of any work-up for a failed knee replacement. Though these are not specific for obvious infection, they are instructive as to associated issues with the implants, such as loosening, malalignment, or polyethylene wear. Knee implants may have extensive radiolucent lines on imaging when a chronic infection has compromised the interface between the bone and implant or cement. When the history, exam, and radiographs are not conclusive, surgeons tend to rely heavily on laboratory data to determine if a knee is infected.

Several studies have highlighted the value in laboratory evaluation of the serum erythrocyte sedimentation rate (ESR) and C-reactive protein (CRP) to screen for infection. In the early postoperative period both will be elevated, though the CRP will normalize within a few weeks while the ESR may take several months to return to baseline values.[75,76] Neither test is specific for infection as they are merely markers for inflammation, so other inflammatory conditions can cause these markers to be elevated. However, if both the ESR and CRP are normal, the likelihood of infection is very low.[77,78] Austin et al[78] found that the combination of these 2 tests, which are inexpensive and readily available, provide an excellent screening tool for infection with a sensitivity of 96% and negative predictive value of 95%. In the face of abnormal results, further investigation is warranted recognizing the poor specificity of the tests that, when combined, was only 56%.[78] In the case of abnormal inflammatory lab markers or clinical suspicion for infection, knee aspiration for synovial fluid analysis can be invaluable. The literature presents conflicting recommendations for interpreting values from synovial fluid.[79-81] Recent data suggest that an aspirate from a painful total knee replacement showing a synovial fluid white blood cell (WBC) count greater than 1100 cells/10^{-3} cm^3 and a neutrophil percentage greater than 64% is highly indicative of a periprosthetic joint infection especially when combined with elevated serum inflammatory markers. When the synovial WBC count and neutrophil percentage are less than those cut-off values, periprosthetic knee infection is almost assuredly not present.[81] It is important to realize that patients with inflammatory conditions were not included in that study and so, in those cases, these values may not apply. Gram stains, though often performed, have a 27% sensitivity for infection and a 79% negative predictive value and are thus not helpful in determining the presence of infection.[82] The use of radionuclide scans has had some interest as a diagnostic tool for periprosthetic joint infection, but they are plagued with poor specificity, as reviewed by Bauer et al.[83] To summarize, current evidence suggests that clinical suspicion should be combined with evaluation of serum inflammatory markers and synovial fluid analysis for WBC count and neutrophil percentage as the best diagnostic modalities for periprosthetic knee infections.

Because no currently available test absolutely rules out an infection, intraoperative assessment is valuable for knees that are undergoing revision arthroplasty. This evaluation requires intraoperative tissue culture and stat frozen section for review by the pathologist. Morgan et al[82] showed that intraoperative gram stain really had no role in the diagnostic dilemma between infected or noninfected. Culture results are often considered the gold standard, but can be affected by recent antibiotic usage resulting in false-negatives or by careless handling resulting in false-positives. Most surgeons consider a positive culture with the same bacterial species from 2 separate samples clinically significant.[69] However, consultation with a local infectious disease specialist is wise whenever there is a positive intraoperative culture. The problem is that these results are not immediately available for making critical intraoperative decisions. Intraoperative frozen sections, therefore, provide the last piece of immediate data useful to the surgeon. Though there is some controversy on this topic, 5 or more neutrophils per high-powered (400x) field in 3 or more fields obtained from capsular tissue and not the fibrinous peri-implant membrane is suggestive of infection.[83] Obtaining multiple deep tissue specimens improves the sensitivity of this test.[83]

The growing concerns of drug-resistant and increasingly virulent organisms have not spared the arthroplasty arena. An increase in the prevalence of multiple drug-resistant organisms infecting joint replacements has been reported.[84] One of the more commonly seen pathogens is methicillin-resistant *Staphylococcus aureus* (MRSA). This can be either hospital or community acquired. Little data are available to guide surgeons regarding this trend. There has been interest in screening programs and expanded prophylactic measures, such as antibiotic-laden cement for primary arthroplasty or broader spectrum preoperative antibiotics for susceptible hosts.[85] However, good data to define the benefit of these measures are lacking. What seems to be true is that infections with resistant organisms may portray worse outcomes and a more difficult process for eradication.[85] As more information is gathered on these organisms, improved guidance on management and novel treatment modalities may assist surgeons in battling total knee infections.

The treatment algorithm for a periprosthetic knee infection depends on the particular circumstances of each case. Early postoperative infections, when recognized and dealt with expeditiously, may respond well to aggressive débridement and irrigation as well as exchange of modular components as appropriate. Arthroscopic lavage is probably not sufficient in these circumstances.[86] Acute hematogenous infections may be treated in a similar way to the early postoperative infection if historical information can confirm that the symptoms are acutely related to a bacteremic event. The gold standard for management of a late chronic infection remains a two-stage revision with the first stage involving débridement, removal of implants, irrigation, and placement of an anti-biotic-impregnated spacer. The interval prior to second-stage reimplantation involves intravenous antibiotics and should include close coordination with an infectious disease specialist. In the face of particularly virulent or resistant bacteria, two-stage revision may be a better course of action for acute hematogenous or early postoperative infections as well. Patient factors may give support to other treatment modalities, such as antibiotic suppression, single-stage revision, or amputation. For the foreseeable future, the prevalence of periprosthetic knee infections requires arthroplasty surgeons to gain familiarity with its diagnosis and management.

OTHER SOURCES OF PAIN AND DYSFUNCTION

The previously noted modes of failure constitute a thorough list of how some knee replacements fail to provide the patient with acceptable pain control and function. However, some cases will present where the patient seems to have a well-functioning and technically sound knee replacement, yet the patient is dissatisfied with the result. Other sources of pain or limitation should be considered prior to embarking on another surgery, as this may not represent a failed knee as much as a failure in patient selection. Specifically, thorough evaluation of sources of referred pain is warranted. It may also be worth revisiting patient expectations and desired activity levels to ensure they are consistent with current knee implant capabilities. Reticence in proceeding to revision surgery is wise if there is no definable cause of the failure despite a thorough investigation.

SUMMARY

Arthroplasty surgeons face an increasing burden of revision TKAs with the aging population and increased frequency of knee replacements. Each surgeon must utilize a systematic method for understanding how knee replacements fail. This allows optimization of revision surgery outcomes. Often, the various modes are intertwined in each particular case. For example, subtle alignment variations may lead to pain associated with patellar tracking abnormalities and early component wear, which eventually results in osteolysis and component loosening with increased pain and, potentially, a new sense of knee instability. However, breaking out the modes of failure into technical factors (instability, stiffness, extensor mechanism complications, and component loosening), implant factors, traumatic complications, and infection helps the surgeon define each patient's problem in a manner that can guide management decisions. This form of problem solving involves critical analysis and creative thinking, but that is the science and art of revision surgery.

REFERENCES

1. Vince KG, Droll K, Chivas D. New concepts in revision total knee arthroplasty. *J Surg Orthop Adv.* 2008;17(3):165-172.
2. Fehring TK, Odum S, Griffin WL, Mason JB, Nadaud M. Early failures in total knee arthroplasty. *Clin Orthop Relat Res.* 2001;(392):315-318.
3. Sharkey PF, Hozack WJ, Rothman RH, Shastri S, Jacoby SM. Insall Award paper. Why are total knee arthroplasties failing today? *Clin Orthop Relat Res.* 2002;(404):7-13.
4. Bozic KJ, Kurtz SM, Lau E, et al. The epidemiology of revision total knee arthroplasty in the United States. *Clin Orthop Relat Res.* 2010;468(1):45-51.
5. Vince KG, Abdeen A, Sugimori T. The unstable total knee arthroplasty: causes and cures. *J Arthroplasty.* 2006;21(4 suppl 1):44-49.

6. Bottros J, Gad B, Krebs V, Barsoum WK. Gap balancing in total knee arthroplasty. *J Arthroplasty.* 2006;21(4 suppl 1):11-15.

7. Sierra RJ, Berry DJ. Surgical technique differences between posterior-substituting and cruciate-retaining total knee arthroplasty. *J Arthroplasty.* 2008;23(7 suppl):20-23.

8. Mihalko WM, Miller C, Krackow KA. Total knee arthroplasty ligament balancing and gap kinematics with posterior cruciate ligament retention and sacrifice. *Am J Orthop (Belle Mead NJ).* 2000;29(8):610-616.

9. McAuley JP, Engh GA, Ammeen DJ. Treatment of the unstable total knee arthroplasty. *Instr Course Lect.* 2004;53:237-241.

10. Parratte S, Pagnano MW. Instability after total knee arthroplasty. *Instr Course Lect.* 2008;57:295-304.

11. Schwab JH, Haidukewych GJ, Hanssen AD, Jacofsky DJ, Pagnano MW. Flexion instability without dislocation after posterior stabilized total knees. *Clin Orthop Relat Res.* 2005;440:96-100.

12. Fehring TK, Valadie AL. Knee instability after total knee arthroplasty. *Clin Orthop Relat Res.* 1994;(299):157-162.

13. Laubenthal KN, Smidt GL, Kettelkamp DB. A quantitative analysis of knee motion during activities of daily living. *Phys Ther.* 1972;52(1):34-43.

14. Ritter MA, Lutgring JD, Davis KE, Berend ME. The effect of postoperative range of motion on functional activities after posterior cruciate-retaining total knee arthroplasty. *J Bone Joint Surg Am.* 2008;90(4):777-784.

15. Ritter MA, Lutgring JD, Davis KE, Berend ME, Pierson JL, Meneghini RM. The role of flexion contracture on outcomes in primary total knee arthroplasty. *J Arthroplasty.* 2007;22(8):1092-1096.

16. Kim J, Nelson CL, Lotke PA. Stiffness after total knee arthroplasty. Prevalence of the complication and outcomes of revision. *J Bone Joint Surg Am.* 2004;86-A(7):1479-1484.

17. Gandhi R, de Beer J, Leone J, Petruccelli D, Winemaker M, Adili A. Predictive risk factors for stiff knees in total knee arthroplasty. *J Arthroplasty.* 2006;21(1):46-52.

18. Schiavone Panni A, Cerciello S, Vasso M, Tartarone M. Stiffness in total knee arthroplasty. *J Orthop Traumatol.* 2009;10(3):111-118.

19. Emerson RH Jr, Ayers C, Higgins LL. Surgical closing in total knee arthroplasty. A series followup. *Clin Orthop Relat Res.* 1999;11(368):176-181.

20. Arnout N, Victor J, Cleppe H, Soenen M, Van Damme G, Bellemans J. Avoidance of patellar eversion improves range of motion after total knee replacement: a prospective randomized study. *Knee Surg Sports Traumatol Arthrosc.* 2009;17(10):1206-1210.

21. Kim YH, Kim JS, Kim DY. Clinical outcome and rate of complications after primary total knee replacement performed with quadriceps-sparing or standard arthrotomy. *J Bone Joint Surg Br.* 2007;89(4):467-470.

22. Lombardi AV Jr, Viacava AJ, Berend KR. Rapid recovery protocols and minimally invasive surgery help achieve high knee flexion. *Clin Orthop Relat Res.* 2006;452:117-122.

23. Lavernia C, Cardona D, Rossi MD, Lee D. Multimodal pain management and arthrofibrosis. *J Arthroplasty.* 2008;23(6 suppl 1):74-79.

24. Jerosch J, Aldawoudy AM. Arthroscopic treatment of patients with moderate arthrofibrosis after total knee replacement. *Knee Surg Sports Traumatol Arthrosc.* 2007;15(1):71-77.

25. Haidukewych GJ, Jacofsky DJ, Pagnano MW, Trousdale RT. Functional results after revision of well-fixed components for stiffness after primary total knee arthroplasty. *J Arthroplasty.* 2005;20(2):133-138.

26. Hutchinson JR, Parish EN, Cross MJ. Results of open arthrolysis for the treatment of stiffness after total knee replacement. *J Bone Joint Surg Br.* 2005;87(10):1357-1360.

27. Babis GC, Trousdale RT, Pagnano MW, Morrey BF. Poor outcomes of isolated tibial insert exchange and arthrolysis for the management of stiffness following total knee arthroplasty. *J Bone Joint Surg Am.* 2001;83-A(10):1534-1536.

28. Rand JA, Morrey BF, Bryan RS. Patellar tendon rupture after total knee arthroplasty. *Clin Orthop Relat Res.* 1989;7(244):233-238.

29. Schoderbek RJ Jr, Brown TE, Mulhall KJ, et al. Extensor mechanism disruption after total knee arthroplasty. *Clin Orthop Relat Res.* 2006;446:176-185.

30. Patel J, Ries MD, Bozic KJ. Extensor mechanism complications after total knee arthroplasty. *Instr Course Lect.* 2008;57:283-294.

31. Cadambi A, Engh GA. Use of a semitendinosus tendon autogenous graft for rupture of the patellar ligament after total knee arthroplasty. A report of seven cases. *J Bone Joint Surg Am.* 1992;74(7):974-979.

32. Emerson RH Jr, Head WC, Malinin TI. Reconstruction of patellar tendon rupture after total knee arthroplasty with an extensor mechanism allograft. *Clin Orthop Relat Res.* 1990;11(260):154-161.

33. Eisenhuth SA, Saleh KJ, Cui Q, Clark CR, Brown TE. Patellofemoral instability after total knee arthroplasty. *Clin Orthop Relat Res.* 2006;446:149-160.

34. Engh GA, Parks NL, Ammeen DJ. Influence of surgical approach on lateral retinacular releases in total knee arthroplasty. *Clin Orthop Relat Res.* 1996;(331):56-63.

35. Matsueda M, Gustilo RB. Subvastus and medial parapatellar approaches in total knee arthroplasty. *Clin Orthop Relat Res.* 2000;2(371):161-168.

36. Berger RA, Crossett LS, Jacobs JJ, Rubash HE. Malrotation causing patellofemoral complications after total knee arthroplasty. *Clin Orthop Relat Res.* 1998;11(356):144-153.

37. Malo M, Vince KG. The unstable patella after total knee arthroplasty: etiology, prevention, and management. *J Am Acad Orthop Surg.* 2003;11(5):364-371.

38. Yoshii I, Whiteside LA, Anouchi YS. The effect of patellar button placement and femoral component design on patellar tracking in total knee arthroplasty. *Clin Orthop Relat Res.* 1992;2(275):211-219.

39. Hofmann AA, Tkach TK, Evanich CJ, Camargo MP, Zhang Y. Patellar component medialization in total knee arthroplasty. *J Arthroplasty.* 1997;12(2):155-160.

40. Parvizi J, Rapuri VR, Saleh KJ, Kuskowski MA, Sharkey PF, Mont MA. Failure to resurface the patella during total knee arthroplasty may result in more knee pain and secondary surgery. *Clin Orthop Relat Res.* 2005;438:191-196.

41. Calvisi V, Camillieri G, Lupparelli S. Resurfacing versus nonresurfacing the patella in total knee arthroplasty: a critical appraisal of the available evidence. *Arch Orthop Trauma Surg.* 2009;129(9):1261-1270.

42. Burnett RS, Boone JL, McCarthy KP, Rosenzweig S, Barrack RL. A prospective randomized clinical trial of patellar resurfacing and nonresurfacing in bilateral TKA. *Clin Orthop Relat Res.* 2007;464:65-72.

43. Barrack RL, Bertot AJ, Wolfe MW, Waldman DA, Milicic M, Myers L. Patellar resurfacing in total knee arthroplasty. A prospective, randomized, double-blind study with five to seven years of follow-up. *J Bone Joint Surg Am.* 2001;83-A(9):1376-1381.

44. Mockford BJ, Beverland DE. Secondary resurfacing of the patella in mobile-bearing total knee arthroplasty. *J Arthroplasty.* 2005;20(7):898-902.

45. Partington PF, Sawhney J, Rorabeck CH, Barrack RL, Moore J. Joint line restoration after revision total knee arthroplasty. *Clin Orthop Relat Res.* 1999;10(367):165-171.

46. Figgie HE 3rd, Goldberg VM, Heiple KG, Moller HS 3rd, Gordon NH. The influence of tibial-patello-femoral location on function of the knee in patients with the posterior stabilized condylar knee prosthesis. *J Bone Joint Surg Am.* 1986;68(7):1035-1040.

47. Koh YG, Kim SJ, Chun YM, Kim YC, Park YS. Arthroscopic treatment of patellofemoral soft tissue impingement after posterior stabilized total knee arthroplasty. *Knee.* 2008;15(1):36-39.

48. Lonner JH, Lotke PA. Aseptic complications after total knee arthroplasty. *J Am Acad Orthop Surg.* 1999;7(5):311-324.

49. Gandhi R, Tsvetkov D, Davey JR, Mahomed NN. Survival and clinical function of cemented and uncemented prostheses in total knee replacement: a meta-analysis. *J Bone Joint Surg Br.* 2009;91(7):889-895.

50. Tew M, Waugh W. Tibiofemoral alignment and the results of knee replacement. *J Bone Joint Surg Br.* 1985;67(4):551-556.

51. Fang DM, Ritter MA, Davis KE. Coronal alignment in total knee arthroplasty: just how important is it? *J Arthroplasty.* 2009;24(6 suppl):39-43.

52. Naudie DD, Ammeen DJ, Engh GA, Rorabeck CH. Wear and osteolysis around total knee arthroplasty. *J Am Acad Orthop Surg.* 2007;15(1):53-64.

53. Gupta SK, Chu A, Ranawat AS, Slamin J, Ranawat CS. Osteolysis after total knee arthroplasty. *J Arthroplasty.* 2007;22(6):787-799.

54. Schmalzried TP, Shepherd EF, Dorey FJ, et al. The John Charnley Award. Wear is a function of use, not time. *Clin Orthop Relat Res.* 2000;12(381):36-46.

55. Griffin WL, Scott RD, Dalury DF, Mahoney OM, Chiavetta JB, Odum SM. Modular insert exchange in knee arthroplasty for treatment of wear and osteolysis. *Clin Orthop Relat Res.* 2007;464:132-137.

56. Griffin WL, Fehring TK, Pomeroy DL, Gruen TA, Murphy JA. Sterilization and wear-related failure in first- and second-generation press-fit condylar total knee arthroplasty. *Clin Orthop Relat Res.* 2007;464:16-20.

57. Bal BS, Greenberg D, Li S, R Mauerhan D, Schultz L, Cherry K. Tibial post failures in a condylar posterior cruciate substituting total knee arthroplasty. *J Arthroplasty.* 2008;23(5):650-655.

58. Berry DJ. Epidemiology: hip and knee. *Orthop Clin North Am.* 1999;30(2):183-190.

59. Parvizi J, Jain N, Schmidt AH. Periprosthetic knee fractures. *J Orthop Trauma.* 2008;22(9):663-671.

60. Lesh ML, Schneider DJ, Deol G, Davis B, Jacobs CR, Pellegrini VD Jr. The consequences of anterior femoral notching in total knee arthroplasty. A biomechanical study. *J Bone Joint Surg Am.* 2000;82-A(8):1096-1101.

61. Gujarathi N, Putti AB, Abboud RJ, MacLean JG, Espley AJ, Kellett CF. Risk of periprosthetic fracture after anterior femoral notching. *Acta Orthop.* 2009;80(5):553-556.

62. Herrera DA, Kregor PJ, Cole PA, Levy BA, Jonsson A, Zlowodzki M. Treatment of acute distal femur fractures above a total knee arthroplasty: systematic review of 415 cases (1981-2006). *Acta Orthop.* 2008;79(1):22-27.

63. Sheth NP, Pedowitz DI, Lonner JH. Periprosthetic patellar fractures. *J Bone Joint Surg Am.* 2007;89(10):2285-2296.

64. Chalidis BE, Tsiridis E, Tragas AA, Stavrou Z, Giannoudis PV. Management of periprosthetic patellar fractures. A systematic review of literature. *Injury.* 2007;38(6):714-724.

65. Kurtz SM, Lau E, Schmier J, Ong KL, Zhao K, Parvizi J. Infection burden for hip and knee arthroplasty in the United States. *J Arthroplasty.* 2008;23(7):984-991.

66. Jamsen E, Huhtala H, Puolakka T, Moilanen T. Risk factors for infection after knee arthroplasty. A register-based analysis of 43,149 cases. *J Bone Joint Surg Am.* 2009;91(1):38-47.

67. Kurtz SM, Ong KL, Lau E, Bozic KJ, Berry D, Parvizi J. Prosthetic joint infection risk after TKA in the Medicare population. *Clin Orthop Relat Res.* 2010;468(1):52-56.

68. Fitzgerald RH Jr, Nolan DR, Ilstrup DM, Van Scoy RE, Washington JA 2nd, Coventry MB. Deep wound sepsis following total hip arthroplasty. *J Bone Joint Surg Am.* 1977;59(7):847-855.

69. Segawa H, Tsukayama DT, Kyle RF, Becker DA, Gustilo RB. Infection after total knee arthroplasty. A retrospective study of the treatment of eighty-one infections. *J Bone Joint Surg Am.* 1999;81(10):1434-1445.

70. Tsukayama DT, Estrada R, Gustilo RB. Infection after total hip arthroplasty. A study of the treatment of one hundred and six infections. *J Bone Joint Surg Am.* 1996;78(4):512-523.

71. Weiss AP, Krackow KA. Persistent wound drainage after primary total knee arthroplasty. *J Arthroplasty.* 1993;8(3):285-289.

72. Vince K, Chivas D, Droll KP. Wound complications after total knee arthroplasty. *J Arthroplasty.* 2007;22(4 suppl 1):39-44.

73. Malinzak RA, Ritter MA, Berend ME, Meding JB, Olberding EM, Davis KE. Morbidly obese, diabetic, younger, and unilateral joint arthroplasty patients have elevated total joint arthroplasty infection rates. *J Arthroplasty.* 2009;24(6 suppl):84-88.

74. Peersman G, Laskin R, Davis J, Peterson M. Infection in total knee replacement: a retrospective review of 6489 total knee replacements. *Clin Orthop Relat Res.* 2001;11(392):15-23.

75. White J, Kelly M, Dunsmuir R. C-reactive protein level after total hip and total knee replacement. *J Bone Joint Surg Br.* 1998;80(5):909-911.

76. Bilgen O, Atici T, Durak K, Karaeminogullari, Bilgen MS. C-reactive protein values and erythrocyte sedimentation rates after total hip and total knee arthroplasty. *J Int Med Res.* 2001;29(1):7-12.

77. Della Valle CJ, Sporer SM, Jacobs JJ, Berger RA, Rosenberg AG, Paprosky WG. Preoperative testing for sepsis before revision total knee arthroplasty. *J Arthroplasty.* 2007;22(6 suppl 2):90-93.

78. Austin MS, Ghanem E, Joshi A, Lindsay A, Parvizi J. A simple, cost-effective screening protocol to rule out periprosthetic infection. *J Arthroplasty.* 2008;23(1):65-68.

79. Parvizi J, Ghanem E, Menashe S, Barrack RL, Bauer TW. Periprosthetic infection: what are the diagnostic challenges? *J Bone Joint Surg Am.* 2006;88(suppl 4):138-147.

80. Mason JB, Fehring TK, Odum SM, Griffin WL, Nussman DS. The value of white blood cell counts before revision total knee arthroplasty. *J Arthroplasty.* 2003;18(8):1038-1043.

81. Ghanem E, Parvizi J, Burnett RS, et al. Cell count and differential of aspirated fluid in the diagnosis of infection at the site of total knee arthroplasty. *J Bone Joint Surg Am.* 2008;90(8):1637-1643.

82. Morgan PM, Sharkey P, Ghanem E, et al. The value of intraoperative Gram stain in revision total knee arthroplasty. *J Bone Joint Surg Am.* 2009;91(9):2124-2129.

83. Bauer TW, Parvizi J, Kobayashi N, Krebs V. Diagnosis of periprosthetic infection. *J Bone Joint Surg Am.* 2006;88(4):869-882.

84. Ip D, Yam SK, Chen CK. Implications of the changing pattern of bacterial infections following total joint replacements. *J Orthop Surg (Hong Kong).* 2005;13(2):125-130.

85. Parvizi J, Bender B, Saleh KJ, Brown TE, Schmalzried TP, Mihalko WM. Resistant organisms in infected total knee arthroplasty: occurrence, prevention, and treatment regimens. *Instr Course Lect.* 2009;58:271-278.

86. Waldman BJ, Hostin E, Mont MA, Hungerford DS. Infected total knee arthroplasty treated by arthroscopic irrigation and debridement. *J Arthroplasty.* 2000;15(4):430-436.

The opinions and assertions contained herein are the private views of the authors and are not to be construed as official or reflecting the views of the Department of the Army or Department of Defense.

3

Revision Total Knee Arthroplasty
A Reference Summary

Vamsi K. Kancherla, MD and Scott M. Sporer, MD, MS

INTRODUCTION AND EPIDEMIOLOGY

Despite the long-term clinical success of total knee arthroplasty (TKA) with reported survivorship of greater than 95% at 15 years[1,2] and improvements in implant design, a small percentage of patients will experience clinical failure presenting with pain and impaired function. The revision rate has been estimated to be less than 3% within the first 2 years of index arthroplasty.[3] By 2030, the demand for primary TKAs is projected to grow by 673% to 3.48 million procedures, while the demand for knee revisions is expected to double by 2015 and grow by 601% through 2030.[4] The prevalence of revision TKA is increasing due to increased volume of total knee replacements, modifications in surgical technique, implant longevity, broadened surgical indications, and improved life expectancy. Consequently, surgeons face an increased number of complex knee revision surgeries. Extensive bone loss, instability, extensor mechanism dysfunction, and peri-articular arthrofibrosis are frequent challenges encountered during surgery. Hence, a systematic approach to patients requiring revision knee surgery can optimize the chance of a successful outcome.

DIFFERENTIAL DIAGNOSIS: WHAT IS THE ETIOLOGY?

The etiologies of dysfunction and pain after total knee replacement can be numerous[5-7]; therefore, it is important to approach the diagnosis in a systematic fashion. A logical approach employs a thorough history, physical examination, and diagnostic modalities while being keenly aware of the differential diagnosis of the painful TKA. The etiologies can be grouped into 2 large categories: extrinsic (extra-articular) or intrinsic (intra-articular) (Tables 3-1 and 3-2). Furthermore, as treatment of the infected TKA is fundamentally different than the patient with aseptic failure, every patient who presents with a failed or otherwise painful TKA must be evaluated for the presence of a deep periprosthetic infection. Even if the cause of failure seems obvious, concomitant infection

Jacofsky DJ, Hedley AK, eds.
*Fundamentals of Revision Knee Arthroplasty:
Diagnosis, Evaluation, and Treatment* (pp 31-58).
© 2013 SLACK Incorporated.

TABLE 3-1. EXTRINSIC (EXTRA-ARTICULAR) ETIOLOGIES

1. Hip pathology
2. Lumbar spine
    a. Stenosis
    b. Radiculopathy
3. Neuroma
4. Complex regional pain syndrome
5. Vascular claudication

6. Soft tissue inflammation
    a. Pes bursitis
    b. Patellar tendonitis
    c. Quadriceps tendinitis
7. Periprosthetic fractures
    a. Tibial stress fractures
    b. Patellar stress fractures
    c. Traumatic fractures

TABLE 3-2. INTRINSIC (INTRA-ARTICULAR) ETIOLOGIES

1. Infection
2. Instability
    a. Axial
    b. Flexion
    c. Global
3. Malalignment
    a. Axial
    b. Flexion
    c. Global
4. Aseptic loosening
5. Polyethylene wear
6. Osteolysis
7. Implant fracture
8. Arthrofibrosis

9. Soft tissue impingement
10. Patellar clunk
11. Popliteus tendon impingement
12. Component overhang/excess cement
13. Extensor mechanism dysfunction
    a. Patellar instability
    b. Patellar fracture
    c. Patellar pain
        i.   Unresurfaced patella
        ii. Lateral facet impingement
        iii. Patella baja
        iv. Excessive composite thickness
    d. Quad/patellar tendon rupture

could be present and substantially change the treatment plan. If at all possible, diagnosis should be made preoperatively for appropriate patient counseling on treatment options.

History and Physical Examination

The history is critical in evaluating the patient. Both aspects of the patient's past medical history and the history surrounding the index arthroplasty may lead the surgeon to a high index of suspicion for a septic (Table 3-3) or an aseptic etiology.

The Patient's History

1.   Were wound healing problems evident at the time of the index arthroplasty?
    ■ Were antibiotics given?
    ■ Was there an extended hospital stay?
    ■ Did he or she have an early return to the operating room?
    ■ Was there chronic drainage after the index arthroplasty?

TABLE 3-3. PATIENT RISK FACTORS FOR INFECTION

1. Diabetes mellitus	6. Prior ipsilateral knee surgery
2. History of septic arthritis of the native knee	7. Malnourished
3. Inflammatory arthritis	8. Renal insufficiency
4. Skin disorders (eg, psoriasis)	9. Otherwise immunocompromised

---

2. Has there been pain since the index procedure (other than preoperative pain)?
- Early postoperative pain
  - ☐ Suspect infection (Are there wound healing problems or drainage?)
  - ☐ Wrong indication (Is pain unchanged from preoperative pain?)
  - ☐ Soft tissue impingement
- Late onset pain
  - ☐ Instability—Starts after 1 to 2 years and can be progressive.
  - ☐ Suspect loosening
  - ☐ Wear
  - ☐ Osteolysis
  - ☐ Hematogenous or chronic infection
- Pain characterization, location, and radiation
  - ☐ Suspect extra-articular source if pain radiates
- Is the patient's pain associated with weightbearing (mechanical) versus rest?
3. Is there a history of a recent systemic illness or other bacteremia?
- Suggests a hematogenous infection
- Specifically ask about dental work or dental problems
4. Was there an early failure of an otherwise well done TKA (especially less than 2 years postoperatively)?

The Physical Exam

- Visual inspection (Particular attention should be paid to prior incisions.)
- Careful palpation (Is swelling or point tenderness present?)
- Effusion (Effusions are typical of instability and can often be bloodstained.)
- Tibiofemoral joint stability
  - ☐ Extension
  - ☐ Mid-flexion
  - ☐ Ninety-degree flexion (flexion instability[8])
    - Posterior stabilized design—Exaggerated anterior drawer test
    - Cruciate-retaining design—Exaggerated posterior and anterior drawer
- Patellofemoral joint stability
  - ☐ Palpation of patella and retinaculum
  - ☐ Carefully evaluate patellar tracking through entire range of motion
    - Patellar clunk syndrome typically observed near 30 to 45 degrees as knee extends from flexed position; more commonly seen in a posterior stabilized design
    - Patellar clunk less common with modern femoral designs[9]
  - ☐ Passive and active motion assessed

- Evaluation of gait and range of motion
  - □ Flexion contracture/extensor lag
- Thorough neurovascular examination
  - □ Quadriceps and vastus medialis oblique strength
  - □ Assessment of quality and symmetry of pulses
- Adjacent joints
  - □ Always examine the ipsilateral hip!
  - □ Lumbar spine
  - □ Foot and ankle
    - Planovalgus deformity can be a contributing factor to failure of the cruciate-retaining TKA[10]
- Other
  - □ Evidence of a present or prior sinus tract?
  - □ Are you going to have problems closing the wound at revision?
    - Dense adherent skin in the area of the tubercle
    - Get a plastic/hand surgeon involved early!
    - Consider medial gastrocnemius flap

Diagnostics

Plain Radiographs

- Required: Weightbearing anteroposterior, lateral, and Merchant views
- Ideal if possible: Preoperative x-rays, serial x-rays, full-length hip-to-ankle views
- Anteroposterior view assessment
  - □ Polyethylene wear, osteolysis, and radiolucent lines
  - □ Periosteal reaction/early lytic lesions are very suspicious for infection
  - □ Tibial component subsidence, overhang, and position change
- Lateral view assessment
  - □ Femoral component prosthetic interface/femoral component size and position
  - □ Patella/patella tendon
  - □ Tibial component slope/sagittal plane subsidence
- Merchant view assessment
  - □ Patellar tilt/malalignment/loosening/composite thickness
- Stress radiographs
  - □ Assess for coronal plane instability when indicated
- Fluoroscopic evaluation
  - □ Facilitates evaluation of cementless total knee replacement interfaces

Advanced Imaging

Nuclear Imaging Studies

- Radionuclide scans are helpful in the diagnosis of:
  - □ Aseptic loosening: indium[111]—white blood cell (WBC) imaging of a painful left TKA shows uptake around both the femoral and tibial components, suggestive of infection (Figure 3-1A). Corresponding technetium-99m sulfur colloid study

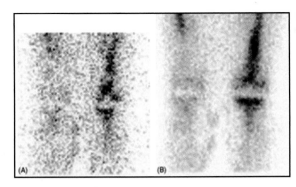

Figure 3-1. Indium[111] WBC scan and technetium-99m sulfur colloid scan. (Reprinted with permission of the *European Journal of Radiology*, 54[2]. Miller TT, Imaging of knee arthroplasty. Pages 164-177. Copyright 2005, with permission of Elsevier.)

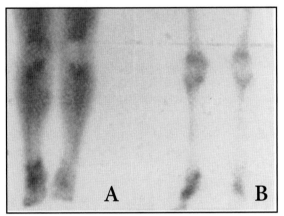

Figure 3-2. Three-phase bone scintigraphy.

(Figure 3-1B) shows spatially matching uptake of the sulfur colloid, thus demonstrating that the uptake of the white cells in Figure 3-1A is merely due to hematopoietically marrow and not due to infection. If the white cell study had been performed without the sulfur colloid study, it would have been incorrectly misinterpreted as infection.[3]

☐ Infection: Bone scintigraphy is useful for excluding infection but has limited value detecting it. Evaluation of indium scanning may lead to a high false-positive rate that is thought to be due to marrow packing.[11] The addition of technetium-99m-labeled sulfur colloid scanning still has limited clinical utility. It has been suggested that positive indium WBC scan and sedimentation rate are the most predictive variables for detecting septic prostheses.[12]

☐ Complex regional pain syndrome (CRPS): CRPS I stage II (Figure 3-2). Blood-pool (Figure 3-2A) and delayed images (Figure 3-2B) demonstrate increased uptake throughout the symptomatic right lower extremity, especially the knee, ankle, and joints of the foot. Sensitivity and specificity of 3-phase bone scintigraphy is variable, however, the sensitivity can increase with disorder progression. Amount of uptake correlates to prognosis; increased uptake can increase likelihood of a positive response to therapy.[13]

☐ Periprosthetic stress fractures: Although most fractures are diagnosed with use of radiographs, a technetium-99m bone scan may be employed to determine whether a fracture is old or new, or to diagnose occult fractures. Bone scans may be positive for up to 2 years following a periprosthetic fracture.

■ Three-phase technetium-99m bone scan

    ☐ May show increased uptake in index TKA indefinitely

    ☐ Uptake around 89% tibial, 63% femoral implants more than 1 year after index TKA[14]

- □ Limits usefulness when performed alone since it cannot distinguish infection from aseptic loosening[3]
- □ Normal bone scan has 95% negative predictive value for excluding both infection and aseptic loosening[3]
- Indium[111]-labeled leukocyte scan
  - □ Accuracy of 78% when used alone for infection
  - □ When combined with technetium-99m, sulfur colloid marrow scans improve accuracy to 88% to 95%[15]
  - □ However, this is still a second-line test as there are less expensive, easier ways to diagnose infection
- Computed tomography
  - □ Less expensive and quicker than magnetic resonance imaging (MRI)
  - □ More accurately defines extent of osteolytic lesions
  - □ Assess femoral and tibial component rotation
    - Femoral component rotation compared to transepicondylar axis
    - Tibial component rotation compared to medial third of tibial tubercle
    - Excessive internal rotation associated with patellar instability,[16] lateral flexion laxity, and poorer clinical function[17]
- MRI
  - □ Expensive and takes hours to complete study
  - □ MRI with metal artifact suppression
    - Can detect osteolysis better than plain radiographs[18-20]
    - Good correlation to operative findings, thus allowing more accurate, quantitative predictions for bone graft requirements and selection of prosthetic if surgical intervention is deemed necessary[20]

Laboratory Tests

- Erythrocyte sedimentation rate (ESR) and C-reactive protein (CRP) are mandatory in the evaluation of the painful total joint replacement
  - □ The single easiest, best, and most cost-effective screening test for infection
  - □ Very rarely normal in the face of infection
    - If ESR is less than 30 mm/hr *and* CRP is less than 10 mg/dL, infection is *very unlikely*[21,22]
    - If one or both are abnormal, joint aspiration should be done to determine if infection is present

Aspiration of the Knee Joint

- Joint aspiration is required if:
  - □ There is high clinical suspicion of sepsis
  - □ It is a high-risk patient
  - □ If either ESR and/or CRP are elevated

- The aspirated fluid should be sent for culture, a synovial fluid WBC count, and a differential
  - Culture
    - Patients should be off antibiotics for a minimum of 2 weeks for the culture results to be accurate
    - Sent for aerobic, anaerobic cultures; consider fungal/acid-fast bacili if prior aspirates negative
    - Repeat the aspiration if your clinical suspicion is high
  - Synovial fluid WBC count
    - Has been shown to be probably ***the best single test!***
    - Inexpensive, ubiquitous, and objective
    - Can be done pre- or intraoperatively (result in approximately 30 minutes)
    - Optimal cut-off value is controversial to a point
      - Reported range of 1100 to 3000 WBC/mm^3
      - Definitely ***not*** the 50,000 WBC/mm^3 for a native knee
  - Synovial fluid WBC count differential
    - Has been shown to be a very good test
    - Optimal cut-off value 60% to 80%
    - Greater than 90% ***very*** suspicious
- Joint aspiration criteria for sepsis
  - Synovial leukocyte count of greater than 1100 cells/uL ***and*** differential greater than 64% indicates sepsis is very likely (98.6%)[21]

Lidocaine Injection

- Can be a very useful adjunct to confirm intra-articular and extra-articular pathology, particularly:
  - Aseptic loosening
  - Soft tissue impingement
  - Pes anserine bursitis

Arthroscopy

- Very limited use and indications
- Some have reported successful arthroscopic lysis of adhesions with manipulation for arthrofibrosis outside the 3 months postoperative window
- Others have established clinical success in arthroscopic evaluation and subsequent débridement in soft tissue impingement, such as patellar clunk[23] and popliteus tendon impingement[24]
- Diagnostic lidocaine injection is helpful prior to arthroscopy

Intraoperative Tests: Appearance, Gram Stain/Culture, Frozen Section

- Intraoperative appearance is not a reliable test!
- Intraoperative gram stains are not reliable!
  - May be helpful in cases where gross purulence is identified to guide empiric treatment
  - Cannot be the only test you use to evaluate a patient for infection
  - Can be falsely positive! Crystal formation in gram's dye can look like gram-positive cocci

TABLE 3-4. CRITERIA FOR INFECTION (OPTION 1)

- At least one positive culture (on solid media, not broth)
- Positive permanent histopathology consistent with infection
- Intraoperative appearance consistent with infection (eg, gross pus)

TABLE 3-5. CRITERIA FOR INFECTION (OPTION 2)

- Elevated CRP
- Positive joint aspiration culture
- Positive intraoperative culture
- Intraoperative appearance consistent with infection (eg, gross pus)
- Elevated ESR

- Intraoperative frozen sections
  - □ Can be reliable
    - Pathologist needs to be interested and dedicated (try to get one person to interpret all of your cases)
    - Meet with him or her to decide on the criteria for infection so you are "speaking the same language"
  - □ Criteria for infection are controversial
    - Average of 10 polymorphonuclear leukocytes (PMNs) in the 5 most cellular fields (Lonner criteria)[25]
    - PMNs in fibrin do *not* count!
- As there is no gold standard for diagnosing infection, the precise criteria for diagnosing infection remain elusive. A combination of tests most definitively makes the diagnosis. We have used the following criteria:
  - □ Two positive cultures with the same organisms *or* 2 of the 3 criteria in Table 3-4
  - □ Parvizi et al has recommended a similar combination of tests with a diagnosis of infection being made by identifying 3 of the 5 criteria in Table 3-5[26]

Algorithm: Septic Versus Aseptic

See Figure 3-3.

Classification for an Infected Knee

See Table 3-6.

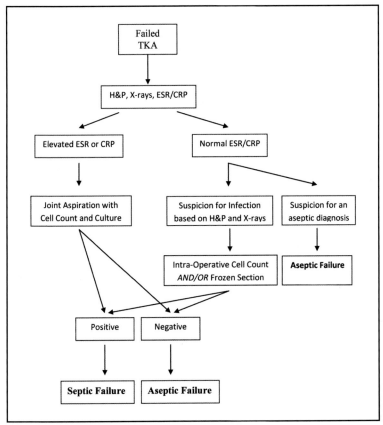

Figure 3-3. An algorithmic approach to diagnosis.

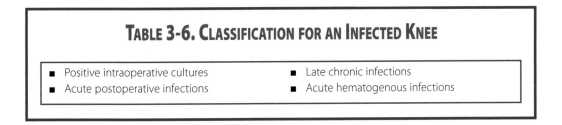

TABLE 3-6. CLASSIFICATION FOR AN INFECTED KNEE

- Positive intraoperative cultures
- Acute postoperative infections
- Late chronic infections
- Acute hematogenous infections

TREATMENT PROTOCOL

Preoperative Planning

The "10 Commandments" of Revision Knee Surgery

1. What is the diagnosis? Why am I revising this knee?
    - It is imperative that a diagnosis is made before surgery. Surgical exploration for a painful knee will rarely provide symptomatic improvement. If you do not know why you are operating on a patient, ***stop!***

2.   What other comorbidities does my patient have?

- Associated medical comorbidities such as malnutrition, diabetes, and lymphedema should be optimized before revision surgery. There may be situations such as Charcot arthropathy, neuromuscular disease, or concomitant infection where revision surgery is contraindicated.

3.   What implants are currently in place?

- Previous surgical records will help identify the current implants. This step is vital since many companies have implants that look similar radiographically. Knowing the implants can also ensure that the correct polyethylene liner is available, and that the options for additional constraint are known if the components are planned to be retained. Some implants will also demonstrate a characteristic mode of failure.

4.   What is the condition of the soft tissue surrounding the knee?

- Wound healing following revision knee surgery is of paramount concern. Previous surgical incision may dictate surgical approach. If there is concern, plastic surgery consultation should be considered.

5.   How will I remove the current implants?

- Varying implants may have devices to assist with component removal. Determining preoperatively what will be required is essential. At a minimum, surgeons should have a reciprocating and sagittal saw, flexible osteotomes, and a device to impact against the component. If there is a large amount of cement in the tibial canal, long osteotomes or ultrasonic cement removal devices should be considered.

6.   How can I reconstruct the tibial or femoral bone loss?

- Plain radiographs historically underestimate the degree of bone loss surrounding the femoral and tibial component.[27] Bone loss can either be cavitary (which is frequently supportive) or segmental (which is frequently nonsupportive). Options for bone loss reconstruction include bone cement, cancellous allograft, structural bulk allograft, metal augments, and custom implants.[28] In general, surgical options that minimize the removal of additional bone should be utilized. The Anderson Orthopaedic Research Institute Bone Defect Classification is helpful in defining the severity of bone loss intraoperatively[29]:
  - Type I: Minor femoral or tibial defects with intact metaphyseal bone not compromising the stability of a revision implant
  - Type II: Damaged metaphyseal bone requiring femoral or tibial bone reconstruction (cement, augment, or bone graft)
    - A: Defects in one femoral or tibial condyle
    - B: Defects in both femoral or tibial condyles
  - Type III: Deficient metaphyseal segment compromising a major portion of either femoral condyle or tibial plateau

7.   What is the condition of the extensor mechanism?

- The extensor mechanism must be protected during revision surgery. It is important to know the function of the extensor mechanism prior to surgery. A preoperative extensor lag may be due to relative shortening of the leg secondary to component loosening and subsequently a loss of resting tension. This type of extensor lag can improve with revision surgery. Situations with a chronic quadriceps or patellar tendon dysfunction may require a concomitant extensor mechanism allograft at the time of surgery.

8. How can I obtain stability?

- Obtaining stability of the knee in both the coronal and sagittal planes is crucial. Attempts should be made to use the least amount of constraint possible. A standard posterior stabilized polyethylene insert can frequently be used in revision surgery once the knee is realigned. However, components with an extended post are helpful if unilateral coronal plane instability exists or a slight flexion-extension mismatch occurs. A more constrained hinge type device can be used in patients with marked flexion-extension mismatch, recurvatum, or global instability.

9. Is the joint line reconstituted?

- Restoring the appropriate height of the joint line will improve the kinematics of the knee. Patella baja can be encountered during surgery and may be an intrinsic contracture of the patellar ligament. In general, distal femoral augmentation is required in revision surgery to avoid elevating the joint line and inducing an artificial patella baja. The joint line can be assessed by looking for the meniscal scar, height from the fibular head, and where the superior pole of the patella is in relation to the superior aspect of the trochlear groove.

10. What special concerns may exist postoperatively?

- Postoperative care following revision surgery is crucial. If compromised skin was present at the time of surgery or if the extensor mechanism was deficient, excessive knee flexion should be avoided. While terminal flexion is important, many patients lack full extension prior to surgery. As a result, hamstring stretching should be encouraged immediately.

Surgical Indications

Absolute Indications

- Progressive osteolysis with impending fracture
- Periprosthetic femur/tibia fracture with loose implant
  - ☐ Assess femoral component
    - If femoral component is well fixed, attempt to retain implant and obtain rigid fixation with either a retrograde nail or peri-articular locking plate. Locking plates with variable fixed angles are helpful to maximize fixation into the distal fragment.
    - If femoral component is loose, femoral revision is required. Bone loss can be reconstructed with metal augments or distal femoral allograft/distal femoral replacing arthroplasty with long stem extension in order to obtain proximal fixation. If allograft prosthetic composite is used, maintain host collateral ligament attachments and secure via screw with washer to allograft.
  - ☐ Assess tibial component for loosening. Most fractures below well-fixed implant can be treated nonoperatively. Long tibial stem extension can be used to bypass fracture if tibial component is loose.
- Septic joint arthroplasty: One-stage exchange, two-stage exchange, or irrigation and débridement with polyethylene liner exchange should be considered depending upon the acuity of the infection. Standard of care in the United States for chronic infection is two-stage exchange.

Relative Indications

- Aseptic loosening with pain
- Progressive osteolysis
- Component malposition

> ## TABLE 3-7. ETIOLOGIES FOR A CHALLENGING EXPOSURE
>
> | | |
> |---|---|
> | ■ Arthrofibrosis | ■ The presence of patella baja |
> | ■ The presence of osteoporotic or osteolytic bone | ■ Obesity or a markedly muscular lower extremity |

Contraindications

- "Surgical exploration" for chronic pain
- Incision and drainage for chronic infection
- Combination of arthrofibrosis, deficient extensor mechanism, and infection; consider arthrodesis

Exposure

The Skin Incision

Principles of exposure of the revision knee begin with tenets regarding prior skin incisions. The majority of the time a single incision is present, and generally this incision can be reasonably used for the patient's revision surgery. Although these incisions maybe straight and directly anterior, medialized, or curvilinear, a single previous primary TKA incision generally allows adequate and reasonably easy exposure for the subsequent revision surgery.

If multiple incisions are present:

- Transverse and oblique incisions should generally be crossed at the most obtuse angle possible in order to minimize the potential for wound healing complications at the corners created by this intersection.
- If multiple longitudinal incisions are present, the blood supply from the medial to the lateral side of the knee, as well as its lymphatic drainage, generally would favor the use of the more lateral incision.
- However, if all incisions are greater than 2 years of age and do not involve a surrounding soft tissue flap, they generally can be chosen based upon their location and based upon which incision would be the most advantageous for component removal and revision surgery.
- One must be sure to protect the extensor mechanism throughout the procedure, as fibrosis, osteolysis in the region of the tibial tubercle, and multiple prior surgical procedures could all put the extensor mechanism at risk for iatrogenic avulsion.
- The exposure must allow for the following:
  - Adequate exposure of the implant
  - Adequate débridement of osteolysis as indicated
  - Adequate visualization of remaining bone stock and surgical field
  - Must be adequate for reimplantation of components
- Given the increased incidence of wound healing complications in the revision setting, one should always err on the side of a slightly longer incision if undue tension will be placed on skin edges if incision extension is not performed. Exposure should generally move from simple to complex surgical techniques.

Specific reasons for difficulty in exposing the revision knee include the presence of those listed in Table 3-7.

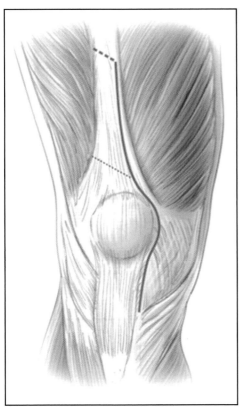

Figure 3-4. Illustration depicting a medial parapatellar arthrotomy (solid line) and quadriceps snip modification (blue dashed line). It is important to keep the longitudinal incision in the tendon and to extend it proximally to the top of the tendon before creating an oblique incision (quadriceps snip) at the proximal extent of the tendon. A transverse or oblique incision across the quadriceps tendon closer to the patella (black dashed line) must be avoided, as this may be associated with postoperative extensor mechanism disruption. (Reprinted with permission of Nelson CL, Kim J, Lotke PA. Stiffness after total knee arthroplasty. *J Bone Joint Surg Am.* 2005;87:264-270.)

Medial Parapatellar Arthrotomy

The medial parapatellar arthrotomy is the workhorse of revision TKA exposure.

- During the exposure, previous sutures should be removed as part of the débridement whenever possible
- After the medial parapatellar arthrotomy is performed, the medial and lateral gutters must be freed of fibrotic tissue in order to assist with mobilization of the extensor mechanism
- The supraparapatellar pouch may be cleared of all scar tissue
- In cases of arthrofibrosis and stiffness, a quadricepsplasty is beneficial to free the extensor mechanism from the anterior aspect of the femur to assist with mobilization of soft tissue
- A copious medial release is always performed when component revision is required
  - Allows subluxation of the tibia anteriorly for the removal of the polyethylene liner
  - This is often referred to as a *medial collateral ligament slide*
  - Once the polyethylene insert is removed, this improves the ability to mobilize the soft tissues, and in many cases this is all the exposure necessary for revision surgery
- Consider lateral arthrotomy if incision is placed laterally or if previous lateral arthrotomy was performed to avoid patellar osteonecrosis

Quadriceps Snip

As the complexity of the exposure increases due to arthrofibrosis or due to the patient's body habitis, the next step is the performance of a quadriceps snip (Figure 3-4).

- An oblique apical extension of the arthrotomy that moves in a proximal and lateral direction, exiting the quadriceps tendon laterally and splitting the fibers of the vastus lateralis obliquus
- This will assist with patellar eversion, knee flexion, and lateralization and mobilization of the extensor mechanism
- It is important to perform the quadriceps snip via exiting the quadriceps tendon prior to the musculotendinous junction of the rectus femoris muscle
- Proximal extension of the arthrotomy beyond the tendon prior to the oblique snip will lead to transection of rectus femoris fibers and should be avoided
- In the majority of cases, the quadriceps snip and medial collateral ligament slide is adequate exposure for the performance of revision knee surgery
- As the closure is essentially identical to a normal capsular closure, and as there is no change in postoperative rehabilitation or outcome, the quadriceps snip may be used liberally to improve exposure

V-Y Turndown

In rare cases, a V-Y turndown might be required. This is very rarely used and is generally reserved for severe quadriceps tendon contracture.

- Should never be used in the case of a multiply operated knee, a history of quadriceps fibrosis, or infection such as seen at the time of reimplantation
- A fibrotic extensor mechanism may fail at the closure of the V-Y turndown, and quadriceps necrosis has been reported after this exposure
- Additionally, even in those with an initially contracted extensor mechanism that requires lengthening for adequate range of motion, an extensor lag is often seen postoperatively in patients undergoing the V-Y turndown approach

Tibial Tubercle Osteotomy

More commonly, an extended tibial tubercle osteotomy can be performed to further improve exposure. Table 3-8 details when this approach is most useful.

The tibial tubercle osteotomy (Figure 3-5) is generally a long osteotomy that is greater than 8 cm in length.

- A proximal shelf of bone is ideally left to prevent proximal migration of the osteotomy fragment
- In practice, however, significant osteolysis, or the need to move the tibial tubercle proximally, often obviates one's ability leave a structurally sound proximal shelf
- The osteotomy is made along the proximal and medial aspect of the tubercle and is hinged about the lateral side with osteotomes
- The soft tissue sleeve about the lateral side is ideally left intact, and the osteotomy is generally fixed with 3 or 4 wires at the time of closure
- Often these wires can be predrilled prior to the osteotomy being hinged open
- In patients with reasonable bone stock, rehabilitation postoperatively can be unaltered after tibial tubercle osteotomy
- Although symptomatic hardware may be seen, nonunions are extremely rare after tibial tubercle osteotomy in the aseptic setting

TABLE 3-8. REASONS FOR TIBIAL TUBERCLE OSTEOTOMY

- The removal of a cemented tibial stem
- In the presence of patellar ligament contracture
- Patella baja requiring proximalization
- In cases of extensor mechanism maltracking and tibial tubercle malposition that requires correction

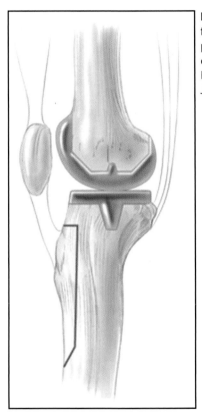

Figure 3-5. Illustration depicting a tibial tubercle osteotomy site from the lateral view, emphasizing the transverse nature of the proximal extent of the osteotomy and the oblique nature of the distal extent of the osteotomy. (Reprinted with permission of Nelson CL, Kim J, Lotke PA. Stiffness after total knee arthroplasty. *J Bone Joint Surg Am.* 2005;87:264-270.)

Medial Femoral Peel

If a tibial tubercle osteotomy is not required, but improved exposure of the components is required due to significant arthrofibrosis, a medial femoral peel maybe performed. This provides outstanding exposure of the femoral component—and often more importantly—exposure to the posterior aspect of the condyles and posterior capsule.

- Typically required during reimplantation for infection if static spacers have been used or in patients where significant contraction of the medial side of the knee has occurred
- Although this can be performed laterally as well, the authors find this to be most helpful on the medial side
- The medial femoral peel can be performed with a cautery by subperiosteum removal of the origin of the medial collateral ligament and the soft tissues around the medial side of the knee
- It is imperative that one keeps the entire medial sleeve, from the region of the extensor mechanism proximally to the superficial medial collateral ligament distally, intact

- Keeping the sleeve intact is critical to the maintenance of medial-sided stability
- Generally, no alteration of rehabilitation after surgery is required

Medial Epicondylar Osteotomy

A medial epicondylar osteotomy can be performed in more severe cases, but generally is not required unless a malunion is present.

- Should a medial epicondylar osteotomy be required, one should make certain that the following is true:
  - Significant osteolysis is not present in the region of the medial condyle or significant uncontained femoral bone deficiency can result. This would make reconstruction and subsequent repair of the osteotomy difficult.

Authors Preference for Exposure

In general, the approach for revision surgery is a generous medial collateral ligament release to the posteromedial or posterior aspect of the tibia, in conjunction with a possible quadriceps snip.

- A tibial tubercle osteotomy is the authors' preferred extensile approach for the removal of a cemented tibial stem or in the presence of patella baja that requires correction
- In cases of severe arthrofibrosis or stiffness, such as seen in reimplantation TKA, a medial femoral peel can be quite useful

Component Removal

After adequate exposure has been performed, the bone-cement or bone-implant interfaces of all 3 components should be exposed well with a needle-nose rongeur.

- A total synovectomy is generally performed
- The components are evaluated for the presence of loosening, malposition, or impingement
- Determining which component should be removed is obviously dependent upon these findings, and perhaps more importantly the diagnosis leading to the indication for revision surgery

The modular polyethylene liner is generally removed with either an implant-specific device or a small osteotome.

- A small osteotome can be impacted between the tibial baseplate and the polyethylene insert and the insert removed without difficulty
- In cases where the tibia tray will be preserved, one should use caution not to damage the locking mechanism or severely damage the tibial tray to prevent increased backside wear after liner exchange

Component removal can be performed with osteotomes, a Gigli saw, ultrasonic equipment, or the use of a small oscillating saw. A thin and narrow blade should be utilized to help steer the blade around pegs of the tibia keel, and to also help prevent inadvertent damage to surrounding soft tissues.

The femoral component is addressed first to improve later access to the tibia.

- The interface is disrupted with a small oscillating saw
- A slap hammer and extraction device can be placed distally or a stepped impactor be placed on the anterior flange if the implant has been loosened sufficiently
- A Gigli saw is quite popular for removal of components and can be effective in most cases
  - However, one must be cautious with the use of a Gigli saw, as it will generally follow the path of least resistance. Even with the most meticulous attention to detail, it can often inadvertently remove portions of bone from the trochlear region of the femur

- Consider retaining well-fixed cement once the component is removed to minimize additional bone loss
- Following femoral component removal, release additional soft tissue along the posterior aspect of the knee to allow tibial subluxation

Begin the tibial component extraction by removing any tibial screws and attempt to disassemble stemmed or modular tibial trays.

- The independent removal of modular tibial components will allow the prosthesis-cement interface of the stem to be disrupted before the tibial stem extension is removed
- Consider placing the knee in full extension to allow exposure to the lateral aspect of the knee
- Generally, the area between the tray and the proximal aspect of the tibial tubercle contains significant fibrotic tissue, but this can be exposed and freed with a curved osteotome or cautery if one locates the true margins of the proximal tubercle
- When extracting the tibial component, take care not to damage the posterior tibial plateau when hitting along the undersurface of the anterior tibial baseplate
- In the case of a cemented stem, a tibial tubercle osteotomy, as described above, can be performed if necessary.
  - However, often attempted impaction of the tibial tray may allow removal of the component, leaving the cement behind. Should this occur, cement removal can be performed with or without a tibial tubercle osteotomy, and may require use of ultrasonic equipment and specialized osteotomes

Should long, well-fixed, cemented stems be present on the femoral or tibial side, windows can be created about the tibial diaphysis or femoral diaphysis to assist with dislodging the implant.

- Rarely, a metal cutting tool such as a high-speed diamond wheel or a high-speed metal-cutting burr can be utilized to cut around the stem to allow removal of the articular tibia or femoral component while leaving the stem in place for later removal
- If you believe this will be required, trephines should be available that approximate the size of the stem in order to assist with stem removal. Subsequent cement removal can be performed as described previously

The patellar component should be retained unless it is loose, demonstrates severe wear, or is unable to be used with the new femoral component

- If the patellar component requires extraction, disrupt the implant-cement interface with the use of a sagittal saw and retain well-fixed cement
- Cementless patellar components requiring removal may require the pegs of the patella to be transected with a metal-cutting burr. Often these pegs can be retained and a cemented patella can still be placed
- If a metal-cutting device is utilized in the surgical bed, the use of sterile ultrasonic jelly placed as a coating over sponges that surround the implant can help minimize the uncontrolled spread of metal debris throughout the field

Reconstruction

Tibial Preparation

Once the tibial and femoral components have been successfully removed, begin with recreation of the joint line height and the reconstruction of tibial defects.[30] The goal of revision surgery is to provide a stable implant while retaining as much host bone as possible. The authors prefer to initially address the tibia, as the platform created will affect both the flexion and extension spaces. Bone loss encountered at the time of revision may be accommodated by cement, cancellous allograft, structural cortical allograft, metal augments, cones, or custom implants. Custom implants are rarely used due to their expense as well their inability to be modified intraoperatively. Most knee revisions will have some degree of cavitary bone loss within the proximal tibia. These defects can generally be ignored and filled with cement, assuming a stemmed tibial implant is used.[31] Impaction bone grafting or the placement of metal augments will provide support for the tibial baseplate if only a thin cortical rim is present.[32] Bulk allografts, metal augments, and tumor prosthesis should be considered when larger structural defects are present within the proximal tibia.[33] Tumor prosthesis is generally reserved for severe bone loss in elderly low-demand patients. Bulk allograft can be used if a segmental defect is present that involves a large portion of the tibial plateau. Metal augmentation has gained popularity due to its ease of insertion and ability to be easily customized intraoperatively.[34]

Stem extensions can be used during both the tibial and femoral reconstruction. Bone loss is inevitably present and can affect component stability. Stem extensions will transfer stress from the deficient proximal tibia more distally to the intact diaphyseal bone.[35] Stem extension will also provide additional surface area for fixation and can also assist with component orientation. The optimal length of a tibial or femoral stem extension remains controversial. In general, the stem extension should engage diaphyseal bone and should bypass any meta-diaphyseal defects. Stem fixation can either be fully cemented or a hybrid technique where the tibial baseplate is cemented and the stem extension is tightly press-fit into the canal.

Advantages of noncemented stems include the ability to use the stem to determine alignment, as they are canal filling, and their ability to be more easily removed if necessary in the future. Disadvantages of noncemented stems include the difficulty of their use in deformed tibial bone, the potential for end-of-stem pain, and their inability to fully offload the tibial plateau due to their lack of true fixation.

Cemented stems allow improved surface area for cement interdigitation, but result in much more difficulty during component removal and do not assist in component orientation.

It is important to re-establish optimal knee kinematics and stability.[36] The landmarks frequently used to assess the joint line may be absent during revision surgery due to bone loss and soft tissue damage. Historical landmarks to determine the appropriate joint line include the previous meniscal scar, one finger/1 cm above the fibular head, one finger/1 cm below the inferior pole of the patella. It is also important to examine the contralateral extremity as the height above the fibular head may be variable and the height of the patella may be altered due to patella baja.

Component Selection

- Consider a modular implant if the femoral component is retained. This will allow placement of the tibia in relative extension and minimize the need to completely sublux the tibia.
- Full block augments allow easier reconstruction than hemi blocks or wedges. This technique is preferred if this does not result in excessive bone resection.
- Use the least constrained insert. Hinged implants are rarely used except in severe flexion-extension mismatch or to handle knee recurvatum.
- Elongated post (NexGen Legacy Constrained Condylar Knee [LCCK]-type implant [Zimmer, Warsaw, IN]) is generally sufficient for coronal or sagittal imbalance.

Technical Tips

- Sublux rather than evert patella. Place knee in external rotation.
- Resect the proximal tibia with a zero-degree cutting block. This will allow the boom to be placed in any orientation. Incorporate posterior tibial slope via implant design rather than bone resection.

- Use a long stem extension to determine alignment and downsize to a shorter stem in most situations.
- Use an offset tibial stem to allow the implant to be placed anteriorly and laterally compared to the tibial canal in most patients.

Femoral Preparation

Femoral reconstruction begins once secure tibial fixation occurs and the joint line has been restored. It is important to begin with a thorough posterior capsular release before bone defects are addressed. Tight posterior capsular structures will result in an apparent loose flexion gap and a tight extension gap. This can lead to the inadvertent elevation of the joint line. Similar to the tibia, most femoral revisions will require the use of a femoral stem extension. The degree of component valgus is dictated by the manufacturer and is generally between 5 and 6 degrees. Consequently, a press-fit femoral stem extension can be used to determine femoral component orientation. Most femoral revision will require augmentation of the distal femur to lower the joint line due to distal femoral bone loss. Additionally, many revisions will require the use of a posterior lateral augment to avoid inadvertent internal femoral rotation. The transepicondylar axis is a useful landmark to ensure appropriate component rotation. Severe bone loss of the femur can be addressed with bulk structural allografts or the use of metal augmentation. While allografts have been used successfully in the past, metal augmentation is frequently used due to its relative ease of use, lack of disease transmission, and the avoidance of subsequent bone resorption.

Component Selection

- Avoid undersizing the femoral component. The "footprint" of the femur may appear small due to bone loss.
- Unlinked constrained implant can be used for the majority of patients with severe bone loss. Consider standard posterior stabilized polyethylene liner. Avoid overconstraint if knee is well balanced.
- Use distal femoral augments in most patients to avoid joint line elevation.

Technical Tips

- Use a long stem extension to determine alignment. Once the alignment is established, use a shorter, thicker stem.
- Consider offset stem to improve bone coverage. An offset stem can also allow adjustment of the implant posteriorly to improve flexion stability[37] or laterally to improve patellar tracking.
- Be careful of stress riser if total hip arthroplasty is on the ipsilateral side. Use a short stem with a minimum of 3 cortical diameters between implants.

Patellar Preparation

The patella should be assessed during knee revision.[38] The implant should be retained if the patella is well fixed and the component is compatible with the revision femoral component. The removal of a well-fixed implant may result in bone loss and subsequent patella fracture. If the implant is loose, incompatible with the femoral component, or shows severe wear, it must be removed.

A sagittal saw can be used to remove the articular portion of the implant while a high-speed burr can be used to remove the posts and cement. If a metal-backed implant is used, the well-fixed pegs can be retained and a new patella can be cemented in place. In some situations, the patellar remnant will be less than 10 mm and will not accept an implant. In these situations, the patella should be left unresurfaced or a "gull wing" osteotomy can be used to improve patella tracking.[39]

TABLE 3-9. ASSESSMENT OF STABILITY

	EXTENSION (TIGHT)	EXTENSION (NORMAL)	EXTENSION (LOOSE)
FLEXION (TIGHT)	Thinner tibial component Resect additional tibia	Smaller femoral component Increase posterior tibial slope Translate femur anteriorly with offset stem	Smaller femoral component with augment to distal femur
FLEXION (NORMAL)	Posterior capsular release Remove posterior osteophytes Resect additional distal femur	No change needed	Augment distal femur
FLEXION (LOOSE)	Larger femoral component with posterior augment Resect additional distal femur	Larger femoral component with posterior augment Translate femur posterior with offset stem	Thicker tibial component

Technical Tips

- Retain well-fixed cement and pegs during patellar revision
- Place patellar component laterally to assist patellar tracking

Assessment of Stability

Once the femoral and tibial component trials have been inserted, the knee can be brought through a range of motion and the stability of the knee can be assessed (Table 3-9). It is imperative that the knee reach terminal extension and that the patella tracks centrally throughout a range of motion. The stability of the knee is assessed in full extension, mid-range flexion, and deep knee flexion.[40] The 3 types of knee instability that exist are anterior-posterior, varus-valgus, and global instability. Most instability patterns can be addressed without excessive constraint. A higher tibial post is generally sufficient in situations of unidirectional instability. A hinge knee is reserved for marked flexion-extension mismatch as well as uncontrolled recurvatum. Longer stem extensions should be considered as the degree of constraint increases.

Technical Tips

- Offset femoral stems can be used to improve patella tracking through lateralizing the femur and improve flexion stability by translating the femoral component posteriorly.

Component Insertion

The technique of component insertion depends upon the mode of stem fixation. If a fully cemented stem is chosen, a canal restrictor should be utilized to allow cement pressurization and avoid distal extravasation. Cement is usually applied to the tibial and femoral components as well as along the metaphyseal region when a noncemented stem is used.[41,42] Small holes can be created in cortical bone to improve cement interdigitation and subsequent fixation. It is crucial to examine the rotation of the tibial component during insertion, as inadvertent internal rotation is common. In general, the rotation of the tibial component should be between the medial and middle one-third of the tibial tubercle. Cement with antibiotics should be considered on all revisions in order to minimize the risk of postoperative infection.

Management of Infection at the Site of a Total Knee Arthroplasty

Treatment of the infected TKA is most easily determined based on the classification of the infection as originally described by Segawa et al.[43]

Positive Intraoperative Cultures

This class includes patients where the cause of failure was thought to be aseptic; however, one or more of the intraoperative cultures comes back as positive. The most extensive research on the topic was recently published by Barrack et al.[44] They identified 41 such cases out of cohort of 692 consecutive revision TKAs from 3 centers.

- Twenty-nine were deemed to be falsely positive based on only one culture being positive and no other evidence of infection
  - Five were treated with antibiotics and 24 were not
  - None of these patients developed later signs of infection
- Twelve patients were felt to have an infection
  - Eleven were treated with antibiotics and one was not
  - Two of these 12 developed a deep infection within 1 year
- Based on their results, they felt that a single positive culture did not require treatment

It is wise to have an outside individual (typically an infectious disease specialist) review the case and help you make the decision to treat or not to treat.

The routine use of antibiotic-loaded cement is recommended for revision TKA, just in case the cultures do come back unexpectedly positive (also recommended given their higher risk of infection overall). Further, consider continued prophylactic antibiotics for 3 days until the final culture results are known. Vancomycin is used for prophylaxis for revision TKA, as prior work from the authors' center has shown that approximately one-third of the organisms that are responsible for deep infections are resistant to cefazolin.[45]

Acute Postoperative Infections

The treatment of an acute postoperative infection has become more controversial in the past few years. Traditionally, an acute postoperative infection has been defined as within the first 4 to 6 weeks postoperatively.

Classically, we have believed that treatment with débridement and exchange of the modular polyethylene liner, followed by 6 weeks of intravenous antibiotics (and in most cases a prolonged course of oral antibiotics), would be successful in approximately 50% of cases. However, more recent work shows that the results are probably much worse, particularly in patients who are infected with resistant and/or slime-producing organisms (such as *Staphylococcus*).

- Deirmengian et al: 92% failure rate with incision and drainage and component retention for patients with *Staphylococcus aureus* (1 of 13)[46]
- Bradbury et al: 84% failure rate, 73% eventual resection for Rx of methicillin-resistant *S aureus* (MRSA) acute postoperative infections with incision and drainage and component retention[47]

Serious consideration should be given to a two-stage exchange, particularly if either *S aureus* or an otherwise resistant organism is known to be the infecting organism.

Figure 3-6. (A) Anteroposterior and (B) lateral views of a static spacer. Threaded Steinmann pins have been coated with antibiotic-loaded cement (3 g vancomycin plus 1.2 g tobramycin per package of cement) and are used to bridge the joint with additional cement placed in the tibiofemoral articulation. Note a thick layer of cement was placed below the extensor mechanism to prevent adhesion to the distal femur and facilitate exposure at the time of reoperation.

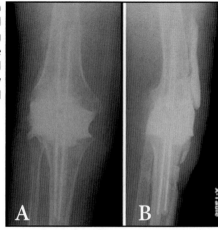

Late Chronic Infections

Débridement with component retention has a dismal failure rate for late chronic infections and should not be performed.

Late chronic infections are most commonly treated in North America by a two-stage exchange protocol. This is based on the results of several studies that show a cure rate of approximately 90%.

The first stage of a two-stage exchange is to remove all components and all cement. Obvious but critical, and a common cause of recurrent infection is failure to completely remove cement.

- Intraoperative x-rays and the use of a canal light can be helpful
- Intramedullary canals should be opened and débrided as one-third will have positive cultures
- Irrigate with 10 L or more using pulsatile lavage
- Place an antibiotic-loaded spacer
    □ Three to 6 g of antibiotics per package of cement
    □ Combining more than one antibiotic seems to increase elution
    □ Usually vancomycin plus tobramycin

The spacer can either be static or articulating (controversial which to choose). Most of the retrospective studies that have compared the use of the 2 suggest the following:

- The cure rates for infection are similar
- Operative times and exposure are easier with the use of an articulating spacer
- A static spacer may be associated with more bone loss between stages
- Knee scores may be higher with use of an articulating spacer

When using a static spacer (Figure 3-6), you are basically creating a temporary knee fusion of sorts.

- The use of a small "puck" of cement is **not** recommended
    □ Rarely provides enough stability
    □ Does not deliver antibiotics to the canals
    □ Can migrate out of the joint damaging the extensor mechanism
- Cement should extend into the metaphysis and antibiotic-loaded dowels should be placed into the medullary canals
- Consider application of a cast (including the foot) postoperatively

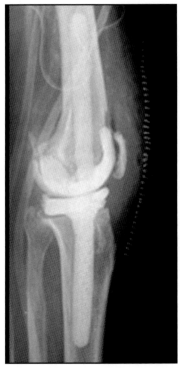

Figure 3-7. Postoperative lateral radiograph showing use of an all-cement articulating spacer using plastic molds. Note the use of antibiotic-loaded cement dowels in the femur and tibia. The tibial dowel is incorporated into the tibial component to prevent it from dislodging. Made using 3 g vancomycin and 1.2 g tobramycin per package of cement.

Articulating spacers (Figure 3-7) can be constructed in a number of ways:
- Autoclave the femoral component and cement in a new polyethylene tibial component
  - Components then loosely cemented into place with high-dose antibiotic cement
  - "Hoffman" technique
- Use of plastic molds to create your own spacer made fully of cement
  - Use of dowels in the canals recommended
  - Knee can dislocate (the authors usually limit range of motion with a hinged knee brace; 0 to 60 degrees or so)
  - Construct spacer with high-dose antibiotic cement
- Use of a pre-formed "off-the-shelf" spacer (one example is the InterSpace Knee [Exactech Incorporated, Gainesville, FL])
  - Concern that the spacer itself is made with a small amount of antibiotics
  - Spacer is then loosely cemented into place using high-dose antibiotic cement
  - Use of dowels in the canals is recommended

The patient is then treated with a 6-week course of organism-specific intravenous antibiotics with the help of an infectious disease consultant
- Weekly ESR and CRP, although it is unclear how useful these numbers are
- ESR and CRP are unpredictable markers of infection resolution with many patients who have a "cured" infection, having persistent elevations of the ESR and/or CRP
- See the patient 2 weeks after antibiotics have been discontinued
  - Recheck ESR and CRP (in order to determine if they go up once off of antibiotics)
  - Aspirate the knee and send for cell count and culture
  - Return to operating room the following week (once final culture results are known)

Performing the two-stage reimplantation
- Get a frozen section
- Débride all bony surfaces and the canals again
- Pulsatile lavage with 10 L or more again
- Use a standard dose of premixed antibiotic cement
- Use a "hybrid cementing technique" (cement metaphysis of component just past the modular junction and press-fit the stem in the canal) although stems can be fully cemented into place
- Incorporate intravenous antibiotics until the final cultures are negative
- Stop oral antibiotics at this time, although many experienced surgeons the authors know place the patient on oral antibiotics for an extended period of time (and sometimes for life!)

One-stage exchange has been more popular in Europe. The recommendations for this protocol include an infection with a known, sensitive, gram-positive organism in a healthy host with a good soft tissue envelope.
- Thorough débridement and cleanse with pulsatile lavage
- Use of standard dose antibiotic-loaded cement is critical
- Intravenous antibiotics following is the optimal course, though not usually specified
- Long-term oral suppression afterward?

Acute Hematogenous Infections

It is difficult to know when hematogenous infections started. They are classically associated with an obvious source of bacteremia (eg, recent dental work), fever, and acute pain in the joint. They can be easily confused with a late chronic infection. Little is presently available in the literature on diagnosis and treatment.

Treatment usually with débridement, liner exchange, and component retention *if* the components are well fixed and the soft tissue envelope is good.
- Followed by 6 weeks of intravenous antibiotics
- Oral antibiotics for a year or more, potentially indefinitely

POSTOPERATIVE MANAGEMENT AND REHABILITATION

Deep Vein Thrombosis Prophylaxis

It is well understood that total joint arthroplasty predisposes patients to developing clots, specifically deep vein thrombosis (DVT) and pulmonary embolism (PE). This complication cannot only cause significant discomfort for the patient, but can also lead to symptomatic and/or fatal PE. Patients undergoing primary TKA have exhibited rates of symptomatic PE as high as 8% when no prophylaxis has been administered.[48] As a result, the use of venous thromboembolic (DVT and PE) prophylaxis, most commonly pharmacologic prophylaxis, has become the standard of care for patients undergoing elective total joint arthroplasty.[48]

Most of the current prophylactic recommendations are based on the presence or absence of DVT. However, the correlation between the presence of a DVT and the risk of PE is low and inconsistent. Therefore, DVT may not be an accurate surrogate marker for the patient at risk after total joint surgery.[49] Furthermore, the risk of fatal PE following primary hip or knee replacement has been consistently reported to be between 0.1% and 0.2%, regardless of the chemoprophylactic agent employed for prophylaxis.[47] The inclusion of asymptomatic DVT as a clinical endpoint has been the basis for the American College of Chest Physicians anticoagulation guidelines and the

TABLE 3-10. POSTOPERATIVE MANAGEMENT

PHYSICAL THERAPY	1. For range of motion, strength, stability, and pain control. 2. Most surgeons recommend routine rehabilitation for quadriceps snip. For quadriceps turndown or tubercle osteotomy, no range of motion for 2 weeks and no active extension for 2 to 6 weeks.
KNEE IMMOBILIZER	1. For preserving knee motion and avoiding flexion contracture formation. 2. Use in the immediate postoperative period in patients that have had a femoral nerve block. The femoral nerve block results in quadriceps weakness and patients are at risk of falling.
CONTINUOUS PASSIVE MOTION DEVICE	1. The effects of continuous passive motion on knee range of motion are too small to justify its use. There is weak evidence that continuous passive motion reduces the subsequent need for manipulation under anesthesia.[50,51] 2. Some surgeons believe patients do better psychologically if they know their knee can move.
FOLLOW-UP	1. Two weeks for suture removal, 6 weeks for motion check and radiographs, 3 months, and then annually. 2. If the patient does not have 90 degrees of motion at 6 weeks, start physical therapy 5 times per week for 2 weeks, followed by another office visit. 3. If the patient has not regained motion, the surgeon should consider manipulation under anesthesia.

fundamental difference from the American Academy of Orthopaedic Surgeons guidelines, which focus on symptomatic DVT, PE, and bleeding risk with concomitant risk stratification.

The Surgical Care Improvement Project (SCIP) guidelines were created to develop a "standard of care" for DVT prophylaxis after total joint arthroplasty. In summary, surgeons need to be aware that the SCIP guidelines recommend low molecular weight heparin, fondaparinux (pentasaccharide), and/or warfarin for TKA patients. As well, aspirin and pneumatic compression devices are acceptable.[48] Prophylaxis should continue for 4 weeks unless contraindicated.

Pain Control

Postoperative pain control is crucial to a successful outcome following revision knee arthroplasty. Regional anesthesia with a concomitant multimodal pain pathway has resulted in improved postoperative pain scores. Patients with a history of extensive narcotic abuse or complex regional pain syndrome should be evaluated by a pain specialist prior to surgical intervention. Patients undergoing revision surgery due to arthrofibrosis should also be monitored closely to ensure pain does not interfere with their postoperative rehabilitation. An indwelling epidural catheter can be used in patients with poor postoperative pain tolerance.

Antibiotics

See as per aforementioned.

Other

See Table 3-10.

COMPLICATIONS

With index revisions, component survivorship is roughly 82% at 12 years and good to excellent results occur 50% to 80% of the time. Complications occur 15% to 30% of the time, and of index revisions, 12.0% fail at an average of 40.1 months. Revision knee arthroplasty is more likely to fail in younger patients and in those who underwent polyethylene exchanges.[52] The most common etiology is continued or new infection, which occurs in 4% of patients. This is roughly 10 times higher than should occur in primary knees.[53] Furthermore, revisions for infection are 4 times more likely to fail than revisions for aseptic loosening. The majority of TKA failures tend to occur in the first 2 years after revision.[54]

- Infection (25.2% to 44.1% of all complications)[54]
- Stiffness (22.6% of all complications)[54]
- Mechanical loosening (16.1% of all complications)[55]
- Implant failure/breakage (9.7% of all complications)[55]
- Dislocation (7.1% of all complications)[55]
- Hematoma formation (3.9% of all complications)[54]
- Periprosthetic osteolysis (3.2% of all complications)[55]
- Knee instability (2.9% to 13% of all complications)[54]
- Periprosthetic fracture (1.5% of all complications)[55]
- Wound complications: If conservative measures fail, then handle aggressively with skin graft, gastrocnemius flap, or free flap. Consider early consultation with plastic surgeon.
- DVT: Treat with anticoagulation protocol
- Myositis ossificans (formation of heterotopic bone): Treat with indomethacin and/or radiation
- Pulmonary embolus
- Leg length discrepancy
- Extensor mechanism problem
- Neurovascular injury (popliteal vessels, peroneal nerve, tibial nerve)
- Anesthesia complications

SUMMARY

Ultimately, the decision to attempt a knee revision is dependent upon the surgeon's comfort level and familiarity with the given clinical scenario. It is crucial that the surgeon understand the failure mode and anticipate potential challenges during both component removal and subsequent reconstruction. Appropriate preoperative planning will ultimately ensure that the appropriate instrumentation and components are available to maximize the chance of a successful clinical outcome.

REFERENCES

1. Ranawat CS, Flynn WF Jr, Saddler S, Hansraj KK, Maynard MJ. Long-term results of the total condylar knee arthroplasty. A 15-year survivorship study. *Clin Orthop Relat Res.* 1993;1(286):94-102.
2. Ritter MA, Berend ME, Meding JB, Keating EM, Faris PM, Crites BM. Long-term followup of anatomic graduated components posterior cruciate-retaining total knee replacement. *Clin Orthop Relat Res.* 2001;7(388):51-57.
3. Miller TT. Imaging of knee arthroplasty. *Eur J Radiol.* 2005;54:164-177.

4. Kurtz S, Ong K, Lau E, Mowat F, Halpern M. Projections of primary and revision hip and knee arthroplasty in the United States from 2005 to 2030. *J Bone Joint Surg Am.* 2007;89:780-785.

5. Fehring TK, Odum S, Griffin WL, Mason JB, Nadaud M. Early failures in total knee arthroplasty. *Clin Orthop Relat Res.* 2001;11(392):315-318.

6. Mulhall KJ, Ghomrawi HM, Scully S, Callaghan JJ, Saleh KJ. Current etiologies and modes of failure in total knee arthroplasty revision. *Clin Orthop Relat Res.* 2006;446:45-50.

7. Sharkey PF, Hozack WJ, Rothman RH, Shastri S, Jacoby SM. Insall Award paper. Why are total knee arthroplasties failing today? *Clin Orthop Relat Res.* 2002;11(404):7-13.

8. Pagnano MW, Hanssen AD, Lewallen DG, Stuart MJ. Flexion instability after primary posterior cruciate retaining total knee arthroplasty. *Clin Orthop Relat Res.* 1998;11(356):39-46.

9. Clarke HD, Fuchs R, Scuderi GR, Mills EL, Scott WN, Insall JN. The influence of femoral component design in the elimination of patellar clunk in posterior-stabilized total knee arthroplasty. *J Arthroplasty.* 2006;21:167-171.

10. Meding JB, Keating EM, Ritter MA, Faris PM, Berend ME, Malinzak RA. The planovalgus foot: a harbinger of failure of posterior cruciate-retaining total knee replacement. *J Bone Joint Surg Am.* 2005;87 (suppl 2):59-62.

11. Joseph TN, Mujtaba M, Chen AL, Maurer SL, Zuckerman JD, Maldjian C, Di Cesare PE. Efficacy of combined technetium-99m sulfur colloid/indium-111 leukocyte scans to detect infected total hip and knee arthroplasties. *J Arthroplasty.* 2001;16:753-758.

12. Bernard L, Lubbeke A, Stern R, et al. Value of preoperative investigations in diagnosing prosthetic joint infection: retrospective cohort study and literature review. *Scand J Infect Dis.* 2004;36:410-416.

13. Intenzo CM, Kim SM, Capuzzi DM. The role of nuclear medicine in the evaluation of complex regional pain syndrome type I. *Clin Nucl Med.* 2005;30:400-407.

14. Rosenthall L, Lepanto L, Raymond F. Radiophosphate uptake in asymptomatic knee arthroplasty. *J Nucl Med.* 1987;28:1546-1549.

15. Scher DM, Pak K, Lonner JH, Finkel JE, Zuckerman JD, Di Cesare PE. The predictive value of indium-111 leukocyte scans in the diagnosis of infected total hip, knee, or resection arthroplasties. *J Arthroplasty.* 2000;15:295-300.

16. Berger RA, Crossett LS, Jacobs JJ, Rubash HE. Malrotation causing patellofemoral complications after total knee arthroplasty. *Clin Orthop Relat Res.* 1998;11(356):144-153.

17. Romero J, Stahelin T, Binkert C, Pfirrmann C, Hodler J, Kessler O. The clinical consequences of flexion gap asymmetry in total knee arthroplasty. *J Arthroplasty.* 2007;22:235-240.

18. Potter HG, Nestor BJ, Sofka CM, Ho ST, Peters LE, Salvati EA. Magnetic resonance imaging after total hip arthroplasty: evaluation of periprosthetic soft tissue. *J Bone Joint Surg Am.* 2004;86-A:1947-1954.

19. Sofka CM, Potter HG, Figgie M, Laskin R. Magnetic resonance imaging of total knee arthroplasty. *Clin Orthop Relat Res.* 2003;1(406):129-135.

20. Vessely MB, Frick MA, Oakes D, Wenger DE, Berry DJ. Magnetic resonance imaging with metal suppression for evaluation of periprosthetic osteolysis after total knee arthroplasty. *J Arthroplasty.* 2006;21:826-831.

21. Ghanem E, Parvizi J, Burnett RS, Sharkey PF, Keshavarzi N, Aggarwal A, Barrack RL. Cell count and differential of aspirated fluid in the diagnosis of infection at the site of total knee arthroplasty. *J Bone Joint Surg Am.* 2008;90:1637-1643.

22. Schinsky MF, Della Valle CJ, Sporer SM, Paprosky WG. Perioperative testing for joint infection in patients undergoing revision total hip arthroplasty. *J Bone Joint Surg Am.* 2008;90:1869-1875.

23. Lucas TS, DeLuca PF, Nazarian DG, Bartolozzi AR, Booth RE Jr. Arthroscopic treatment of patellar clunk. *Clin Orthop Relat Res.* 1999;10(367):226-229.

24. Allardyce TJ, Scuderi GR, Insall JN. Arthroscopic treatment of popliteus tendon dysfunction following total knee arthroplasty. *J Arthroplasty.* 1997;12:353-355.

25. Della Valle CJ, Bogner E, Desai P, et al. Analysis of frozen sections of intraoperative specimens obtained at the time of reoperation after hip or knee resection arthroplasty for the treatment of infection. *J Bone Joint Surg Am.* 1999;81:684-689.

26. Morgan PM, Sharkey P, Ghanem E, et al. The value of intraoperative Gram stain in revision total knee arthroplasty. *J Bone Joint Surg Am.* 2009;91:2124-2129.

27. Nadaud MC, Fehring TK, Fehring K. Underestimation of osteolysis in posterior stabilized total knee arthroplasty. *J Arthroplasty.* 2004;19:110-115.

28. Whittaker JP, Dharmarajan R, Toms AD. The management of bone loss in revision total knee replacement. *J Bone Joint Surg Br.* 2008;90:981-987.

29. Engh GA, Ammeen DJ. Bone loss with revision total knee arthroplasty: defect classification and alternatives for reconstruction. *Instruct Course Lect.* 1999;48:167-175.

30. Dennis DA, Berry DJ, Engh G, et al. Revision total knee arthroplasty. *J Am Acad Orthop Surg.* 2008;16:442-454.

31. Bush JL, Wilson JB, Vail TP. Management of bone loss in revision total knee arthroplasty. *Clin Orthop Relat Res.* 2006;452:186-192.

32. Lonner JH, Lotke PA, Kim J, Nelson C. Impaction grafting and wire mesh for uncontained defects in revision knee arthroplasty. *Clin Orthop Relat Res.* 2002;11(404):145-151.

33. Engh GA, Ammeen DJ. Use of structural allograft in revision total knee arthroplasty in knees with severe tibial bone loss. *J Bone Joint Surg Am.* 2007;89:2640-2647.

34. Long WJ, Scuderi GR. Porous tantalum cones for large metaphyseal tibial defects in revision total knee arthroplasty: a minimum 2-year follow-up. *J Arthroplasty.* 2009;24:1086-1092.

35. Bourne RB, Finlay JB. The influence of tibial component intramedullary stems and implant-cortex contact on the strain distribution of the proximal tibia following total knee arthroplasty. An in vitro study. *Clin Orthop Relat Res.* 1986;7(208):95-99.

36. Porteous AJ, Hassaballa MA, Newman JH. Does the joint line matter in revision total knee replacement? *J Bone Joint Surg Br.* 2008;90:879-884.

37. Mahoney OM, Kinsey TL. Modular femoral offset stems facilitate joint line restoration in revision knee arthroplasty. *Clin Orthop Relat Res.* 2006;446:93-98.

38. Maheshwari AV, Tsailas PG, Ranawat AS, Ranawat CS. How to address the patella in revision total knee arthroplasty. *Knee.* 2009;16:92-97.

39. Rorabeck CH, Mehin R, Barrack RL. Patellar options in revision total knee arthroplasty. *Clin Orthop Relat Res.* 2003;11(416):84-92.

40. Ries MD, Haas SB, Windsor RE. Soft-tissue balance in revision total knee arthroplasty. Surgical technique. *J Bone Joint Surg Am.* 2004;86-A (suppl 1):81-86.

41. Haas SB, Insall JN, Montgomery W 3rd, Windsor RE. Revision total knee arthroplasty with use of modular components with stems inserted without cement. *J Bone Joint Surg Am.* 1995;77:1700-1707.

42. Peters CL, Erickson J, Kloepper RG, Mohr RA. Revision total knee arthroplasty with modular components inserted with metaphyseal cement and stems without cement. *J Arthroplasty.* 2005;20:302-308.

43. Segawa H, Tsukayama DT, Kyle RF, Becker DA, Gustilo RB. Infection after total knee arthroplasty. A retrospective study of the treatment of eighty-one infections. *J Bone Joint Surg Am.* 1999;81:1434-1445.

44. Barrack RL, Jennings RW, Wolfe MW, Bertot AJ. The Coventry Award. The value of preoperative aspiration before total knee revision. *Clin Orthop Relat Res.* 1997;12(345):8-16.

45. Fulkerson E, Valle CJ, Wise B, Walsh M, Preston C, Di Cesare PE. Antibiotic susceptibility of bacteria infecting total joint arthroplasty sites. *J Bone Joint Surg Am.* 2006;88:1231-1237.

46. Deirmengian C, Greenbaum J, Stern J, et al. Open debridement of acute gram-positive infections after total knee arthroplasty. *Clin Orthop Relat Res.* 2003;11(416):129-134.

47. Bradbury T, Fehring TK, Taunton M, et al. The fate of acute methicillin-resistant *Staphylococcus aureus* periprosthetic knee infections treated by open debridement and retention of components. *J Arthroplasty.* 2009;24:101-104.

48. Sheth NP, Lieberman JR, Della Valle CJ. DVT prophylaxis in total joint reconstruction. *Orthop Clin North Am.* 2010;41:273-280.

49. Lotke PA, Lonner JH. Deep venous thrombosis prophylaxis: better living through chemistry—in opposition. *J Arthroplasty.* 2005;20:15-17.

50. Harvey LA, Brosseau L, Herbert RD. Continuous passive motion following total knee arthroplasty in people with arthritis. *Cochrane Database Syst Rev.* 2010;3:CD004260.

51. Lenssen TA, van Steyn MJ, Crijns YH, et al. Effectiveness of prolonged use of continuous passive motion (CPM), as an adjunct to physiotherapy, after total knee arthroplasty. *BMC Musculoskelet Disord.* 2008;9:60.

52. Suarez J, Griffin W, Springer B, Fehring T, Mason JB, Odum S. Why do revision knee arthroplasties fail? *J Arthroplasty.* 2008;23:99-103.

53. Wheeless C, Berend M. Revision total knee arthroplasty. *Wheeless' Textbook of Orthopaedics*; 2010.

54. Mortazavi SM, Molligan J, Austin MS, Purtill JJ, Hozack WJ, Parvizi J. Failure following revision total knee arthroplasty: infection is the major cause. *International Orthopaedics.* 2011;35:1157-1164.

55. Bozic KJ, Kurtz SM, Lau E, et al. The epidemiology of revision total knee arthroplasty in the United States. *Clin Orthop Relat Res.* 2010;468:45-51.

Surgical Exposure in Revision Total Knee Arthroplasty

Robert M. Cercek, MD

Careful preoperative planning and performance of the surgical approach are key first steps toward a successful outcome in revision total knee arthroplasty (TKA). The surgical approach chosen must not only expose the knee joint but also provide complete exposure of the surgical implants and the implant-cement-bone interface. It must also allow adequate visualization of the remaining bone stock and provide access for complete débridement of all osteolytic lesions. Finally, it must permit proper visualization and access for implantation of the revision components. The exposure must avoid damage to the important surrounding anatomic structures. These structures include the medial and lateral collateral ligaments, the extensor mechanism, and the neurovascular structures in close proximity to the knee.

Prior surgical procedures and subsequent postoperative changes can greatly alter the native anatomy of the knee. The surgical exposure is more challenging in knees that have undergone more than one prior surgical procedure, in knees with severe flexion contractures or arthrofibrosis, as well as in knees with osteopenic or osteolytic bone, patella baja, and/or in obese patients. It is not always possible in revision TKA to achieve adequate exposure with routine exposure techniques. In these situations, visualization of the surgical field must be improved with more extensile surgical techniques. There is a greater risk of extensor mechanism disruption in revision TKA.[1] A more extensile exposure should be performed early if necessary in order to avoid this complication, as it clearly results in poorer long-term function.[2]

Enhancement of the surgical exposure in revision TKA falls into 2 general categories. The first category includes proximal soft tissue techniques, such as extension of the quadriceps incision, which allows retraction of the extensor mechanism laterally and distally. The second category includes distal techniques, such as a tibial tubercle osteotomy, which allows the extensor mechanism and tibial tubercle to retract laterally. The proximal soft tissue procedures minimize the risk of mechanical complications associated with the distal techniques; however, the proximal procedures may compromise the blood supply to the extensor mechanism and the patella. The tibial tubercle osteotomy, while associated with a risk of mechanical complications, allows for excellent visualization of the knee and permits bone-to-bone healing, which may be superior to soft tissue healing.

Jacofsky DJ, Hedley AK, eds.
Fundamentals of Revision Knee Arthroplasty:
Diagnosis, Evaluation, and Treatment (pp 59-74).
© 2013 SLACK Incorporated.

Figure 4-1. The extraosseous peri-patellar anastomotic ring, which is supplied by 6 main arteries. LSG = lateral superior genicular, LIG = lateral inferior genicular, ATR = anterior tibial recurrent, SG = supreme genicular, MSG = medial superior genicular, MIG = medial inferior genicular. (Reprinted with permission of Ayers DC, Dennis DA, Johanson NA, Pellegrini VD Jr. Common complications of total knee arthroplasty. *J Bone Joint Surg Am.* 1997;79:278-311.)

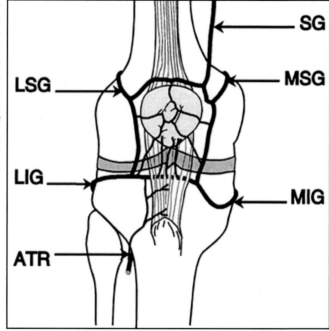

RELEVANT ANATOMY

The surgeon must have a thorough understanding of the anatomy of the knee prior to embarking on revision TKA. This begins with the blood supply to the skin surrounding the knee. The cutaneous blood supply is distinct from the blood supply to the patella; there is little communication between the two. The patella is separated from the skin by the prepatellar bursa, through which few blood vessels pass. Microanatomic studies of the skin surrounding the knee have shown that the majority of the blood supply arises from the medial aspect of the knee.[3] Perforating vessels arise from the saphenous and descending genicular arteries, and these vessels give rise to an anastamosis of vessels located just superficial to the deep fascia. From the anastamosis, blood vessels then travel superficially through the subcutaneous fat to supply the epidermis. While the medial vessels normally provide the majority of the blood supply to the anastamosis, the lateral vessels will increase their contribution to the plexus when the medial vessels have been compromised, such as after the anteromedial surgical approach. However, there are few anastamoses in the dermal/epidermal layer. Therefore, wide dissection superficial to the deep fascia can compromise the blood supply to the skin. Close parallel incisions can also compromise the epidermal blood supply.

The patella also receives its blood supply from an arterial anastamosis. Vessels contributing to this plexus include the descending genicular artery, the medial and lateral genicular arteries, and the anterior tibial recurrent artery (Figure 4-1). The plexus forms multiple branches anterior to the patella, which in turn give rise to vessels that penetrate the patella inferiorly and anteriorly to provide the intraosseous blood supply. The medial parapatellar arthrotomy disrupts the contribution of the medial vessels to the anastamosis. The inferior lateral geniculate artery will also be sacrificed during excision of the lateral meniscus. In addition, excision of the suprapatellar and infrapatellar fat pads place the superior lateral genicular artery and branches of the anterior tibial recurrent artery at risk. Finally, the superior lateral genicular artery runs deep to the synovium in the same plane as the vastus lateralis muscle. It travels just distal to the distal-most muscle fibers. Careful dissection in this area during a lateral release may allow preservation of the vessel, thereby maintaining a collateral blood supply to the patella.[4]

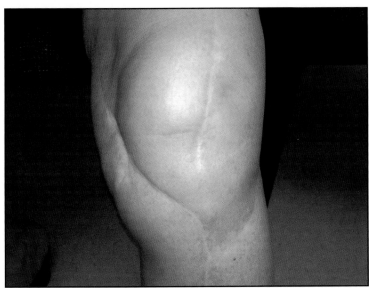

Figure 4-2. Multiple prior incisions may be encountered in the revision setting. Generally the most lateral incision that provides adequate exposure to the knee should be used. (Reprinted with permission of David J. Jacofsky, MD.)

The surgeon must also be familiar with the ligamentous and capsular structures medially, laterally, and posteriorly surrounding the knee. The medial collateral ligament travels from the medial epicondyle of the femur to the medial aspect of the tibia, with a broad insertion 2 cm distal to the joint line. The superficial aspect has a more distal insertion, and blends with the insertion of the pes anserinus tendons anteriorly and the semimembranosus tendon posteriorly. The deep aspect of the medial collateral ligament is a condensation of fibers within the joint capsule and inserts directly into the tibia at the level of the joint.[5] The lateral collateral ligament travels from the lateral epicondyle of the femur to the fibular head. It lies superficial to the popliteus tendon and the joint capsule. The posterior joint capsule originates from the distal femur above the level of the condyles and runs deep to the medial and lateral heads of the gastrocnemius to attach on the posterior aspect of the proximal tibia. The posterior cruciate ligament originates on the medial aspect of the intercondylar notch of the femur and runs posterolaterally to insert on the posterior aspect of the tibia. It is commonly absent secondary to prior surgical procedure(s). If preserved, it is usually attenuated at the time of revision surgery. Care should be taken when excising any retained posterior cruciate ligament to not inadvertently penetrate the posterior joint capsule.

The femoral artery becomes the popliteal artery as it passes through the adductor hiatus, and the popliteal artery then travels distally just posterior to the joint capsule. It is tethered to the posterior capsule by the genicular arteries, which travel anteriorly. Therefore, flexion of the knee will not distract the artery away from the posterior joint capsule. If necessary for exposure or balancing, dissection around the posterior capsule should be performed very carefully. The safest approach is a subperiosteal elevation of the posterior capsule directly off the femoral condyles.

The tibial nerve lies posterior to the artery and is therefore less likely to be injured. The popliteal vein lies between the two. The peroneal nerve lies on the lateral aspect of the joint, traveling posterior to the biceps tendon as it inserts onto the fibular head. It lies superficial to the lateral collateral ligament. It is at less risk to direct injury from exuberant surgical dissection, but it is more vulnerable to a traction or compression injury.

SUPERFICIAL APPROACH

There is a greater risk of wound healing problems and wound infection in the revision setting.[6] Conditions placing patients at an increased risk include multiple prior surgical procedures (Figure 4-2), restricted preoperative range of motion, rheumatoid arthritis, a history of corticosteroid use or other immunocompromised state, and a history of prior infection. Many of these factors are outside of the surgeon's control. This underscores the importance of preoperative planning in the revision setting. The location of previous scars should be closely examined. The general health of the skin and the capillary return at the edges of the scar(s) should be inspected. The venous return should be assessed distally, as poor venous return may lead to tissue ischemia at the wound edges due to venous engorgement. If difficultly with wound closure or delayed wound healing is anticipated, preoperative consultation with a plastic surgeon may be advisable.

Most often, only a single prior longitudinal incision will be present, and this can generally be utilized for the revision surgery. The incision may be straight and anterior, straight and medialized, or curvilinear. It is helpful to mark the incision on the skin with a permanent marker prior to surgical preparation, as it may not be visible after the application of the surgical drapes. If a transverse or oblique incision was used, it should be crossed at the most obtuse angle possible to minimize wound healing complications at the corners created by this intersection. If multiple prior longitudinal incisions were made, generally the most lateral incision giving appropriate exposure should be used, as the dominant fascial perforators arise from the medial aspect of the knee. However, if all incisions are greater than 2 years old and did not involve a surrounding soft tissue flap, it is generally safe to utilize the incision most advantageous for the revision surgery. In some cases, the previous skin incisions will not allow reasonable access to the joint, and a new incision must be made. If possible, a minimum 6-cm skin bridge between incisions should be maintained.

The ideal incision is centered over the patella proximally, and is angled slightly medial as it is carried distally, to end 1 cm medial to the tibial tubercle. If the prior incision overlies the tubercle, this should be used; however, deep dissection should be performed very cautiously, as the patellar tendon will likely be invested in significant scar tissue. Extension of the incision into native tissue beyond the distal end of the scar will assist in the development of tissue planes. The incision should be made sufficiently long to avoid undue tension on the skin edges. The superficial soft tissues should be handled with extreme care throughout the procedure, utilizing minimal pressure from forceps and retractors. Dissection is then carried out deep to the deep fascia in order to preserve the blood supply to the skin; unnecessary undermining of tissue should be avoided. Deeper dissection is then performed around the extensor mechanism, which is identified and separated from the surrounding scar. It is often difficult to identify the tissue planes within the scar; once again, extending the approach into virgin tissue will help facilitate proper identification of tissue planes and subsequent dissection. Vessels encountered during the approach are cauterized, as a postoperative hematoma can lead to wound breakdown by compromising the bloody supply to the skin.

CAPSULAR APPROACH: THE MEDIAL PARAPATELLAR ARTHROTOMY

The extensor mechanism is not adequately exposed until the medial border of the patella, the quadriceps tendon, the patellar tendon, and the tibial tubercle are all clearly identified. Only then should the capsular incision be made. In most revision cases, the medial parapatellar arthrotomy is performed; however, a previous lateral arthrotomy may dictate a repeat lateral approach in order to avoid patellar osteonecrosis.[7] There are multiple variations on the medial arthrotomy, including the standard medial parapatellar approach, the Insall approach, the von Langenbeck approach, and the subvastus approach (Figure 4-3). Insall's classic anterior approach[8] is made by dividing the medial third of the quadriceps tendon from the lateral two-thirds longitudinally. The incision is then continued distally over the patella in a relatively straight fashion. The quadriceps expansion is peeled subperiosteally from the anterior surface of the patella until the medial border of the

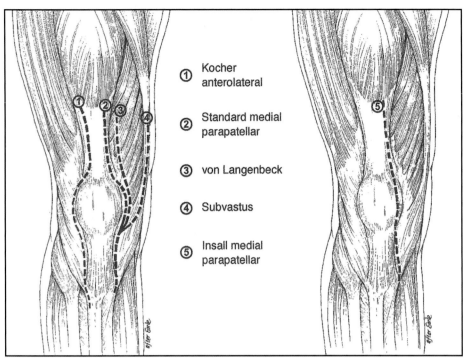

1. Kocher anterolateral
2. Standard medial parapatellar
3. von Langenbeck
4. Subvastus
5. Insall medial parapatellar

Figure 4-3. Capsular incisions used for revision total knee arthroplasty. All can be reached by subfascial dissection, but this should be kept to a minimum to prevent skin necrosis. (© 1998 American Academy of Orthopaedic Surgeons. Reprinted with permission of the *Journal of the American Academy of Orthopaedic Surgeons*, Volume 6[1], page 59 with permission.)

patella is reached. The incision is then extended distally along the medial border of the patellar tendon. The standard medial parapatellar approach uses the same proximal and distal dissections as described by Insall, but at the level of the patella, the dissection is curved around the medial border of the patella, and the retinaculum is incised between the patella and the fibers of the vastus medialis.[9] Either approach may be safely employed in the revision setting.

The von Langenbeck approach is similar to the medial parapatellar approach distally, but the more proximal aspect of the dissection is carried out through the fibers of the vastus medialis.[10] This exposure is not recommended, especially for revision surgery, as the repair of the vastus medialis can be disrupted postoperatively, resulting in lateral patellar maltracking and extensor mechanism dysfunction. The subvastus approach also uses the same distal interval as the medial parapatellar approach, but the proximal dissection is carried out medial and deep to the fibers of the vastus medialis, lifting the muscle as needed off the intermuscular septum. The muscle fibers are bluntly freed from the medial intermuscular septum and elevated laterally.[11] This approach also is not recommended for revision surgery, as intraoperative lateral patellar retraction will place severe tension on the insertion of the patellar tendon, increasing the risk of extensor mechanism rupture.

The anterolateral approach is a "mirror image" of the medial parapatellar approach. Proximally, the quadriceps tendon is splint along the lateral one-third. The approach then curves around the lateral aspect of the patella, and continues distally along the lateral course of the patellar tendon. It may be difficult to subluxate the patella medially with this approach. Extending the approach in an extensile fashion also involves a great deal of soft tissue dissection and undermining of the skin, with potential devascularization of the soft tissue sleeve. This approach should play a limited

Figure 4-4. The medial and lateral gutters should be recreated during exposure in the revision setting. (Reprinted with permission of David J. Jacofsky, MD.)

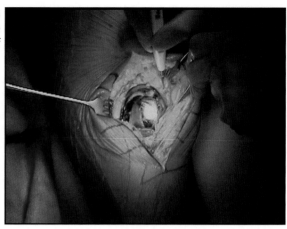

role in revision surgery. Primary indications include a prior lateral arthrotomy and patients with a severe, fixed valgus deformity. The primary surgical approach for most revision cases will therefore be a medial parapatellar arthrotomy with apical or distal extension, as needed, for visualization and access.

In most revision cases, the capsular incision alone will not provide sufficient access to safely remove the retained implant. Further soft tissue dissection must still be performed. The medial and lateral gutters should carefully be freed and recreated (Figure 4-4). The dissection is taken down to the level of the collateral ligaments. The suprapatellar pouch is freed of scar tissue to assist with mobilization of the extensor mechanism. There is often significant fibrotic tissue located between the quadriceps mechanism and the anterior aspect of the femur, which will limit knee flexion. Sharp dissection should be performed to remove scar tissue without damage to the extensor mechanism or collateral ligaments.

The soft tissue adhesions between the anterior aspect of the tibia and the patellar tendon proximal to the level of the tubercle should also be released. This will assist in improving patellar mobilization. This should be performed very cautiously in order to prevent iatrogenic injury to the extensor mechanism. Patellar subluxation (as opposed to eversion) is generally sufficient to allow adequate exposure to the knee. The "meniscus" of scar encircling the patella and/or patellar component should be identified and excised sharply. A plane can be identified proximally between the organized fibers of the quadriceps tendon and the disorganized scar tissue, and this is then extended distally around the patella. The extensor mechanism must be protected throughout the procedure, as fibrosis, osteolysis in the region of the tibial tubercle, and multiple prior surgical procedures place the extensor mechanism at risk for iatrogenic avulsion.

The exposure is then continued distally around the proximal tibia. Sharp subperiosteal dissection is performed on the medial tibial cortex at the insertion of the superficial medial collateral ligament. This dissection is extended medially and posteriorly to the level of the insertion of the semimembranosus tendon in the midcoronal plane (Figure 4-5). Care should be taken to maintain a continous medial soft tissue sleeve, including the fibers of the deep medial collateral ligament. As the dissection is extended posteriorly, continuous external rotation of the tibia facilitates exposure and relaxes the insertion of the patellar tendon. Tibial external rotation and anterior subluxation will then allow greater flexion of the knee and lateral patellar subluxation. This copious posteromedial release is often referred to as the *medial collateral ligament slide*, and in many cases is sufficient exposure for revision surgery.[12]

The polyethylene liner should then be removed, which will further decrease the tension on the patellar tendon and improve the mobility of the soft tissues. The patellar tendon insertion should

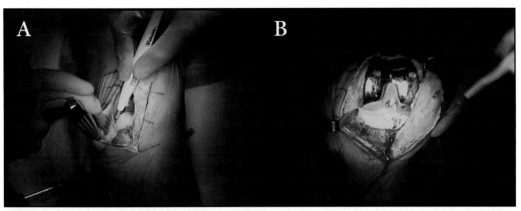

Figure 4-5. (A) The medial collateral ligament slide is carried posteromedially in a subperiosteal fashion. (B) Appearance of the medial proximal tibia once the medial collateral ligament slide has been performed. (Reprinted with permission of David J. Jacofsky, MD.)

be carefully inspected as the patella is subluxated laterally. If the knee can be flexed to 110 degrees with minimal tension on the patellar tendon, the revision procedure may then proceed without any need for further exposure. Careful preparation of the soft tissues, utilization of patellar subluxation, and removal of the polyethylene insert will maximize success. However, if significant tension is still present on the patellar tendon and/or visualization of the components remains difficult, a more extensile approach should be considered to improve exposure of the knee and prevent iatrogenic injury to the extensor mechanism.

QUADRICEPS SNIP

The quadriceps snip is an excellent first choice for additional exposure. It is used when the standard medial parapatellar approach fails to give adequate exposure of the joint. The procedure was first described by Insall, and various modifications have subsequently been described.[13] At the proximal end of the medial parapatellar incision, the dissection is extended in an oblique fashion proximally and laterally, exiting the quadricep tendon laterally and splitting the fibers of the vastus lateralis. The quadriceps snip should exit the quadriceps tendon distal to the musculotendinous junction of the rectus femoris muscle (see Figure 3-4). Proximal extension of the arthrotomy beyond the tendon prior to the oblique snip will lead to transection of a portion of the rectus femoris fibers and should be avoided. When performed properly, the musculotendinous bridge of vastus medialis and vastus lateralis is maintained. It is of critical importance that none of the structures contributing to knee extension are transversely divided during the exposure.

The quadriceps snip will improve patellar eversion and mobilization of the extensor mechanism. The knee is once again flexed, while carefully observing the insertion of the patellar tendon. If the patella still cannot be sufficiently subluxated or everted, excision of additional scar tissue may assist in the exposure. If a lateral release is performed, a bridge of tissue consisting of the vastus lateralis insertion into the quadriceps tendon must be maintained.

The closure of a quadriceps snip is performed in routine fashion, similar to a normal capsular closure, and no change in postoperative rehabilitation is necessary. Numerous studies have demonstrated equivalent results for patients undergoing either a standard medial parapatellar arthrotomy or a quadriceps snip.[12-15] The quadriceps snip has few associated complications and should generally be the first technique employed when a more extensile exposure is required in revision TKA.

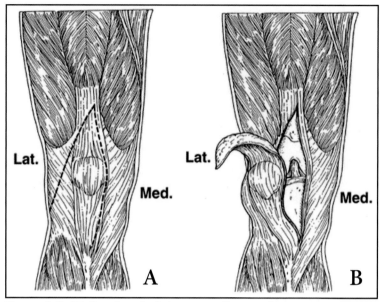

Figure 4-6. (A) Drawing depicting a patellar turndown transecting the rectus tendon, the vastus lateralis tendon, and the lateral retinaculum. The incision is outlined by dotted lines. (B) The completed incision. (Reprinted with permission of Barrack RL. Specialized exposure for revision total knee arthroplasty: quadriceps snip and patellar turndown. *J Bone Joint Surg Am.* 1999;81:138-141.)

V-Y Turndown

The classic V-Y patellar turndown was first described by Coonse and Adams in 1943.[16] The approach starts at the proximal aspect of the quadriceps tendon. The incision is carried distally through the central aspect of the quadriceps tendon, stopping 2 cm proximal to the patella. Two oblique limbs are then extended distally, traveling medial and lateral to the patella. The patella and patellar tendon are then reflected distally to obtain knee exposure. This turndown minimizes the need for soft tissue retraction, thereby reducing the level of trauma to the surrounding knee structures. It requires a broad-based distal flap to maintain an adequate blood supply to the extensor mechanism, and a routine medial parapatellar arthrotomy cannot be converted into a Coonse-Adams approach. Thus, the surgeon must choose whether or not to perform this technique at the commencement of the retinacular approach.

Due to these limitations, the traditional Coonse-Adams approach was subsequently modified by Insall. The knee is first approached in a standard medial parapatellar fashion. If adequate exposure cannot be achieved, or if tension on the quadriceps tendon is excessive, a second quadriceps tendon incision is then performed. This second incision extends distally at a 45-degree angle from the superior pole of the initial parapatellar incision. The dissection is then carried distally through the tendinous insertion of the vastus lateralis, the lateral retinaculum, and the upper portion of the iliotibial tract (Figure 4-6). The modified V-Y patellar turndown may compromise the blood supply to the patella; the second limb should be always be ended short of the inferior lateral geniculate artery to lessen this risk. Scott and Siliski[17] modified the approach by taking the lateral limb of the incision underneath the edge of the vastus lateralis through the tendinous insertion into the retinaculum, rather than through the retinaculum itself. The blood supply to the patella is then possibly maintained through the superior lateral genicular artery—as well as the vessels within the remaining fat pad—which supply the inferior pole of the patella. Controversy exists, however, whether preservation of the superior lateral genicular artery has any clinical significance after TKA.[18]

At the time of wound closure, the apex of the incision and the medial vertical incision are always repaired. The oblique lateral retinacular incision, however, can be left open as a lateral retinacular release to enhance patellar tracking. In the case of a severe quadriceps tendon contracture, a V-Y advancement of the tendon can be performed at the time of closure. Rehabilitation protocols after the modified V-Y patellar turndown technique have varied. Initial recommendations included immobilization for 2 to 6 weeks to allow the repair to heal. This also included several weeks of protected weightbearing. Other authors have recommended a more aggressive approach, including full weightbearing and use of a continuous passive motion machine.[17]

Multiple studies have shown significantly lower functional knee scores after a V-Y patellar turndown.[14,17,19] A persistent extension lag of 10 to 30 degrees is a common result. Studies have also demonstrated persistent weakness in knee extension, even when there is near normal range of motion. These findings are present even in patients in whom an initially contracted extensor mechanism required lengthening in order to achieve an adequate range of motion. Due to the complications associated with this technique, the indications for a traditional V-Y turndown are now very limited. This includes the rare scenario in which a quadriceps snip is not sufficient for exposure, and severe osteopenia or osteolysis of the proximal tibia precludes the option of a tibial tubercle osteotomy. The turndown should not be performed in a knee with multiple previous operations, a history of quadriceps fibrosis, or a previous infection (eg, during reimplantation). A fibrotic extensor mechanism may also fail at the closure of the V-Y turndown, and avascular necrosis of the patella has been reported after this procedure.[20]

MEDIAL FEMORAL PEEL

If greater exposure of the knee is still required after the quadriceps snip, a medial femoral peel can be performed. This technique was first described by Windsor and Insall in the mid-1980s.[21] The peel may be indicated when there is significant contracture of the medial side of the knee, such as during reimplantation following infection, the use of static spacer, or with a fixed flexion contracture. The joint is first approached in standard fashion. The copious medial release of the proximal tibia (the medial collateral ligament slide) is performed, and the origin of the medial collateral ligament and the soft tissues around the medial femoral condyle are then further elevated subperiosteally with electrocautery (Figure 4-7). It is imperative to keep the entire medial soft tissue sleeve intact from the region of the extensor mechanism proximally to the superficial medial collateral ligament distally, as this maintains stability of the medial side of the knee. The posterior capsule is then carefully elevated subperiosteally, resulting in complete exposure of both the femoral component and the posterior aspect of the femoral condyles. A lateral subperiosteal peel can also be performed, if necessary. The femoral peel—combined with the medial subperiosteal dissection of the proximal tibia—allows the knee to be flexed and extended without danger of damaging or tearing the surrounding soft tissue structures. When the incision is closed, the medial soft tissue sleeve will fall back to its normal position around the distal femur and proximal tibia, and if properly performed, no alteration or postoperative rehabilitation is required.

The medial femoral peel is not without complication, however. When the release is performed circumferentially (ie, medially, laterally, and posteriorly), this may result in devascularization of the distal femur due to the extensive nature of the dissection. In addition, exuberant dissection may result in varus-valgus instability, thereby requiring the use of an implant with increased

Figure 4-7. Appearance of the knee upon completion of the medial collateral ligament peel in a patient with severe arthrofibrosis. Note that the medial soft tissue sleeve has been maintained in continuity. (Reprinted with permission of David J. Jacofsky, MD.)

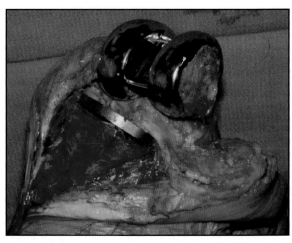

articular constraint. Lavernia et al reported the results of 116 revision cases in which the femoral peel was performed; while all Knee Society scores improved significantly after surgery, the overall complication rate was 17%.[22]

MEDIAL EPICONDYLAR OSTEOTOMY

The medial epicondylar osteotomy is an alternative to the femoral peel. The knee is approached in routine fashion. If excessive medial contracture is encountered, the superficial medial collateral ligament and the soft tissues superior to the medial epicondyle are then raised as a continuous flap, and a 1-cm thick wafer of bone is hinged off the medial epicondyle and adductor tubercle with an osteotome. The medial epicondyle is preserved as a bony fragment within the soft tissue flap. The dissection is then carried out posteriorly and laterally around the femur and tibia, and the joint is opened by externally rotating the knee and hinging the knee into valgus. At the conclusion of the case, the osteotomized epicondyle is reattached with a screw or suture anchors. The remainder of the closure is performed in standard fashion, and the postoperative protocol is unchanged.

The medial epicondylar osteotomy is generally not required unless a malunion of the distal femur is present. Should it be required, one must be certain that osteolysis of the medial femoral condyle is minimal, as an osteotomy in the face of extensive osteolysis may result in a large uncontained femoral bone defect. In a series of 93 cases involving an epicondylar osteotomy, Engh and Ammeen reported a substantial incidence of the epicondyle healing via fibrous union (46%), although this was not associated with symptoms such as focal tenderness, restricted motion, or pain.[23] The authors reported excellent patient satisfaction, knee stability, motion, and deformity correction. Engh and Ammeen promote the procedure as less damaging to the medial-sided ligamentous structures than the medial femoral peel and the medial collateral ligament slide, although many experienced surgeons disagree, especially in the face of poor bone stock.

TIBIAL TUBERCLE OSTEOTOMY

The tibial tubercle osteotomy is an alternative method used to obtain additional exposure in revision TKA. It is especially useful in the presence of patella baja, for the removal of a cemented tibial stem, and in cases of extensor mechanism maltracking and tibial tubercle malposition that require correction. The osteotomy can be technically challenging, however, and there are potentially serious complications associated with this technique. The advantages to tibial tubercle osteotomy include bone-to-bone healing, superior exposure compared to proximal soft tissue techniques, ability to proximalize the patella if baja is encountered, and potential preservation of the patellar blood supply. Disadvantages of the technique will be reviewed next.

The tibial tubercle osteotomy was first described for use in TKA by Dolin in 1983.[24] He performed an osteotomy 4.5 cm long, which was repaired at the conclusion of the case with a single screw. There was concern for failure of this fixation and subsequent escape of the osteotomy fragment. Whiteside modified the technique to include a longer osteotomy fragment, 8 to 10 cm in length.[25] The superficial surgical approach and subcutaneous exposure are carried out in routine fashion. If the knee cannot be sufficiently flexed to allow adequate exposure after all scar tissue has been excised and the gutters have been released, a tibial tubercle osteotomy can then be performed.

To perform the osteotomy, the incision is extended distally along the medial aspect of the tibial shaft. The periosteum is incised 1 cm medial to the tubercle for a length of 8 to 10 cm. The medial cortex of the tibia is cut with an oscillating saw from medial to lateral. If bone stock allows, a step-cut should be made proximally to minimize the risk of proximal migration of the bone fragment (see Figure 3-5). However, extensive promimal tibial osteolysis, or the need to advance the tibial tubercle proximally, often obviates one's ability to leave a structurally sound proximal shelf in the revision setting. The proximal aspect of the osteotomy should be 2 cm wide and 1 to 2 cm thick. The osteotomy is thinned to a wedge distally, tapering to just a few millimeters at the distal tip. The proximal and distal ends of the osteotomy are completed with curved osteotomes, and the osteotomes are used to hinge the bone fragment laterally. The lateral cortex is not exposed, and the periosteum and lateral compartment musculature are retained as a lateral soft tissue hinge. If properly performed, the osteotomy fragment should move laterally, rather than proximally, when complete.

At the time of closure, the osteotomy is repaired with either screws or cerclage wires. While a recent biomechanical study demonstrated 2-screw fixation to have higher load-to-failure than 3 cerclage wires,[26] either method has sufficient strength to withstand physiologic loads. Closure with cerclage wires allows for the use of canal-filling tibial stems. Two or 3 wires are passed around the lateral edge of the tibial tubercle and back onto the tibial crest (Figure 4-8). The wires are angled distally as they pass from the osteotomy fragment to the tibial shaft, in order to tether the osteotomy fragment distally. Long-stemmed revision tibial components should be used, bypassing the distal extent of the osteotomy by at least 2 cortical diameters. When the patient has reasonable bone stock, no alteration in postoperative rehabilitation is necessary. This includes full weightbearing and early range of motion as tolerated.

Initial studies on the use of the tibial tubercle osteotomy in revision TKA reported varying results. Whiteside found a complication rate of 7% in his series of 136 revision cases involving a tibial tubercle osteotomy.[25] His complications included fixation failure, painful hardware, tibial shaft fracture, and a postoperative extension lag. He urged caution when performing the osteotomy in patients with diabetic Charcot neuropathy and advised against postoperative manipulation under anesthesia for arthrofibrosis following the osteotomy. Wolff et al found a higher complication rate of 35% in their series.[27] Their complications included superficial skin necrosis, deep wound necrosis, deep infection, proximal displacement of the osteotomized fragment, and tibial shaft fracture. They also demonstrated higher complication rates in patients with rheumatoid arthritis and a higher union rate with the use of cortical lag screw fixation.

The tibial tubercle osteotomy continues to be an active area of ongoing research. Contemporary series report a complication rate of 5% to 10%.[28-30] The procedure results in good or excellent Knee Society scores in 73% to 87% of cases.[28,30] Deane et al recently reported on fixation of the osteotomy fragment with Ethibond suture in order to decrease the risk of hardware-related complications. They reported no fixation failures or proximal migration of the osteotomy fragment.[31] Chalidis and Ries also recently reviewed their series of 87 tibial tubercle osteotomies in revision

Figure 4-8. (A) Cerclage wires are passed through the osteotomy fragment at the time of osteotomy repair. (B) Appearance of the osteotomy once the repair is complete. (Reprinted with permission of David J. Jacofsky, MD.)

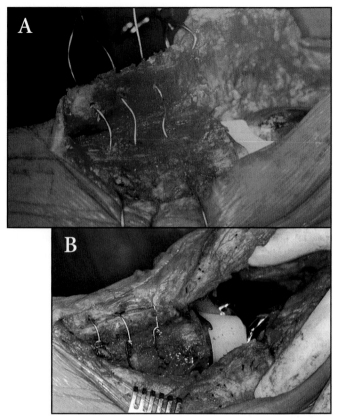

TKA.[32] They specifically investigated whether extension of the osteotomy into the intramedullary canal or a repeat osteotomy affected the healing rate of the osteotomy. They found bony union in all cases, although the time to union was significantly longer for the intramedullary osteotomy group compared to the extramedullary osteotomy group (21 versus 12 weeks). Repeat osteotomy was not associated with delayed bony union. Neither intramedullary extension nor repeat osteotomy was found to increase the complication rate for the procedure.

QUADRICEPSPLASTY

Judet first described his quadricepsplasty technique at the annual meeting of the British Orthopaedic Society in 1959.[33] He developed the procedure for the treatment of the post-traumatic stiff knee. He described a 2-incision technique; the first was a medial parapatellar incision to access and mobilize the patella and suprapatellar pouch, and the second incision was made along the posterolateral thigh, in order to elevate the vastus lateralis and vastus intermedius from the femoral shaft and the lateral intermuscular septum. The Judet quadricepsplasty has subsequently been modified for use in revision TKA in the presence of severe arthrofibrosis and joint stiffness.[34] In these cases, the extensor mechanism is often severely scarred and extensively adherent to the anterior femur.

The modified Judet quadricepsplasty is performed through the standard anterior incision. A blunt periosteal elevator (such as a Cobb) is used to carefully and progressively elevate the vastus intermedius directly off the femoral shaft, the vastus lateralis off the femoral shaft and the lateral intermuscular septum, and the vastus medialis off the femoral shaft and the medial intermuscular septum. Care must be taken during medial exposure, as the femoral neurovascular bundle lies in close proximity to the medial intermuscular septum. The quadricepsplasty can be carried proximally along the entire length of the femoral shaft if necessary in order to free the fibrotic extensor mechanism from the anterior femur.[35] Postoperative mobilization is critical in order to prevent recurrent adhesive scar tissue formation.

Judet developed a postoperative scoring system based on the improvement of knee flexion. Postoperative flexion greater than 100 degrees is rated excellent, 80 to 100 degrees is good, 50 to 80 degrees is fair, and less than 50 degrees is poor. He reported on a series of 53 knees with a broad distribution of postoperative results among all 4 categories. His only reported complication was wound edge necrosis. Subsequent studies have confirmed a low incidence of associated complications, and according to Judet's criteria, the majority of cases result in good or excellent results.[35-37]

SUMMARY

A thorough understanding of the local anatomy of the knee will assist the surgeon greatly during revision TKA. This will help minimize unnecessary injury to the extensor mechanism, the collateral ligaments, and the vital neurovascular structures. The skin incision should be carefully chosen, and skin flaps should be made full thickness, deep to the fascia, to minimize wound-healing complications. A complete excision of the scar deep to the extensor mechanism, as well as recreation of the medial and lateral gutters, will greatly assist in mobilization of the extensor mechanism and subsequent joint exposure. The need for more extensile exposure techniques will be minimized with careful preparation of the soft tissues, utilization of patellar subluxation, and early removal of the modular polyethylene insert.

When exposure of the knee and retained components is still inadequate, more advanced exposure techniques are then employed. These should be applied early in the procedure, whenever possible, before unnecessary damage to the extensor mechanism has occurred. The authors' recommended approach for the majority of revision procedures is a generous medial collateral ligament release to the posterior aspect of the tibia in conjunction with a quadriceps snip. This can be performed routinely, with no adverse effect on the long-term outcome. A tibial tubercle osteotomy is a useful extensile approach for the removal of a cemented tibial stem or the correction of patella baja. In cases of severe arthrofibrosis, such as during reimplantation TKA after the use of a static spacer, a medial femoral peel and/or a modified Judet quadricepsplasty may be required. The medial epicondylar osteotomy can be performed as surgeon preference allows. There is little indication for the use of the V-Y patellar turndown technique, as this has largely been abandoned in favor of the more successful modern exposure techniques. Understanding the basic principles of these advanced surgical exposure techniques is crucial toward maximizing the likelihood of a successful surgical outcome in revision TKA.

REFERENCES

1. Parker DA, Dunbar MJ, Rorabeck CH. Extensor mechanism failure associated with total knee arthroplasty: prevention and management. *J Am Acad Orthop Surg.* 2003;11(4):238-247.
2. Schoderbek RJ Jr, Brown TE, Mulhall KJ, et al. Extensor mechanism disruption after total knee arthroplasty. *Clin Orthop Relat Res.* 2006;446:176-185.
3. Colombel M, Mariz Y, Dahhan P, Kenesi C. Arterial and lymphatic supply of the knee integuments. *Surg Radiol Anat.* 1998;20(1):35-40.
4. Pawar U, Rao KN, Sundaram PS, Thilak J, Varghese J. Scintigraphic assessment of patellar viability in total knee arthroplasty after lateral release. *J Arthoplasty.* 2009;24(4):636-640.

5. Wymenga AB, Kats JJ, Kooloos J, Hillen B. Surgical anatomy of the medial collateral ligament and the posteromedial capsule of the knee. *Knee Surg Sports Traumatol Arthrosc.* 2006;14(3):229-234.

6. Jamsen E, Huhtala H, Puolakka T, Moilanen T. Risk factors for infection after knee arthroplasty. A register-based analysis of 43,149 cases. *J Bone Joint Surg Am.* 2009;91(1):38-47.

7. Ogata K, Shively RA, Shoenecker PL, Chang SL. Effects of standard surgical procedures on the patellar blood flow in monkeys. *Clin Orthop Relat Res.* 1987;215:254-259.

8. Insall J. A midline approach to the knee. *J Bone Joint Surg Am.* 1971;53(8):1584-1586.

9. Crenshaw AH. Surgical techniques and approaches. In: Canale ST, Beaty JH, eds. *Campbell's Operative Orthopaedics.* St. Louis, MO: Mosby Elsevier; 2008:37-38.

10. Younger AS, Duncan CP, Masri BA. Surgical exposures in revision total knee arthroplasty. *J Am Acad Orthop Surg.* 1998;6(1):55-64.

11. Hofmann AA, Plater RL, Murdock LE. Subvastus (Southern) approach for primary total knee arthroplasty. *Clin Orthop Relat Res.* 1991;269:70-77.

12. Della Valle CJ, Berger RA, Rosenberg AG. Surgical exposures in revision total knee arthroplasty. *Clin Orthop Relat Res.* 2006;446:59-68.

13. Garvin KL, Scuderi G, Insall JN. Evolution of the quadriceps snip. *Clin Orthop Relat Res.* 1995;321:131-137.

14. Barrack RL, Smith P, Munn B, Engh G, Rorabeck C. The Ranawat Award. Comparison of surgical approaches in total knee arthroplasty. *Clin Orthop Relat Res.* 1998;356:16-21.

15. Meek RM, Greidanus NV, McGraw RW, Masri BA. The extensile rectus snip exposure in revision of total knee arthroplasty. *J Bone Joint Surg Br.* 2003;85(8):1120-1122.

16. Coonse K, Adams JD. A new operative approach to the knee joint. *Surg Gynecol Obstet.* 1943;77:344.

17. Scott RD, Siliski JM. The use of a modified V-Y quadricepsplasty during total knee replacement to gain exposure and improve flexion in the ankylosed knee. *Orthopedics.* 1985;8(1):45-48.

18. Ritter MA, Herbst SA, Keating EM, Faris PM, Meding JB. Patellofemoral complications following total knee arthroplasty: effect of a lateral release and sacrifice of the superior lateral geniculate artery. *J Arthroplasty.* 1996;11:368-372.

19. Trousdale RT, Hanssen AD, Rand JA, Cahalan TD. V-Y quadricepsplasty in total knee arthroplasty. *Clin Orthop Relat Res.* 1993;286:48-55.

20. Smith PN, Parker DA, Gelinas J, Rorabeck CH, Bourne RB. Radiographic changes in the patella following quadriceps turndown for revision total knee arthroplasty. *J Arthroplasty.* 2004;19:714-719.

21. Windsor RE, Insall JN. Exposure in revision total knee arthroplasty: the femoral peel. *Techniques Orthop.* 1988;3:1-4.

22. Lavernia C, Contreras JS, Alcerro JC. The peel in total knee revision: exposure in the difficult knee. *Clin Orthop Relat Res.* 2011;469:146-153.

23. Engh GA, Ammeen D. Results of total knee arthroplasty with medial epicondylar osteotomy to correct varus deformity. *Clin Orthop Relat Res.* 1999;367:141-148.

24. Dolin MG. Osteotomy of the tibial tubercle in total knee replacement. *J Bone Joint Surg Am.* 1983;65:704-706.

25. Whiteside LA. Exposure in difficult total knee arthroplasty using tibial tubercle osteotomy. *Clin Orthop Relat Res.* 1995;321:32-35.

26. Davis K, Caldwell P, Wayne J, Jiranek WA. Mechanical comparison of fixation techniques for the tibial tubercle osteotomy. *Clin Orthop Relat Res.* 2000;380:241-249.

27. Wolff AM, Hungerford DS, Krackow KA, Jacobs MA. Osteotomy of the tibial tubercle during total knee replacement. A report of twenty-six cases. *J Bone Joint Surg Am.* 1989;71:848-852.

28. Mendes MW, Caldwell P, Jiranek WA. The results of tibial tubercle osteotomy for revision total knee arthroplasty. *J Arthroplasty.* 2004;19(2):167-174.

29. van den Broek CM, van Hellemondt GG, Jacobs WC, Wymenga AB. Step-cut tibial tubercle osteotomy for access in revision total knee replacement. *Knee.* 2006;13(6):430-434.

30. Young CF, Bourne RB, Rorabeck CH. Tibial tubercle osteotomy in total knee arthroplasty surgery. *J Arthroplasty.* 2008;23(3):371-375.

31. Deane DR, Ferran NA, Ghandour A, Morgan-Jones RL. Tibial tubercle osteotomy for access during revision knee arthroplasty: Ethibond suture repair technique. *BMC Musculoskelet Disord.* 2008;9:98.

32. Chalidis BE, Ries MD. Does repeat tibial tubercle osteotomy or intramedullary extension affect the union rate in revision total knee arthroplasty? *Acta Orthopaedica.* 2009;80(4):426-431.

33. Judet R. Mobilisation of the stiff knee. *J Bone Joint Surg Br.* 1959;41:856-857.

34. Aglietti P, Windsor RE, Buzzi R, Insall JN. Arthroplasty for the stiff or ankylosed knee. *J Arthroplasty.* 1989;4(1):1-5.

35. Ebraheim NA, DeTroye RJ, Saddemi SR. Results of Judet quadricepsplasty. *J Orthop Trauma.* 1993;7(4):327-330.

36. Alici T, Buluc L, Tosun B, Sarlak AY. Modified Judet's quadricepsplasty for loss of knee flexion. *Knee.* 2006;13(4):280-283.

37. Masse A, Biasibetti A, Demangos J, Dutto E, Pazzano S, Gallinaro P. The Judet quadricepsplasty: long-term outcome of 21 cases. *J Trauma.* 2006;61(2):358-362.

Component Removal in Revision Total Knee Arthroplasty

Curtis W. Hartman, MD and Craig J. Della Valle, MD

Implant removal during revision total knee arthroplasty (TKA) is a necessary step that can vary in complexity depending on the indication for revision and the type of implants being revised. The goal of this chapter is to describe the techniques required to remove implants during revision TKA in an atraumatic fashion and to describe the equipment needed to aid in that process.

PREOPERATIVE PLANNING

Careful planning is a necessary step before any revision arthroplasty. A vigorous attempt should be made to identify the implants being revised by obtaining the implant record from the previous surgery, including the implant stickers (Figure 5-1), especially if a single-component revision is being considered. Occasionally, the implant record is not available. In situations where the identity of the implant is uncertain, one should be cautious in planning a single-component revision, or plan to revise all implants. When the implants have been identified, the implant manufacturer should be contacted for any additional implant removal devices that may be specific to the implant being revised. Knowledge of the implants in place will also alert the surgeon to specific failure modes, allow the surgeon to have appropriate trials available, and anticipate any particular difficulties in component removal.

The radiographs should be carefully scrutinized for any areas of osteolysis, bony deficiency, or deformity that may predispose the patient to intraoperative periprosthetic fracture. The radiographs will provide substantial information with regard to the difficulty of component removal. Serial radiographs demonstrating migration of an implant indicate that the implant is loose and removal in such cases should be relatively straightforward.

Preoperative planning should also give the surgeon an opportunity to order any specialized instrumentation necessary for implant removal. Commonly used instruments in revision TKA include thin flexible osteotomes, a high-speed burr with multiple bit options, offset osteotomes, and a footed impactor. Additionally, cement removal instruments, including angled osteotomes, gouges, taps, cement splitters, reverse cutting hooks, and an ultrasonic device, may be useful if cemented stems are to be removed.

Jacofsky DJ, Hedley AK, eds.
Fundamentals of Revision Knee Arthroplasty:
Diagnosis, Evaluation, and Treatment (pp 75-84).
© 2013 SLACK Incorporated.

Figure 5-1. Implant stickers obtained from the medical record.

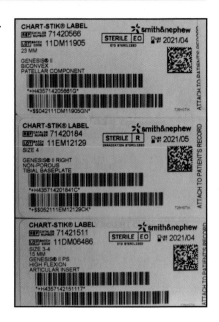

Implant Removal

Revision TKA should begin with a sufficient approach to fully expose the implants to be removed. A discussion on the various extensile exposure techniques is beyond the scope of this chapter but can be reviewed in Chapter 4 of this book. Implant removal should begin with the modular tibial insert, if present. This maneuver will provide additional exposure to the femoral and tibial implants by reducing the soft tissue tension around the knee. As previously described, it is imperative to know the model and manufacturer of the implants being revised. While most polyethylene locking mechanisms can be defeated with an osteotome, some systems may be more complex. Having the appropriate tools available can facilitate the efficiency of the procedure (Figure 5-2).

Primary Femoral Components

The principle of removing cemented femoral components is to fully disrupt the interface between the implant and the underlying cement, remove the implant, and then remove cement from the underlying femur.[1,2] When the femoral component has been adequately exposed, any bone or soft tissue overlying the bone-cement-prosthetic interface should be débrided to clearly visualize this interface. Cemented implants will have varying amounts of cement in the interface.

The cement-prosthetic interface is then disrupted with thin flexible osteotomes, a thin high-speed burr, or a thin saw blade directed parallel to the interface (Figure 5-3). A high-speed pencil-tip burr can be effective in helping to develop this interface, which must be completed with flexible osteotomes. An offset osteotome (Figure 5-4) can be valuable for accessing the interface in the intercondylar notch and on the posterior condyles, which are not easily accessible to traditional flexible osteotomes. An alternative method involves the use of a narrow, reciprocating saw blade to disrupt the cement-prosthetic interface.[3] Regardless of the technique employed to disrupt the interface, the instruments used should stay in the cement-prosthetic interface to avoid damaging the underlying bone.[3]

When the interface has been sufficiently disrupted to develop motion of the implant, it should be removed using direct axial force. This can be accomplished with an attachment on the implant using a mallet or slap hammer. This can also be accomplished with a footed impactor on the exposed surface of the femoral flange (Figure 5-5). One should be cautious to avoid delivering a

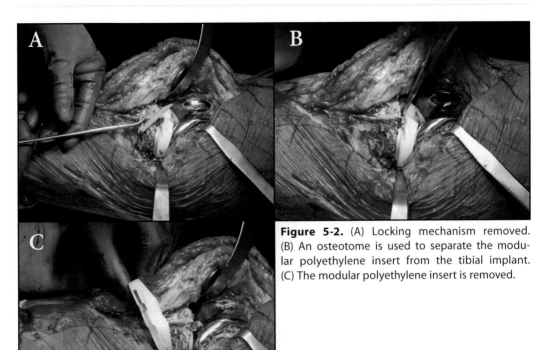

Figure 5-2. (A) Locking mechanism removed. (B) An osteotome is used to separate the modular polyethylene insert from the tibial implant. (C) The modular polyethylene insert is removed.

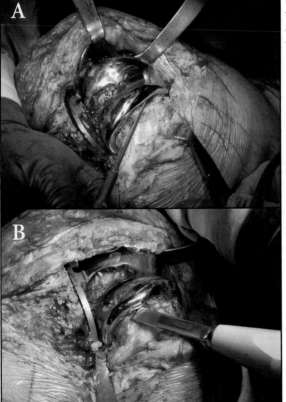

Figure 5-3. (A) The cement-prosthetic interface is disrupted with a high-speed burr. (B) The cement-prosthetic interface is disrupted with a thin osteotome.

Figure 5-4. An offset osteotome is used to access the intercondylar notch.

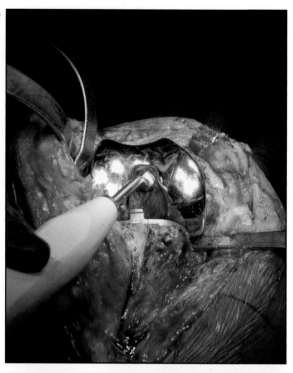

Figure 5-5. A footed impactor is used to deliver axial force.

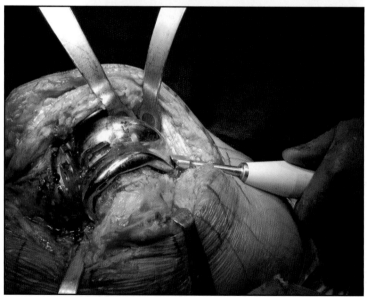

levering-type force (oblique), as this can predispose the patient to distal femoral fracture.[4] The remaining cement is now easily accessible and can be removed; however, well-fixed cement in aseptic revisions can be left if the revision implant is to be cemented and the risk of removal appears to outweigh the benefits.

Revision of cementless implants follow similar principles. The bone-prosthetic interface is adequately exposed and disrupted with instruments directed parallel to the interface. A Gigli saw can be a useful tool for the anterior bone-prosthetic interface. However, caution is necessary with this technique to prevent the saw from drifting into the bone of the anterior femur.[3] When the

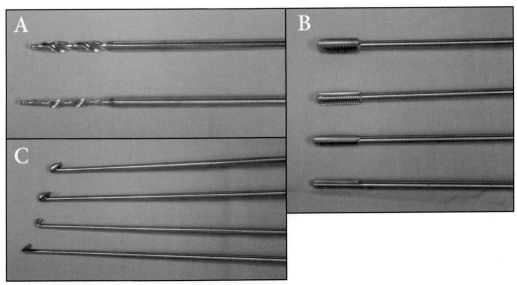

Figure 5-6. Tools used to remove cement include (A) cement drills, (B) cement taps, and (C) reverse hook osteotomes.

interface has been completely disrupted and implant motion is possible, axially directed forces are used to remove the implant.

Stemmed Femoral Components

The presence of a stemmed femoral implant introduces an increasing level of complexity. The preoperative radiographs will determine if the previous surgeon used a technique involving press-fit stems or fully cemented stems. Implants with press-fit stems can be managed in a similar fashion to a primary femoral component, as these stems—while providing additional support—do not typically osseointegrate. Therefore, after disrupting the implant-cement interface, the implant can be removed with axially directed force. Occasionally, a large amount of cement may be present in the intercondylar/metaphyseal portion of the femur, preventing removal without additional exposure. In these cases, a high-speed metal-cutting burr may be used to remove the intercondylar portion of the implant and disrupt the cement mantle.

Cemented stems present a unique challenge to the revision surgeon, as the majority of the implant-cement interface is inaccessible. Removal of these stems should follow the principles discussed previously; namely, disruption of the implant-cement interface followed by axially directed forces to remove the implant. Masri et al[3] have described 3 possible results of this technique:

1. The axial force debonds the implant from the cement, allowing the implant to be removed, leaving an intact cement mantle behind.
2. The axial force causes the cement mantle to debond from the bone and advance as a single unit.
3. The implant-cement construct remains well fixed and cannot be removed without additional exposure.

Surgeons faced with the first situation will have successfully removed a stemmed implant and will have an intact cement mantle to remove. This can be accomplished using several techniques. Combinations of thin osteotomes, cement drills and taps, and reverse cutting hooks (Figure 5-6) are highly effective at removing a well-fixed cement mantle. Additionally, ultrasonic devices have also been shown to be efficient and safe in the removal of well-fixed cement mantles.[1,5-8]

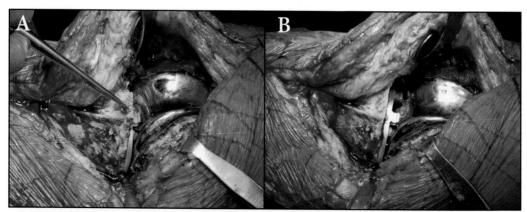

Figure 5-7. Débridement of the bone-cement-prosthetic interface. (A) Before débridement. (B) After débridement.

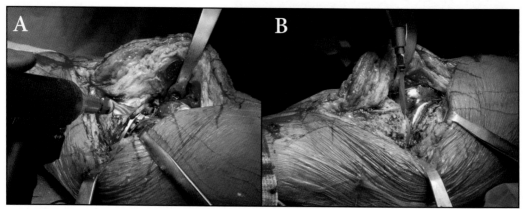

Figure 5-8. Disruption of the cement-prosthetic interface with a reciprocating saw.

Surgeons who encounter the second situation should be cautious with continued extraction, as the implant-cement construct may lead to an intercondylar fracture with progressive force. In this situation, the stem-cement interface should be disrupted with osteotomes so the stem can be removed from the cement and the cement can be removed as in the first situation.

The final situation is the most challenging and requires additional exposure of the cement mantle. This can be accomplished with a cortical window proximal to the stem and distally directed force on the stem with an impactor and mallet. Additionally, a cortical window can be created along the length of the stem to allow access to disrupt the cement-stem interface. Once the stem has been loosened from the cement mantle, the implant is removed as previously described. The presence of an "offsetting" coupler to the implant presents formidable difficulties both with the femoral and the tibial components. An anterior window is usually indicated to fragment the cement mantle to avoid massive bone loss with excessive distal distraction forces.

Primary Tibial Components

The principles of removing tibial implants are essentially identical to the femoral principles: completely disrupt the fixation interface, remove the implant, and remove cement if necessary. Cemented tibial components should have adequate exposure. The interface should be débrided of any bone or soft tissue (Figure 5-7). The prosthetic-cement interface is then disrupted with thin osteotomes or a reciprocating saw (Figure 5-8). The anterior and medial aspects of the tibial

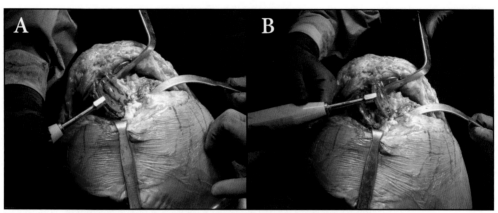

Figure 5-9. Removing the loosened tibial component with a footed impactor.

implant are relatively easy to access; however, the posterior and lateral portions can be more challenging. This fact highlights the importance of adequate exposure, particularly behind the patellar tendon. Once the proximal portion of the implant-cement interface has been completely disrupted, the implant can be dislodged with axially directed force from a footed impactor and mallet (Figure 5-9). A cemented keel typically releases from the cement and the implant is removed, allowing access to the remaining cement.

An all-poly implant is removed by transecting the implant at the proximal bone-cement-implant interface with an oscillating saw. The remaining keel is then removed after loosening from the surrounding cement using osteotomes.

The surgeon should make certain the proper instruments are available to remove any additional means of fixation used with cementless tibial implants. If the surgeon is faced with difficulty removing a cementless tibial tray despite disrupting the interface below the tray, the tray itself can be sectioned with a metal-cutting burr to access the keel or other areas of fixation in the metaphysis that may be preventing safe extraction.

Stemmed Tibial Components

As with the stemmed femoral components, stemmed tibial components can add considerable difficulty to a revision TKA. Tibial components implanted with press-fit stems are removed in a similar fashion to the primary tibial component. The proximal cement-implant interface is disrupted, and an axially directed force is used to dislodge the implant.

Fully cemented stemmed tibial implants can be removed in a similar fashion to the press-fit stemmed tibial implant. However, an extensile exposure is often necessary to access the tibial canal directly. The tibial tubercle osteotomy is a useful technique for this purpose and is described in Chapter 4. Through the osteotomy, the cement-implant interface can be disrupted, allowing removal of the implant. When necessary, the implant can be transected with a high-speed metal-cutting burr, allowing the stem to be removed separately with trephines.

There may be situations where either the tibial tray or femoral component can be electively disengaged from the stem or the stem may inadvertently become disengaged during attempted extraction maneuvers. In these situations either a high-speed burr can be utilized to remove cement around the stem to facilitate extraction or a trephine can be utilized to help remove either a cemented or cementless stem.

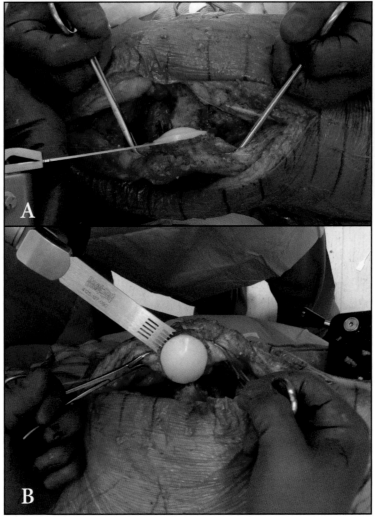

Figure 5-10. Removing an all-polyethylene patella with an oscillating saw blade.

Patellar Components

Because patellar bone stock is limited, extreme patience is required when removing a well-fixed patellar implant to avoid removing so much bone stock that subsequent reconstruction becomes either exceedingly difficult or impossible and to avoid periprosthetic fracture. As described previously, the first step is clearing soft tissue from the interface between the component and the cement mantle or the bony interface so it can be clearly visualized.

All polyethylene designs can be transected at the level of the cement interface with a thin oscillating saw blade (Figure 5-10). The underlying cement is then accessible. The pegs can be removed with a high-speed pencil-tip burr or curette (Figure 5-11). In cases of infection, all cement must be removed, and in some cases it can be very difficult to identify any residual cement. Great care should be taken.

Metal-backed patellar implants require careful disruption of the bone-implant or cement-implant interface with thin, flexible osteotomes or a high-speed pencil-tip burr. The pegs can

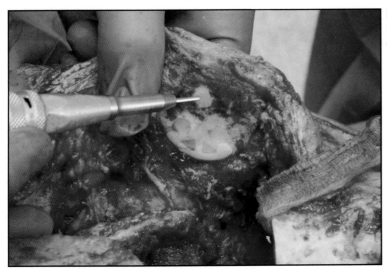

Figure 5-11. Removal of residual cement/polyethylene with a high-speed burr.

then be transected with a metal-cutting wheel. Once the overlying button has been removed, the fixation pegs can be removed with either a high-speed burr to disrupt the interface around the pegs or with a metal-cutting burr to remove the pegs directly.

SUMMARY

Removal of well-fixed implants during revision TKA can pose a challenge to the unprepared surgeon. With adequate preoperative planning, appropriate instrumentation, and patience, most implants can be removed in an atraumatic fashion.

REFERENCES

1. Caillouette JT, Gorab RS, Klapper RC, Anzel SH. Revision arthroplasty facilitated by ultrasonic tool cement removal. Part II: histologic analysis of endosteal bone after cement removal. *Orthop Rev.* 1991;20(5):435-440.
2. Windsor RE, Scuderi GR, Insall JN. Revision of well-fixed cemented, porous total knee arthroplasty. Report of six cases. *J Arthroplasty.* 1988;3(suppl):S87-S94.
3. Masri BA, Mitchell PA, Duncan CP. Removal of solidly fixed implants during revision hip and knee arthroplasty. *J Am Acad Orthop Surg.* 2005;13(1):18-27.
4. Dennis DA, Berry DJ, Engh G, et al. Revision total knee arthroplasty. *J Am Acad Orthop Surg.* 2008;16(8):442-454.
5. Gardiner R, Hozack WJ, Nelson C, Keating EM. Revision total hip arthroplasty using ultrasonically driven tools. A clinical evaluation. *J Arthroplasty.* 1993;8(5):517-521.
6. Klapper RC, Caillouette JT, Callaghan JJ, Hozack WJ. Ultrasonic technology in revision joint arthroplasty. *Clin Orthop Relat Res.* 1992;(285):147-154.
7. Caillouette JT, Gorab RS, Klapper RC, Anzel SH. Revision arthroplasty facilitated by ultrasonic tool cement removal. Part I: in vitro evaluation. *Orthop Rev.* 1991;20(4):353-357.
8. Klapper RC, Caillouette JT. The use of ultrasonic tools in revision arthroplasty procedures. *Contemp Orthop.* 1990;20(3):273-279.

Management of Bone Loss in Revision Total Knee Arthroplasty

R. Michael Meneghini, MD

BACKGROUND

Dealing with bone loss during revision knee replacement remains a challenging clinical problem. Smaller defects have been traditionally and effectively treated with morselized cancellous bone graft,[1,2] cement augmented with screw fixation,[3-6] or the use of modular metal augments that accompany revision knee implant systems.[7,8] Large or massive bone defects require more extensive reconstructive efforts and have been traditionally managed with large structural allografts,[8-17] impaction bone grafting,[18-21] custom prosthetic components,[22] specialized hinged knee components,[23] or, more recently, porous metal metaphyseal cones.[24-27] Despite the multitude of utilized treatment methods, the best reconstructive technique for bone defects during revision knee replacement has not been clearly established.[22]

BONE LOSS ASSESSMENT AND CLASSIFICATION

The critical step in determining the appropriate reconstruction method in revision total knee replacement is to accurately determine the quantity, location, and extent of the bone loss. This is done after meticulous and cautious removal of the failed tibial and femoral implants, with careful attention to existing bone preservation. Once the components are removed, it is important to determine whether the defects are contained or uncontained (segmental). In addition, the location of supportive bone that surrounds the bone loss is essential; it will dictate the type and size of the augmentation that is required. Smaller contained defects can be treated with either cement fill with screw augmentation or morselized allograft fill, particularly in older patients. However, larger uncontained defects typically require larger reconstructive measures such as modular block augments, bulk allograft, or highly porous metal metaphyseal cones.

A common system of categorizing bone defects in revision knee arthroplasty is the Anderson Orthopaedic Research Institute Bone Defect classification.[22] In this bone defect classification, type I defects describe only minor and contained cancellous bony defects within either tibial

Jacofsky DJ, Hedley AK, eds.
Fundamentals of Revision Knee Arthroplasty:
Diagnosis, Evaluation, and Treatment (pp 85-98).
© 2013 SLACK Incorporated.

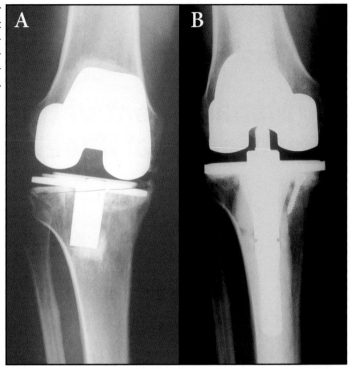

Figure 6-1. (A) Anteroposterior radiograph of tibial bone defect secondary to medial tibial collapse. (B) Lateral radiograph utilizing cement fill with screw augmentation at 12 months follow-up.

plateau or femoral condyle. Type IIA defects include moderate to severe cancellous and/or cortical bone defects of only one tibial plateau or condyle; type IIB defects include moderate to severe cancellous bone defects of both tibial plateaus and/or segmental cortical defects of one tibial plateau or condyles. In type II defects, neither the tibial tubercle on the tibial side nor the epicondyles on the lateral side are deficient. Type III defects describe combined cavitary and segmental bone loss of both tibial plateaus or femoral condyles and involve bone loss below the tubercle or proximal to the epicondyles, respectively.

CEMENT AND SCREWS

The use of cement as a reconstructive augment has the benefits of being simple, inexpensive, and efficient, as the revision knee arthroplasty is already utilizing this material for fixation in most instances. This reconstruction method is typically indicated for smaller, contained defects less than 5 mm in depth,[3,4] although some authors have advocated its use in larger defects with excellent clinical results.[5,6] When cement is used for defects in revision knee arthroplasty, augmentation with bone screws is typically recommended to enhance the biomechanical properties of the construct (Figure 6-1). However, if the patient is young and active, it may be more advantageous to utilize morselized allograft to restore bone stock in these types of defects.

Surgical Technique

The surgical technique begins with the tibial or femoral provisional, or "freshening," cuts. Once these are performed, a more accurate assessment of the defect is possible. A meticulous débridement of the defect is performed with removal of all fibrous tissue, which would impede adequate interdigitation of the cement and create suboptimal fixation. Sclerotic bone surfaces are frequently encountered in revision surgeries and must be roughened with either a small drill or a burr. Once the defect is clearly delineated and prepared, the location of remaining bone is identified for adequate screw fixation. If the defect is of minimal depth, it may be filled with cement alone during cementation of the standard revision tibial or femoral components. If the defects are larger or the surgeon is uncertain, reinforcement with screw augmentation is recommended. Once the bone defect is adequately prepared for cement, titanium self-tapping cancellous bone screws are placed into the host metaphyseal bone and advanced so that the heads are positioned well below the level of the tibial tray or femoral component. Trial implants may be utilized at this point to confirm there is no contact with the screw heads. Once the cement is mixed and in a doughy state, it is placed into the defect and around the screw heads and pressurized by hand. The final prosthesis is then placed and the cement is allowed to cure with removal of the excess cement.

Clinical Results

Satisfactory mid-term results have been reported with the use of screws and cement for bone defects in total knee arthroplasty (TKA). Ritter reported on 57 total knee replacements with large medial tibial defects reconstructed with screws and cement at an average of 6.1 years follow-up.[6] Although nonprogressive radiolucent lines were common and seen in 27% of cases, there were no reported cases of tibial component loosening, component failure, or cement failure. In a subsequent report by Ritter and Harty, 125 TKAs that utilized screws and cement to fill large medial tibial defects secondary to severe varus deformities were reported at a mean of 7.9 years follow-up.[5] The authors reported 2 failures that occurred due to medial tibial collapse at 5 and 10 years, respectively, but no other failures or loosening were observed. However, this was a series of primary knee arthroplasties without the typical stem extensions used in revision knee arthroplasty to augment fixation and prevent medial collapse in the setting of bone deficiency and suboptimal bone quality. In summary, smaller and more contained defects that are encountered in revision knee arthroplasty, particularly in older or less active patients, are appropriate for the use of screws and cement. This is a viable and successful method of reconstruction that is inexpensive, relatively simple, and efficient.

MORSELIZED ALLOGRAFT

Bone loss in revision knee arthroplasty can be treated reliably and successfully with morselized cancellous allograft and has an established clinical track record.[19,28-32] This method is typically reserved for contained defects (Figure 6-2) and is particularly attractive for younger patients in whom restoration of deficient bone stock is a priority given the potential for future reconstructive surgeries. Biologically, morselized cancellous allograft appears to incorporate similarly to cancellous autograft, albeit at a much slower rate. It is beneficial to have a well-vascularized recipient bed in order to facilitate incorporation of the allograft bone. If a highly sclerotic defect is encountered, it may be beneficial to either burr away the sclerotic bone to underlying cancellous and vascular bone or, conversely, use another reconstruction method such as a block augment. Furthermore, if the defect is large and segmental, although some authors have reported adequate results with impaction allografting,[19,29] reconstruction with more robust structural augments such as metal blocks, bulk allograft, or metaphyseal porous metal cones will typically produce more biomechanically stable constructs.

Surgical Technique

As with all the reconstructive techniques, the surgical technique of utilizing morselized allograft to fill contained defects requires the meticulous débridement of the defect with careful attention to removal of all fibrous tissue. Careful attention is paid to preparation of a vascular bed

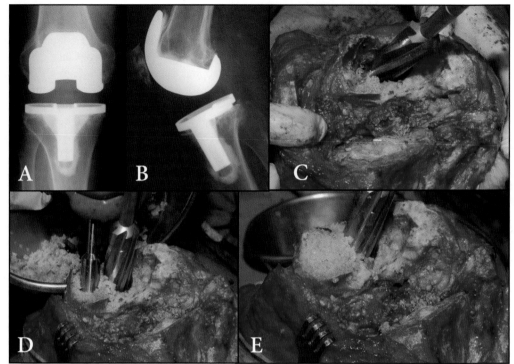

Figure 6-2. (A) Anteroposterior and (B) lateral radiograph of failed total knee replacement with severe femoral bone loss in the lateral condyle secondary to osteolysis. (C-E) Intraoperative pictures of impaction grafting using the intramedullary reamer to facilitate compaction of morselized allograft into the defect.

for allograft incorporation to host bone and long-term bone reconstitution. Once the defect is adequately débrided, prepared, and confirmed to be contained with supporting peripheral structure, the morselized allograft can be inserted into the defect. It is also necessary to grind up any larger pieces into a fine morselized consistency in order to facilitate both biological and structural properties. It is helpful to place an adequately sized reamer or trial stem into the medullary canal and impact the morselized allograft material around the reamer, which facilitates compaction of the graft in order to optimize its ability to provide structural support (see Figures 6-2C to 6-2E). Once this complete, the reamer is removed and the final implant is inserted with an intramedullary stem for supplemental support.

Clinical Results

Mid-term results have been published for the technique of impaction allograft reconstruction in revision TKA. Lotke et al prospectively studied the mid-term results of 48 consecutive revision TKAs with substantial bone loss treated with impaction allografting.[29] At an average follow-up of 3.8 years, no mechanical failures of the revisions were reported, and all radiographs demonstrated incorporation and remodeling of the bone graft. Although the authors concede the technique is time consuming and technically demanding, they advocate impaction grafting as a viable and successful technique for addressing bone loss in revision TKA.[29] Whiteside and Bicalho reported on 63 patients who had revision knee arthroplasty using morselized cancellous allograft to fill large femoral and/or tibial defects.[32] Firm seating of the components on a rim of viable bone and rigid fixation with a medullary stem were achieved in all cases. Fourteen reoperations occurred, and a biopsy specimen was taken from the central portion of the allograft, which revealed evidence of active new bone formation. Evidence of healing, bone maturation, and formation of trabeculae was observed on all radiographs at 1-year follow-up. Two patients required revision surgery for aseptic loosening in this series, and the authors felt both had greatly improved bone stock so that new implants could be applied with minor additional grafting.[32]

STRUCTURAL ALLOGRAFT

Bulk structural allograft has frequently been used to reconstruct large bone defects with the intention of providing mechanical support and reconstituting bone, which are considered advantages of this technique. Bulk allograft is typically indicated for defects that are larger than 1.5 cm in depth and exceed the dimensions of typical metal block augments that accompany most revision total knee systems. The advantage of bulk allograft is the potential for bone reconstitution, particularly in young patients to whom this goal is of great importance with the likelihood of multiple future surgeries and reconstructions. The drawbacks are the potential for graft resorption, collapse, and graft-host nonunion. Patient factors that include health status, physiologic age, bone quality, and activity must be considered when contemplating use of this reconstructive technique over other reconstruction strategies such as porous metal cones.

Surgical Technique

The technique involves shaping the defect to accept a bulk allograft, most commonly a femoral head. The shaping can be done with high-speed burr or acetabular reamers. As with morselized allograft, it is beneficial to ensure that the allograft bone is in contact with vascularized host bone as opposed to the dense and frequently avascular sclerotic bone encountered in many revision knee defects. Once in place, the graft is secured to the host bone with threaded Steinmann pins or screws. It is advantageous to countersink the screw heads to avoid metal-metal contact with the prosthesis and the subsequent galvanic corrosion that can occur. The tibial (or femoral) surface is then shaped accordingly, either freehand or with the knee revision system alignment cutting guides, and supplemental stem fixation with or without cement, which is utilized to bypass the reconstructed defect.

Clinical Results

Recently, Engh and Ammeen reported on a series of 46 revision knee arthroplasties with reconstruction of massive tibial defects using bulk allograft.[17] The authors reported only 4 failures, 2 for infection, at a mean of 95 months follow-up with no evidence of graft collapse. The authors subsequently recommend using bulk allograft for large tibial defects.[17] However, resorption and collapse of the allograft has been a concern from other authors.[7,22] In a series of 52 revision knee replacements with bulk allograft followed prospectively, Clatworthy et al reported that 13 knee replacements failed, yielding a 75% success rate at 97 months follow-up. Five knees had graft resorption, resulting in implant loosening, and 2 knees had nonunion between the host bone and the allograft. The survival rate of the allografts was 72% at 10 years.[9] In a retrospective study from the Mayo Clinic, authors reviewed 65 knees that underwent revision knee arthroplasty with bulk allograft for large bone defects and reported a 10-year revision-free survivorship of 76%. Sixteen patients (22.8%) had failed reconstructions and underwent additional surgery with 8 of 16 due to allograft failure and 3 due to failure of a component unsupported by allograft.[33] While these reports support the use of bulk allograft for severe tibial or femoral bone defects in revision knee arthroplasty, they also highlight the need for a more durable reconstruction method to facilitate long-term success and avoid the complications inherent with allograft, namely graft nonunion, resorption, and subsequent reconstruction failure.

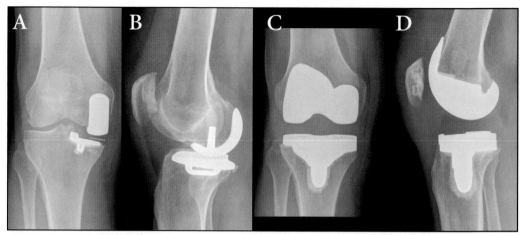

Figure 6-3. (A) Anteroposterior and (B) lateral radiograph of a failed total knee replacement originally performed through a minimally invasive incision with subsequent severe varus tibial component malposition, creating a moderate medial tibial defect and clinical instability. (C) Anteroposterior and (D) lateral radiograph of the revision total knee replacement reconstruction with a block augment and cemented stem extension restoring the mechanical alignment and subsequent stability of the knee.

RECONSTRUCTION WITH MODULAR BLOCKS OR WEDGES

Modular blocks and wedges are indicated in small to moderate segmental tibial and femoral defects (Figure 6-3). Modular metal blocks have the advantages of being versatile, efficient, technically straightforward, and not requiring osseointegration. Therefore, they are particularly useful in older and less active patients, yet have the disadvantage of failing to restore bone stock. The majority of revision total knee systems have numerous shapes and sizes of augments for both the tibia and femur, which facilitates restoration of the joint line and proper balancing of the knee in a relatively efficient manner as well.

Surgical Technique

The surgical technique of using modular metal blocks or wedges is relatively straightforward. Once the location and extent of the defects have been determined, the size and shape of the augment that best fits that defect is selected. In the tibia, wedges or blocks may be used, and the majority of knee revision systems have alignment and cutting guides that prepare the bone for a nearly exact fit with the prosthesis. Although modular tibial wedges were designed to accommodate the frequently encountered defect seen in varus collapse of the medial tibia, there is legitimate concern that wedges subject the interface cement to shear forces, which are not ideal long term with cement. Therefore, many surgeons will remove a bit more bone and convert a wedge-shaped defect into one that will accept a block augment so that the cement interface is subjected to predominantly compressive loads, which are much more favorable to long-term cement survivorship. Furthermore, it has been shown that block augments are superior to wedges biomechanically in creating an overall more stable and rigid tibial construct.[34] It is helpful to use intramedullary instrumentation to align the tibial cut perpendicular to the mechanical axis of the tibia. The associated cutting guide will guide the 1- to 2-mm "skim" or freshening cut on each plateau to perform the least amount of bone removal. This will also facilitate bone preparation to accept the exact size and shape of the augment. It is also important to determine the proper tibial component rotation, which is typically aligned with the medial one-third of the tibial tubercle, so that the sagittal cut of the block augment will seat in the corresponding correct rotational position. Once the cuts are made, sclerotic bone is roughened to facilitate cement interdigitation and the final tibial component with stem extension is placed.

There are several factors that are unique to the femoral component preparation for modular block augments. First, the majority of augments are block-shaped and come in a variety of sizes distally and posteriorly to accommodate the most commonly encountered areas of bone loss. Once the tibial platform is reconstructed, which is typically the initial step in performing a revision TKA, the thickness of these augments can be altered to correctly position the femoral component with regard to the balancing of the flexion and extension gaps. For example, if the extension space is larger than the flexion space, distal augmentation may be used to balance the knee, which emphasizes the importance of determining the correct balance of the knee prior to making any femoral augment cuts. This may compromise the surgeon's ability to properly balance the knee. Conversely, if the flexion gap is larger than the extension gap, which is the more commonly encountered scenario, upsizing the femoral component and using thicker posterior augments to maintain bone contact and fixation will facilitate proper knee balancing. As with the tibia, the correct alignment of the distal femoral cuts should typically be determined with intrameduallary alignment guides, which also have the associated cutting guides for correct placement and sizing of augments. The final and critical step in femoral component position is determining the correct femoral component rotation, which should align the implant with the transepicondylar axis as determined by the medial and lateral epicondyles. Frequently, a larger posterior augment will be required laterally—compared to the medial side—in order to avoid placement of the femoral component in relative internal rotation, which is deleterious for patellar tracking and overall knee balance. Again, once the bone preparation is complete, the final modular augments are applied to the femoral component and implanted with cement to bony surfaces that have been adequately prepared to facilitate cement interlock.

Clinical Results

Several studies have reported successful mid-term results with modular metal augments in revision knee arthroplasty.[35-37] Patel et al reported the 5- to-10-year results of 102 revision knee arthroplasties in patients with type II defects treated with augments and stems, which were studied prospectively.[36] Average follow-up was 7 years, and nonprogressive radiolucent lines were observed around the augment in 14% of knees but were not associated with decreased survivorship or increased failure of the implants. The overall survivorship of the components was 92% at 11 years.[36] Rand prospectively studied 41 consecutive revision TKAs with modular augmentation.[37] Modular augments were used for the distal femur alone in 2 knees, posterior condyles of the femur alone in 16 knees, and both distally and posteriorly in 12 knees. Tibial augmentation was used in 13 knees. At a mean of 3 years follow-up, 96% of the knees demonstrated good to excellent results, and there were no cases of aseptic loosening.[37]

RECONSTRUCTION WITH
POROUS METAL METAPHYSEAL CONES

Highly porous metal metaphyseal cones have recently been developed and used for large tibial and femoral defects and were designed to avoid the incidence of nonunion and resorption associated with bulk allograft reconstructions. Highly porous metals, particularly porous tantalum, are biomaterials that offer several potential advantages over traditional materials and include low stiffness, high porosity, and a high coefficient of friction. The design intent for these porous tantalum metaphyseal cones is to address the variable patterns of severe bone loss encountered during revision knee arthroplasty, in addition to providing mechanical support with biologic integration and avoiding allograft nonunion and resorption. Short-term evidence now exists that supports the use of these implants in the reconstruction of large tibial defects in revision TKA.[24-27]

The indications for the use of the highly porous metaphyseal cones are similar to those traditionally used for bulk allograft and include large contained or uncontained tibial or femoral bony defects in a failed total knee replacement. The size of the defect is typically larger than is appropriately reconstructed with traditional modular blocks or wedges. The defects can be classified with the Anderson Orthopaedic Research Institute Bone Defect classification, and the porous metaphyseal cones are typically indicated for type II and type III defects, which are characterized by moderate to severe cancellous and/or cortical defects. The surgeon should keep in mind, however, that contained defects with a substantial supportive cortical rim may be more appropriate for impaction grafting, particularly in younger patients, and small uncontained defects that are less than 5 to 10 mm in depth and isolated to one tibial plateau will likely be more amenable to standard metal blocks. Alternatively, reconstruction of large tibial or femoral defects in young patients may be more appropriately performed with bulk allograft in an attempt to reconstitute bone stock for future revision surgery. Furthermore, large defects in patients with insufficient bone support or decreased potential for osseointegration may be amenable to reconstruction with custom prostheses or tumor megaprostheses.

Surgical Technique

The quantity and location of remaining cortical and cancellous bone must be noted and considered in the final assessment of whether porous metal metaphyseal cones are indicated to augment the reconstruction. The most common tibial scenario appropriate for the porous metaphyseal cones is typically a severe contained or uncontained medial tibial plateau bony defect with varying amounts of lateral tibial plateau remaining for structural support (Figure 6-4). The most common femoral defect appropriate for porous metal cones is a severe medial and lateral condyle cancellous bone deficiency with an intact, yet minimally supportive, cortical rim. The assessment should include the anticipated size and shape of the porous metaphyseal cone that will be appropriate, with respect to its fit within the tibial or femoral metaphysis as well as its tentative location and placement required to reconstitute the proximal tibial or distal femoral supporting surface. Visual inspection of the metaphyseal region and associated defect is performed with respect to the fit of the porous tantalum cone trial, and a high-speed burr is used to contour the metaphyseal bone to accommodate the porous tantalum cone trial with the maximal bone contact and stability possible.

The appropriate porous tantalum cone size and shape are chosen, and the final implant is impacted in the tibial or femoral metaphysis carefully with size-specific impactors. In order to minimize the chance of intraoperative periprosthetic fracture, the surgeon should be careful of overly aggressive impaction of the final implant. Tibial and femoral metaphyseal bone in the revision setting is typically sclerotic, damaged, mechanically weak, and prone to inadvertent fracture. The frictional coefficient of the actual porous tantalum implant will create greater resistance to insertion and subsequent stability. Once the porous metal cone is in its final and stable position, any areas or voids between the periphery of the porous tantalum cone and the adjacent bone of the proximal tibia are filled with morselized cancellous bone or putty to prevent any egress of bone cement between the cone and host bone during cementation of the stemmed component. Also, the surgeon should be aware that the rotation of the final implant is not dependent on the final rotation of the femoral or tibial components, as the porous metal cones are designed to fit within the defect to reconstitute the metaphyseal platform. There typically is sufficient room within the porous metal cone to allow rotation of the tibial and femoral components into correct position to optimize stability and patellofemoral mechanics; however, this rotational freedom varies among implant systems.

The tibial and/or femoral revision prosthetic component is inserted through the cone using either cementless or cemented stem extensions. With either type of stem fixation,

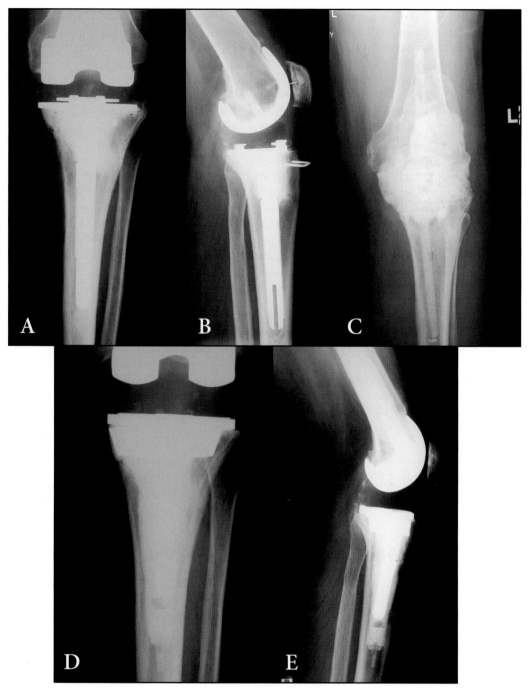

Figure 6-4. (A) Anteroposterior and (B) lateral radiograph of failed total knee replacement with periprosthetic infection in addition to severe medial tibial bone loss due to a prior reconstruction. (C) Anteroposterior radiograph of static antibiotic cement spacer. (D) Anteroposterior and (E) lateral radiograph of the revision total knee replacement demonstrating the porous metal tibial metaphyseal cone bypassed with cemented stem extension.

polymethylmethacrylate is placed between the porous cone and the tray and the proximal keel of the tibial component and/or between the box and augments of the femoral component. It is advantageous to contour and smooth the curing cement around the exterior of any exposed porous tantalum material, such as occurs in the area of uncontained defects, particularly in the vicinity of the medial collateral ligament. This helps minimize the postoperative medial knee pain that can occur due to local irritation of soft tissues that are intended to be mobile, such as the medial collateral ligament, against the high frictional surface of porous tantalum. Once the cement has hardened, the remainder of the surgical procedure is carried out in standard fashion with insertion of the appropriate polyethylene insert and meticulous wound closure.

The postoperative care of revision knee arthroplasty patients who have reconstructions utilizing porous tantalum metaphyseal cones is no different than for those undergoing a standard revision TKA. Patients are allowed to bear weight as tolerated based on the implant stability and quality of reconstruction. If the surgeon achieves an inherently stable porous metaphyseal cone and final implant construct, the patient is allowed to bear weight as tolerated. If it is suspected that the mechanical stability of the construct is tenuous, the patient is kept partial weightbearing for 6 weeks, and radiographs are obtained at that follow-up interval. If there is no evidence of implant or construct migration, the patient is then allowed to progress to weightbearing as tolerated.

Clinical Results

Recently, early outcomes with highly porous metaphyseal cones utilized in large tibial defects for revision TKA have been reported by multiple authors.[24,25] Meneghini et al reported a series of 15 revision knee arthroplasties that were performed with a porous metal metaphyseal tibial cone and were followed for a minimum of 2 years. All tibial cones were found to be osseointegrated radiographically and clinically at final follow-up with no reported failures in this initial series.[25] In a series of 16 revision TKAs with severe tibial defects, Long and Scuderi reported good results with osseointegration of the porous tantalum cone in 14 of 16 cases at a minimum 2-year follow-up. Two metaphyseal cones required removal for recurrent sepsis and were found to be well fixed at surgery.[24] These early results appear equivalent to those obtained with bulk allograft, custom implants, or large modular metal augments at the same time interval. Further clinical and radiographic follow-up will provide insight into the long-term durability of these highly porous augments.

MEGAPROSTHESIS FOR SALVAGE OF SEVERE BONE LOSS

In rare cases of the most severe femoral or tibial bone loss, salvage reconstruction with a megaprosthesis to replace the deficient bone is needed due to the inadequacy of native bone support for reconstruction with any of the previously described techniques. While initial designs reported early failures likely due to the increased constraint in the bearing that transmitted forces to the prosthesis-bone interface, modern rotating hinge designs (see Figure 6-4) have demonstrated improved outcomes and clinical results.[38-41] In general, the indications for use of a distal femoral replacing rotating hinge device are rare and reserved for the most severe cases of bone loss (type III) in more elderly and lower demand patients. One can estimate a distal femoral replacement may be indicated based on the proximal femoral extent of the bone loss. If the bone loss encompasses the medial epicondyle, there is a good chance the medial collateral will be incompetent, which typically necessitates a greater level of varus-valgus constraint in the form of a rotating hinge bearing. Due to the space required for the hinge articulation and bearing, significant bone removal is required. When proximal bone loss is even more pronounced, such as in chronic infection, the most severe osteolysis, severe osteopenia in the face of a distal periprosthetic femur fracture, or if the patient is of advanced age or lower demand, prosthetic replacement of the bone loss may be advantageous in order to facilitate mobilization, avoid the prolonged restricted weightbearing, and avoid the unpredictable union rates associated with bulk allograft. In this case, a rotating hinge distal femoral replacement or proximal tibial replacement may be necessary.

Surgical Technique

Preoperative planning is critical in order to enact the proper leg length restoration, which in a revision total knee replacement to a hinge distal femoral replacement or proximal tibial replacement can affect the extensor mechanism tension and subsequent quadriceps muscle and knee extension strength. Restoration of the joint line and reproduction of the coronal plane anatomy will ensure the optimal extensor mechanism tension and optimize patellar function. Depending on how proximal the incision is required, many of these cases may necessitate a sterile surgical tourniquet. An extended medial parapatellar arthrotomy is typically used, and because a rotating hinge will be used, the superficial medial collateral ligament may be released from the proximal tibia to facilitate exposure, particularly if a proximal tibial replacement is anticipated. Familiarity with the peri-articular neurovascular anatomy is required and an extensive dissection is necessitated. This dissection should be performed meticulously and carefully, avoiding the tendency to stray away from the bone surfaces. Once the femoral or tibial bone is removed, an appropriate clean-up cut is made according to the preoperative plan and restoration of leg length and joint line. The tibial preparation in a distal femoral replacement is performed as in a typical revision total knee replacement, with attention to enacting a stable tibial platform perpendicular to the mechanical axis. With respect to the femoral component, a trial is inserted against a flush cut perpendicular to the anatomic axis of the femur and a trial reduction is performed. When rotating hinge distal femoral or proximal tibial replacements are utilized for severe bone loss in revision total knee replacement, long stems are a requisite to ensure long-term adequate fixation. In younger patients, press-fit stems are available, while in the more common elderly or low-demand patients, cemented stems are preferable in order to gain immediate and adequate fixation for weightbearing and immobilization. Particular attention is paid to the rotation of the femoral component. This correct rotation can be referenced to the linea aspera posteriorly or, if there are residual epicondyles, an approximation to the epicondylar line may be chosen, and finally, confirmation of optimal patellar tracking with the trial implants is critical to ensure optimal outcomes with the final implants and minimization of the deleterious complication of patellar maltracking. Once the final components are in place, attention is turned to closure in standard fashion with meticulous attention to protection of the soft tissues and skin.

Clinical Results

The clinical results of rotating hinge distal femoral replacements have been satisfactory for the salvage of the most severe bone deficiencies and complex revision total knee replacements.[38-41] Springer et al reported on 26 knees that were treated at the Mayo Clinic with an arthroplasty using a modular segmental kinematic rotating hinge prosthesis for non-neoplastic limb salvage.[38] The indications included nonunion of a periprosthetic femur fracture, severe bone loss and ligamentous instability, nonunion of a supracondylar femur fracture, acute periprosthetic fracture, fracture of a previous hinge, and prior resection arthroplasty. The average age of the patients was 72 years, and the average follow-up was 58 months. Improvements in functional scores and motion occurred in the majority. Complications occurred in 8 patients, with the most common complication being deep infection, which occurred in 5 patients.[38] Barrack reported on a series of 23 revision total knee replacements using a second-generation rotating hinge component.[40] Indications for surgery included medial collateral ligament disruption, revision of a previous hinged component with massive bone loss, comminuted distal femur fracture or distal femoral nonunion in elderly patients, extensor mechanism disruption requiring reconstruction in an unstable knee, and ankylosis requiring femoral peel exposure with moderate residual flexion-extension gap imbalance. At the

2- to 9-year follow-up, the author reported that the clinical results, range of motion, and satisfaction were comparable with that of a standard condylar revision knee arthroplasty despite the fact that the cases were more complex.[40]

SUMMARY

Bone loss in revision TKA can be challenging in terms of reconstruction and restoration of function. The techniques range from cement fill with screws, modular augments, morselized or bulk allograft, highly porous metal metaphyseal cones, and megaprosthesis reconstruction with a rotating hinge device. Adhering to the treatment strategies outlined above can guide the practicing surgeon and provide direction to enact the most optimal outcomes in patients with these challenging reconstructions.

REFERENCES

1. Benjamin J, Engh G, Parsley B, Donaldson T, Coon T. Morselized bone grafting of defects in revision total knee arthroplasty. *Clin Orthop Relat Res.* 2001;(392):62-67.
2. Ries MD. Impacted cancellous autograft for contained bone defects in total knee arthroplasty. *Am J Knee Surg.* 1996;9(2):51-54.
3. Aleto TJ, Berend ME, Ritter MA, Faris PM, Meneghini RM. Early failure of unicompartmental knee arthroplasty leading to revision. *J Arthroplasty.* 2008;23(2):159-163.
4. Gross AE. Revision total knee arthroplasty of bone grafts versus implant supplementation. *Orthopedics.* 1997;20(9):843-844.
5. Ritter MA, Harty LD. Medial screws and cement: a possible mechanical augmentation in total knee arthroplasty. *J Arthroplasty.* 2004;19(5):587-589.
6. Ritter MA. Screw and cement fixation of large defects in total knee arthroplasty. *J Arthroplasty.* 1986;1(2):125-129.
7. Bobyn JD, Poggie RA, Krygier JJ, et al. Clinical validation of a structural porous tantalum biomaterial for adult reconstruction. *J Bone Joint Surg Am.* 2004;86-A(suppl 2):123-129.
8. Hockman DE, Ammeen D, Engh GA. Augments and allografts in revision total knee arthroplasty: usage and outcome using one modular revision prosthesis. *J Arthroplasty.* 2005;20(1):35-41.
9. Clatworthy MG, Ballance J, Brick GW, Chandler HP, Gross AE. The use of structural allograft for uncontained defects in revision total knee arthroplasty. A minimum five-year review. *J Bone Joint Surg Am.* 2001;83-A(3):404-411.
10. Mnaymneh W, Emerson RH, Borja F, Head WC, Malinin TI. Massive allografts in salvage revisions of failed total knee arthroplasties. *Clin Orthop Relat Res.* 1990;(260):144-153.
11. Stockley I, McAuley JP, Gross AE. Allograft reconstruction in total knee arthroplasty. *J Bone Joint Surg Br.* 1992;74(3):393-397.
12. Tsahakis PJ, Beaver WB, Brick GW. Technique and results of allograft reconstruction in revision total knee arthroplasty. *Clin Orthop Relat Res.* 1994;(303):86-94.
13. Mow CS, Wiedel JD. Structural allografting in revision total knee arthroplasty. *J Arthroplasty.* 1996;11(3):235-241.
14. Harris AI, Poddar S, Gitelis S, Sheinkop MB, Rosenberg AG. Arthroplasty with a composite of an allograft and a prosthesis for knees with severe deficiency of bone. *J Bone Joint Surg Am.* 1995;77(3):373-386.
15. Ghazavi MT, Stockley I, Yee G, Davis A, Gross AE. Reconstruction of massive bone defects with allograft in revision total knee arthroplasty. *J Bone Joint Surg Am.* 1997;79(1):17-25.
16. Parks NL, Engh GA. The Ranawat Award. Histology of nine structural bone grafts used in total knee arthroplasty. *Clin Orthop Relat Res.* 1997;(345):17-23.
17. Engh GA, Ammeen DJ. Use of structural allograft in revision total knee arthroplasty in knees with severe tibial bone loss. *J Bone Joint Surg Am.* 2007;89(12):2640-2647.
18. Suarez-Suarez MA, Murcia A, Maestro A. Filling of segmental bone defects in revision knee arthroplasty using morsellized bone grafts contained within a metal mesh. *Acta Orthop Belg.* 2002;68(2):163-167.
19. Lonner JH, Lotke PA, Kim J, Nelson C. Impaction grafting and wire mesh for uncontained defects in revision knee arthroplasty. *Clin Orthop Relat Res.* 2002;(404):145-151.

20. Toms AD, Barker RL, Jones RS, Kuiper JH. Impaction bone-grafting in revision joint replacement surgery. *J Bone Joint Surg Am.* 2004;86-A(9):2050-2060.

21. Whiteside LA. Morselized allografting in revision total knee arthroplasty. *Orthopedics.* 1998;21(9):1041-1043.

22. Engh GA, Ammeen DJ. Bone loss with revision total knee arthroplasty: defect classification and alternatives for reconstruction. *Instr Course Lect.* 1999;48:167-175.

23. Jones RE, Skedros JG, Chan AJ, Beauchamp DH, Harkins PC. Total knee arthroplasty using the S-ROM mobile-bearing hinge prosthesis. *J Arthroplasty.* 2001;16(3):279-287.

24. Long WJ, Scuderi GR. Porous tantalum cones for large metaphyseal tibial defects in revision total knee arthroplasty. A minimum 2-year follow-up. *J Arthroplasty.* 2009;24(7):1086-1092.

25. Meneghini RM, Lewallen DG, Hanssen AD. Use of porous tantalum metaphyseal cones for severe tibial bone loss during revision total knee replacement. *J Bone Joint Surg Am.* 2008;90(1):78-84.

26. Meneghini RM, Lewallen DG, Hanssen AD. Use of porous tantalum metaphyseal cones for severe tibial bone loss during revision total knee replacement. Surgical technique. *J Bone Joint Surg Am.* 2009;91(suppl 2 pt 1):131-138.

27. Radnay CS, Scuderi GR. Management of bone loss: augments, cones, offset stems. *Clin Orthop Relat Res.* 2006;446:83-92.

28. Bradley GW. Revision total knee arthroplasty by impaction bone grafting. *Clin Orthop Relat Res.* 2000;2(371):113-118.

29. Lotke PA, Carolan GF, Puri N. Impaction grafting for bone defects in revision total knee arthroplasty. *Clin Orthop Relat Res.* 2006;446:99-103.

30. Samuelson KM. Bone grafting and noncemented revision arthroplasty of the knee. *Clin Orthop Relat Res.* 1988;1(226):93-101.

31. Ullmark G, Hovelius L. Impacted morsellized allograft and cement for revision total knee arthroplasty: a preliminary report of 3 cases. *Acta Orthop Scand.* 1996;67(1):10-12.

32. Whiteside LA, Bicalho PS. Radiologic and histologic analysis of morselized allograft in revision total knee replacement. *Clin Orthop Relat Res.* 1998;12(357):149-156.

33. Bauman RD, Lewallen DG, Hanssen AD. Limitations of structural allograft in revision total knee arthroplasty. *Clin Orthop Relat Res.* 2009;467(3):818-824.

34. Chen F, Krackow KA. Management of tibial defects in total knee arthroplasty. A biomechanical study. *Clin Orthop Relat Res.* 1994;8(305):249-257.

35. Haas SB, Insall JN, Montgomery W 3rd, Windsor RE. Revision total knee arthroplasty with use of modular components with stems inserted without cement. *J Bone Joint Surg Am.* 1995;77(11):1700-1707.

36. Patel JV, Masonis JL, Guerin J, Bourne RB, Rorabeck CH. The fate of augments to treat type-2 bone defects in revision knee arthroplasty. *J Bone Joint Surg Br.* 2004;86(2):195-199.

37. Rand JA. Modularity in total knee arthroplasty. *Acta Orthop Belg.* 1996;62(suppl 1):180-186.

38. Springer BD, Sim FH, Hanssen AD, Lewallen DG. The modular segmental kinematic rotating hinge for nonneoplastic limb salvage. *Clin Orthop Relat Res.* 2004;4(421):181-187.

39. Springer BD, Hanssen AD, Sim FH, Lewallen DG. The kinematic rotating hinge prosthesis for complex knee arthroplasty. *Clin Orthop Relat Res.* 2001;11(392):283-291.

40. Barrack RL. Evolution of the rotating hinge for complex total knee arthroplasty. *Clin Orthop Relat Res.* 2001;11(392):292-299.

41. Barrack RL, Lyons TR, Ingraham RQ, Johnson JC. The use of a modular rotating hinge component in salvage revision total knee arthroplasty. *J Arthroplasty.* 2000;15(7):858-866.

7

Principles and Tenets of Reconstruction in Revision Total Knee Arthroplasty
A Stepwise Approach

John J. Bottros, MD; Michael R. Bloomfield, MD; Trevor G. Murray, MD; Joseph F. Styron, MD, PhD; and Wael K. Barsoum, MD

Revision total knee arthroplasty (TKA) is a successful, cost-effective procedure that improves the quality of life of patients with a failed knee replacement.[1-5] While the rate of primary TKA has increased in recent years, the revision burden has stayed relatively constant at 8.2%.[1] As the American population ages, the rate of primary TKA is expected to further increase exponentially over the next 2 decades, resulting in a proportionate increase in revision TKA, assuming there is a similar revision burden.[6] As the increasing demand for revision TKA burdens the health care delivery system, it will be important for the general orthopedic surgeon to competently manage the failed knee arthroplasty.

PREOPERATIVE EVALUATION

The most common modes of TKA failure include polyethylene wear, aseptic loosening, instability/component malposition, and infection. Less common etiologies include arthrofibrosis, extensor mechanism deficiency, periprosthetic fracture, and osteonecrosis of the patella.[7] Often, more than one etiology may be contributing to the clinical picture of a painful or dysfunctional TKA. In one very large database, infection was the most frequent ICD-9 code given for revision TKA.[8] While the incidence of infection following TKA is low, patients undergoing revision TKA for infection have inferior outcomes compared to their noninfected peers.[9] Any patient with persistent pain after TKA, or new pain with a previously well-functioning arthroplasty, should be carefully evaluated for infection.

A thorough history is the critical first step in determining the failure etiology. The current chief complaints may include pain, stiffness, and/or instability. The patient's symptoms preceding

Jacofsky DJ, Hedley AK, eds.
*Fundamentals of Revision Knee Arthroplasty:
Diagnosis, Evaluation, and Treatment* (pp 99-120).
© 2013 SLACK Incorporated.

Figure 7-1. Preoperative (A) anteroposterior and (B) lateral radiographs showing lucencies around the tibial component indicating loosening.

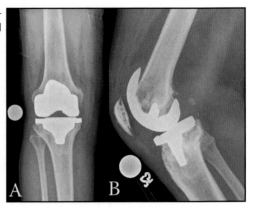

the index arthroplasty should be determined, and if the current symptoms are similar and referable to other anatomic areas (such as the hip or spine), a revision is unlikely to be of benefit. The postoperative course following the primary TKA should be investigated to determine if wound healing issues or drainage were present, which may indicate infection. The timing of symptoms is also important. Early symptoms in a knee that was "never right" after surgery are often due to infection or instability with component malposition. Insidious late-onset pain in a previously well-functioning arthroplasty is often due to loosening, osteolysis, or polyethylene wear and could cause instability. Hematogenous infection should be suspected with acute-onset late pain, particularly with recent open wounds or invasive procedures. Sensations of instability, such as unsteadiness or giving way, can be exacerbated with activities requiring weightbearing in full or mid-flexion, such as squatting or descending stairs. Pain related to instability may manifest as pes anserine or extensor mechanism tendinitis, as these dynamic stabilizers are forced to overcompensate. Instability is also indicated by recurrent effusions.[10] Anterior knee pain may be related to patellar maltracking due to internal rotation of the femoral component or arthrosis of an unresurfaced patella.

A careful physical examination can confirm the working diagnosis suspected by history. Previous incisions are evaluated, and the knee is inspected for warmth, erythema, and effusion. Palpation will elicit areas of tenderness. Range of motion and presence of pain with motion are noted. Stability of the tibiofemoral joint should be tested in full extension, mid-flexion, and with the knee in 90 degrees of flexion while the patient is seated. Patellar apprehension and tracking are assessed throughout the entire range of motion, and quadriceps muscle strength and bulk are noted. It is also important to examine the foot, hip, and lumbar spine to rule out these sources of referred pain. A diagnostic injection of local anesthetic into the knee joint may be considered to differentiate intra- from extra-articular pathology.

Preoperative imaging is critical in determining the etiology of failure and developing an appropriate treatment plan based on the remaining bone stock. Standard knee radiographs are required, including anteroposterior (weightbearing), lateral, and Merchant views. In addition, full-length lower extremity films should be obtained to assess the mechanical axis. The position and alignment of the components, as well as the fixation interfaces, should be scrutinized. The radiographs are also closely evaluated for evidence of polyethylene wear or osteolysis. When compared to previous radiographs, progressive radiolucent lines around the prosthesis are indicative of component loosening (Figure 7-1). In a cemented prosthesis, a complete radiolucent line of 2 mm or more indicates aseptic loosening. In an uncemented knee implant, the criteria are less definite and the surgeon must look for lucencies that are progressive, extensive, or associated with symptoms. Since the angle of the x-ray beam relative to the knee can greatly alter the appearance of radiolucencies, fluoroscopy can be used when clinical suspicion of aseptic loosening exists despite normal radiographs. When instability is suspected, determining ligament balance may require a stress examination under fluoroscopy to further evaluate the type and degree of instability. Computed tomography (CT) imaging is useful for further assessing osteolytic lesions, bone loss, and periprosthetic fracture patterns. CT is also extremely helpful to assess tibial and femoral component rotation when malrotation causing instability or patellofemoral problems is suspected.

The evaluation of a painful TKA should routinely include laboratory studies including peripheral white blood cell (WBC) count and differential, erythrocyte sedimentation rate, and C-reactive protein, to evaluate for periprosthetic infection. A patient with an elevation in any of these markers should have a joint aspiration, which remains the gold standard for diagnosing infection. Synovial WBC counts greater than 2500 cells/mm^3 (with greater than 60% neutrophils) are typically consistent with an infection,[11] although newer literature indicates a threshold of 1700 WBC imparts a higher sensitivity.[12] Gram stain and culture should also be performed. A high red blood cell count in the aspirate (with a proportionate number of WBCs) indicates hemarthrosis and may be an indication of instability.[10] Nuclear medicine studies—such as combined indium[111] leukocyte/technetium-99m sulphur colloid scans—have shown excellent specificity and positive predictive value in the diagnosis of periprosthetic infection.[13] These may be considered if an indolent infection is suspected and the above work-up is equivocal.

Previous operative notes and implant stickers should be obtained for all planned revisions and are especially critical when considering less than a total revision. These are helpful in identifying the current prosthesis, the surgical approach used during the primary TKA, and other prior procedures. This information allows the surgeon to request implant-specific equipment and better anticipate the condition of the joint at the time of surgery.

Patients should be optimized by a medical consultant prior to surgery to minimize the risk of complications during the perioperative period. Diabetics are at increased risk of developing postoperative complications, particularly wound-related problems and infection,[14] which tight glucose control may help to prevent. Other medical comorbidities including hypertension and cardiopulmonary problems, should be well controlled, as patients with these issues have been shown to have worse outcomes following TKA.[15] We also recommend screening for malnutrition in those at elevated risk (substance abusers, the elderly, or obese patients) with laboratory tests including albumin, prealbumin, and total protein levels. A nutrition consultation is warranted in patients with abnormalities to optimize nutritional status and wound healing potential prior to surgery.

PREOPERATIVE PLANNING AND RECONSTRUCTIVE STRATEGY

The technical goals of a revision arthroplasty are to achieve a pain-free, stable joint with restoration of limb alignment (ie, a neutral mechanical axis).[10,16] Therefore, the surgeon's tasks are to reconstruct lost bone stock and re-establish proper ligamentous tension and balance. Revision TKA often has a high failure rate due to ligament imbalance and subsequent implant loosening.[10] To successfully reconstruct the knee, it is of paramount importance to obtain stability in the coronal, sagittal, and transverse planes.[17]

Assess Ligament Integrity and Stability

Ligamentous laxity can occur secondary to bone loss, component loosening or subsidence, late rupture, or iatrogenic injury at the time of initial arthroplasty. The ligaments contract on the concave side of a deformity and stretch on the convex side.[18,19] The literature has shown that soft tissue management alone cannot be used to treat patients with ligamentous instability. This is due to the fact that there is often an element of bony malalignment.[16]

Prosthetic knee instability has been classified into extension space, flexion space, and global (combined) patterns.[18,20] Extension instability with varus and valgus stress is either symmetric (due to excessive distal femur resection relative to the flexion gap) or asymmetric (due to collateral ligament imbalance or insufficiency[21]). Flexion space instability is assessed by applying anterior/posterior and varus-valgus forces to the knee in 90 degrees of flexion. All knee implants without an anterior cruciate ligament will have a small amount of anterior translation with an anterior drawer test. Posterior stabilized (PS) knees with significant anterior translation and cruciate-retaining (CR) knees with exaggerated anterior and posterior translation have an element of flexion instability. A posterior sag sign and quadriceps active test can confirm the presence of flexion instability. Flexion instability can also be symmetric or asymmetric. A symmetrically loose flexion gap usually results from flexion-extension mismatch at the time of the TKA[22] or incompetence of the posterior cruciate ligament in a CR knee.[23] Asymmetry within the flexion gap (medial to lateral) often occurs due to malrotation of the femoral component. If the femur is internally rotated, the lateral dimension is enlarged compared to the medial dimension.[24] Solving this issue requires femoral component revision. In global instability, both the sagittal and coronal planes have been compromised with loose flexion and extension gaps. This scenario is common in patients with a preoperative hyperextension contracture or those with disruption of the extensor mechanism. Global instability can present in the early postoperative period when the polyethylene insert is of insufficient thickness, or late when a result of polyethylene wear.

The options for treatment of instability include isolated polyethylene exchange, single component or total revision, or use of a hinged TKA. It is important for the surgeon to recognize which instability patterns can be treated with less involvement. In a well-fixed, neutrally aligned construct with evidence of late wear of a modular tibial polyethylene, an isolated polyethylene exchange is an acceptable treatment. If mild varus-valgus instability is encountered in this situation, a thicker polyethylene may be used after releasing the concave side to match the stretched convex side. Polyethylene exchange to a thicker component can also be performed for balanced instability due to insufficient polyethylene thickness. Posterior cruciate ligament insufficiency or rupture is a cause of postoperative flexion instability in CR knees and may be treated with an isolated polyethylene exchange to an ultracongruent anteroposterior-constrained insert. Other than these situations, we believe that instability cannot be adequately addressed with a partial revision. Most revisions for instability can be performed using a varus-valgus constrained implant, as discussed below, provided the new components are well aligned and the collateral ligaments are present. In cases of severe instability due to recurvatum, collateral ligament absence, or posterolateral corner insufficiency, a rotating hinge prosthesis is advised.

Assess Bone Loss

It is imperative that the surgeon recognize the severity of bone loss on preoperative imaging in order to plan a stable construct that will accurately re-establish the joint line. Bone defects can be caused by malalignment, subsidence, aseptic loosening, osteonecrosis, stress shielding, or iatrogenic bone loss during implant removal.[25-27] There are several classifications of bone defects, which primarily rely on the location and size and whether or not the defect is contained.

The Anderson Orthopaedic Research Institute classification system distinguishes 3 types of defects based on the radiographic status of the metaphyseal bone of the distal femur and proximal tibia[28]:

- Type I femoral and tibial defects have minimal bone loss with an intact metaphysis and structurally sound cancellous bone. Therefore, the components will have no evidence of subsidence.

- Type II defects have damaged cancellous bone or joint line elevation, and often manifest with component subsidence. For both the tibia and femur, type II defects are further divided into type IIA, which involves one condyle, and type IIB, which involves both condyles.

- Type III defects have severely deficient metaphyseal bone that occurs above the level of the femoral epicondyles or below the level of the tibial tubercle. These defects may compromise the integrity of the collateral ligament or patellar tendon insertions and present with instability or extensor mechanism incompetence.

There is a modified classification proposed by Clatworthy, Gross, and colleagues[29] that is based on intraoperative findings. This classification distinguishes major and minor defects and defines them as contained or uncontained. Minor defects are less than 1 cm^3 and are below the level of the femoral condyles. Major defects are greater than 1 cm^3 and are above the level of the condyles. Contained defects have only cancellous bone loss, with the cortical rim remaining structurally intact. Uncontained defects have missing cortical bone and provide no structural support to that portion of the implant. Many view these classification schemes as useful tools to guide treatment according to the type of defect encountered.[25,26,28,30]

Options in Bone Defect Reconstruction

It is important to ensure that all potentially useful equipment is available at the time of surgery. The surgeon has many reconstructive options for managing bone defects including cement fill (with or without screw reinforcement), morselized or structural bone graft, modular augments and stems, and customized implants.[30-34] In addition to the pattern of bone loss, the surgeon must also weigh patient-related factors such as activity level and age when formulating a treatment plan. In active, younger patients it is a priority to restore bone stock when possible, while bone-replacing implants with augments have proven successful in sedentary and older patients.

Many algorithms for management of bony defects have been described, and most follow a graduated approach. Type I defects that are less than 5 mm can be managed with nonstructural bone graft and standard implants. When these defects approach 1 cm^3, they may be managed with cement filling, without bone grafting or augments. Ritter et al[35,36] describe the use of cement filling with screw stabilization for tibial plateau defects. Other biomechanical studies have found 30% less deflection when using a titanium screw to augment the construct, compared to cement alone. This option should only be used in reconstructions that have varus-valgus stability during trialing.

Type II defects require more structural support than cement alone. These defects often have limited collapse of the femoral condyle or tibial plateau. Modular augments provide a stable, straightforward solution to re-establish the joint line. Once the implant has been removed, precise cuts must be made to provide proper fit of these augments. For distal and posterior femoral defects, we believe augments are excellent tools to both restore the joint line and balance the flexion and extension gaps. In defects that are 30 mm or larger, Werle et al[37] reported that large distal femoral augments had no revisions or radiographic loosening at 37 months follow-up. Tibial plateau wedges and block augments are also useful to reconstruct bone loss and alignment. Pagnano et al[38] had 94% good or excellent results in 25 patients (mean: 5.6-year follow-up) after wedge augmentation for tibial deficiency. However, we believe that tibial block augments should be used instead of wedges to maximize compressive forces and eliminate shearing at the implant interfaces. We believe that stemmed components should be used with augments for additional biomechanical support and fixation surface area and to prevent malalignment.

Type III defects have severe compromise of the supporting metaphyseal bone and therefore require additional support for the prosthesis. Structural allograft is a reconstructive option in these challenging cases, which may restore bone stock for potential future revision.

Femoral head structural allografts have been used to fill cavitary defects and reconstruct isolated femoral condylar loss. Dorr et al[39] treated 24 knees with tibial deficiency using structural allograft; 22 demonstrated unions without collapse at 3- to 6-year follow-up. Bush et al[25] recommend the use structural allograft for defects involving 50% or more of either tibial plateau. Massive defects may require an entire distal femur or proximal tibial allograft. If a structural allograft is to be used, we advocate the use of a cortical step-cut to increase the surface area joining the allograft to host bone. This junction must be bypassed with a long-stem component (cemented or uncemented) to divert stress from the metaphyseal region. Two series demonstrated 86% and 87% good or excellent results at mid-term follow-up.[40-42]

Clatworthy et al[29] presented the largest series of structural allografts performed in 52 revision TKAs. The initial success rate of 92% decreased to 72% by 10 years postoperative, and 23% underwent rerevision at a mean of 71 months. This study raised concern over the longevity of structural allografts, likely due to the failure of allograft revascularization.[43] Hence, we believe structural allograft should be used infrequently and only by experienced surgeons. The surgeon must preserve as much viable host bone as possible and avoid attachment of the collateral ligaments directly to the allograft, as this will likely result in ligamentous insufficiency. The use of structural allograft necessitates a prolonged period of restricted weightbearing, which may not be optimal for less active or elderly patients.

Elderly patients with large defects are better managed with bone-substituting implants to provide immediate stability and more rapid postoperative mobilization. Modular distal femoral and proximal tibial replacements are available with a rotating hinge design. These implants should only be used by surgeons with significant experience in their use. Highly porous tantalum modular augments and structural metaphyseal-filling cones have recently been used in revision TKA. Tantalum is a biocompatible and corrosion-resistant porous metal that is similar to bone in that it possesses high strength and low stiffness.[44] The advantage of tantalum, when compared to allograft, is that its structural properties will not degrade over time. Recent experience has been gained using porous tantalum metaphyseal-filling cones to compensate for femoral and tibial metaphyseal bone loss.[25,31] These cones are manufactured to be press-fit into host bone to allow for bony ingrowth and to provide a platform to which the prosthesis is cemented. We also recommend the use of a stemmed prosthesis when using this technique to bypass the segment and allow for bony ingrowth.

In summary, certain fundamentals apply for every step in the management of severe bone loss. First, it is imperative to maintain a host bone for potential future procedures. Second, the joint line must be restored, which can be done with femoral augments for most mild or moderate defects. Last, structural allograft, metaphyseal-filling implants, or custom prosthesis may be used in situations of substantial bone loss.

Component Selection

Implant stability in TKA is determined by 2 factors: the supporting soft tissue sleeve and the intrinsic constraint of the prosthesis. Soft tissue stability is imparted by the posterior cruciate ligament, collateral ligaments, and capsule. Ideally, as in primary TKA, stability is achieved by the patient's own soft tissues, so minimal implant constraint is needed. Constraint is a continuum and is determined by the geometry and design of the prosthesis. There is a direct relationship between constraint and stresses at the implant-cement-host bone interfaces. These increased forces with more highly constrained devices lead to an increased potential for loosening. The clinical question then becomes how much implant constraint is required to achieve the stability needed (given the condition of the ligaments), with the least amount of force transmitted to the fixation interfaces. Patient factors should also be considered when deciding on constraint, as lower demand patients may tolerate higher levels of constraint without significant clinical consequence.

Cruciate Retaining

Posterior CR implants are the least constraining and thus have a limited role in revision surgery. This implant may be retained when polyethylene exchange for a thicker insert can be performed for balanced instability (varus-valgus and flexion-extension). However, polyethylene exchange for instability should be used on a limited basis, as results are not universally good.[45] CR devices have also been used when revising a unicompartmental arthroplasty to a TKA with relative success.[46] Other than these 2 situations, our preference is to use, at the very least, a PS implant.

Posterior Stabilized Implants

PS implants influence knee biomechanics by substituting a "tibial post and femoral cam" for the posterior cruciate ligament. The protrusion (post) on the tibial insert articulates with a specially shaped bar (cam) on the femoral component. Although the post imparts anteroposterior stability, the design does not provide rotational or varus-valgus control. This prosthesis can only be used when flexion and extension gaps have been balanced and both collateral ligaments are functioning. PS components impart little increased stress to the interfaces because they still allow rotation and do not control coronal plane motion. Caution must be used when flexion gap instability is present, as the post can dislocate posterior to the cam in deep flexion.[47] If the surgeon is unable to establish a balanced flexion gap by the methods described previously, serious consideration should be given to using a more constrained device. However, if the soft tissues are competent and well balanced, acceptable results can be expected when using a PS design in revision surgery.[48-50]

Varus-Valgus Constrained (Total Stabilized/Constrained Condylar Knee)

The next level of constraint includes coronal plane control. These knee implants are termed *varus–valgus constrained*, *total stabilized* (TS), or *constrained condylar* (CC). They consist of a taller, broader post, which reduces rotation and achieves coronal stability. This implant is indicated when varus-valgus instability is caused by attenuated but present collateral ligaments. The increased constraint and lack of physiologic rotation of these devices make it paramount for the surgeon to place the components in the appropriate coronal and rotational alignment as malalignment may predispose the implant to early failure. Subtle flexion and extension mismatch is another indication for a TS implant. However, caution must be used in extreme cases because dislocation of the post can still occur. The trade-off for this increased stability is increased interface stresses. Although these implants perform similarly to less constrained implants in the short term, there is concern about their longevity.[50,51] Stems should always be used when placing a TS implant to disperse the forces between the implant and host bone over a larger surface area.

If there is question as to the need for a TS versus a PS implant, the surgeon can implant a TS femur but use a PS polyethylene insert. The advantage of this technique is 2-fold. First, it limits constraint in hopes of improving longevity of the implant. If the knee becomes unstable postoperatively, the polyethylene can be exchanged for a varus-valgus constrained design, a relatively straightforward operation with low morbidity. This technique should only be used when the surgeon has a very low suspicion of instability during intraoperative trialing. Depending on the implant system used, the post of a TS polyethylene may be compatible with the box of a PS femur, giving the surgeon further intraoperative flexibility. However, we recommend caution when using this technique in the absence of stems.

Hinged Prostheses

The final level of constraint is a linked, or hinged, implant. This design is used when severe bone loss or severe flexion-extension mismatch exists, or when the collateral ligaments are absent. The significant constraint of the implant imparts substantial forces to the implant interfaces, making loosening a significant problem.[52,53] Rotating hinges have been developed to decrease the torsional stresses transmitted to the implant-bone-cement interfaces, resulting in improved outcomes.[54,55]

The hinge is a useful tool for difficult cases, but due to a relatively high complication rate and diminishing results with longer follow-up, they should only be used when absolutely indicated.[56] It is our opinion that hinged implants should only be used by surgeons with significant experience with these prostheses, and thus will not be discussed in detail.

Surgical Technique

Set-Up and Positioning

As with any operative case, the set-up for revision TKA is very important. Given the increased risk of infection with revision procedures, the surgeon must diligently adhere to perioperative antibiotic guidelines.[9] One recent study determined that preoperative antibiotics did not affect culture results in revision TKA for infection.[57] We typically use a cephalosporin (30 minutes prior to incision) or vancomycin (1 hour prior) depending on the patient's infection history and allergies. Hypotensive spinal anesthesia is usually preferred by the senior author (WKB), but for complex revisions, combined spinal-epidural or general anesthesia may be necessary given the anticipated operative time. A urinary catheter is placed to monitor the fluid status during and after surgery. It is important to reexamine the knee after the patient has been anesthetized, as the patient's inability to guard may expose previously subtle findings, which may alter the preoperative plan.

We use a radiolucent operative table for most revisions. Intraoperative radiographs are sometimes necessary to evaluate the adequacy of cement removal, iatrogenic fracture, or stem placement. We place a head extender onto the foot of the bed and move the patient distally to gain radiographic access to the entire femur.

Once the patient is adequately positioned, the surgeon should determine the rotation of the leg and use a small bump under the hip when excessive external rotation is present. A leg holder is placed at the level of the mid-calf with the leg in extension. In most cases, a nonsterile tourniquet is placed as proximal as possible on the thigh. In situations when a stem and/or cement extend proximally into the femur, a sterile tourniquet may be used to enhance access later in the case. The nonoperative leg is padded but left accessible under the drapes to assess leg lengths if a hinged device is being implanted. Before starting, all radiographs are displayed and the surgeon should check to ensure all needed equipment is available.

Exposure

Once the leg is prepped and draped sterile, all old incisions are marked. Ideally, a long midline incision is utilized to optimize exposure and wound healing. If old incisions preclude this due to a narrow skin bridge, the most lateral previous incision should be utilized based on the vascular supply to the prepatellar soft tissues.[58] Horizontal incisions should be crossed perpendicularly to avoid acute angles, which can lead to skin necrosis. Sharp dissection is carried down to the extensor mechanism, taking care not to create a large lateral flap, which can lead to wound healing problems.[59] Any areas of compromised skin should be conservatively excised if the tension on the tissue will permit adequate closure. When soft tissues are severely compromised, a preoperative plastic surgery consult is warranted to help plan the incision, consider rotational or free muscle flaps,[60,61] or possible prerevision soft tissue expansion.[62]

A standard medial parapatellar arthrotomy is used to enter the joint, which can be easily extended when additional exposure is necessary. Distally, the capsulotomy is carried down to the medial border of the tibial tubercle. With the leg in extension, the soft tissues are subperiosteally stripped from the proximal medial tibia. Injury to the medial collateral ligament is avoided by placing a half-inch curved osteotome at the joint line and using it to retract and elevate the medial collateral ligament during the release. The release is continued posterior to the semimembranosus, which helps with balancing as well as exposure, allowing for external rotation of the tibia and thus relieving tension on the extensor mechanism. Next, the fat pad and scar tissue are removed from the infrapatellar region down to the insertion on the tubercle. An aggressive synovectomy is performed, recreating the medial and lateral gutters. It is important to completely free the quad mechanism from the anterior femur by removing the fibrotic scar tissue that tethers it down.

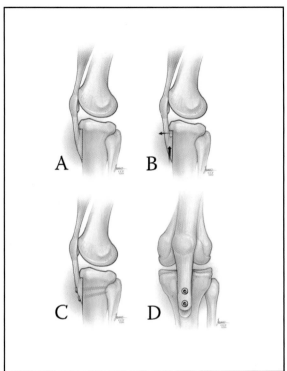

Figure 7-2. Authors' preferred technique for tibial tubercle osteotomy. (A) Planned osteotomy cuts. (B) When patella baja is present, a portion of bone is removed from the proximal osteotomy fragment, which is then translated proximally to restore patellar height. (C, D) The fragment is then fixed in the new position with 2 screws.

Synovial and fibrous tissue removed during the exposure should be evaluated for infection. Frozen section analysis, with a threshold of 5 or 10 WBC per high power field, has been shown to be an accurate predictor of infection.[63,64] Tissue should also be sent for microbiologic cultures, although intraoperative gram stain of synovial fluid and tissue has poor sensitivity and specificity for infection.[64] If infection is suspected, a two-stage revision should be performed with interval placement of an antibiotic-eluting spacer.

At this point, the modular polyethylene insert is removed, which further aids in exposure. The knee is gently flexed, taking care to not avulse the patellar tendon. If there is a concerning amount of stress on the patellar tendon insertion, a staple or pin can be placed through the tendon into the tibia. The patella is subluxated (rather than everted), which helps to minimize risk to the patellar tendon insertion.

If exposure is still inadequate, a quadriceps snip can be performed to help relieve tension on the quadriceps mechanism.[65] This is done by making a 45-degree oblique extension to the arthrotomy, starting distal-medial and continuing proximal-lateral through the quadriceps tendon. This release preserves the continuity of the vastus lateralis with the lateral retinaculum and patella, as well as the vastus medialis and rectus to the medial joint capsule. This allows side-to-side closure of the tendon, has few associated complications, and requires no changes to the postoperative rehabilitation program.[66]

If the exposure is still not adequate despite a quadriceps snip, a V-Y turndown[67] or tibial tubercle osteotomy (TTO)[68] may be performed. Although both techniques release the extensor mechanism and greatly improve exposure, we prefer the TTO because of the improved healing potential (bone-to-bone repair) and the improved biomechanics with regard to tension on the repair. Furthermore, it may aid in the removal of the tibial component and cement, especially in the setting of a tibial stem. The incision is extended distally 7 to 10 cm to allow for visualization of the patellar tendon on the tubercle and the anterior cortex of the proximal tibia. The osteotomy is medially based and made in the coronal plane (Figure 7-2A). We use an oscillating saw starting

2 to 5 mm proximal to the tendon insertion and extend the osteotomy distally about 8 cm. It is tapered from 1 cm deep proximally to a thin wafer distally, leaving the lateral cortex intact. A small osteotome is used at the proximal end of the osteotomy parallel to the joint line, creating a bony block to help prevent migration of the fragment after fixation. A broad osteotome is then used to open the osteotomy, leaving a lateral soft tissue hinge of anterior compartment muscle. If patella baja exists, we remove 2 to 5 mm of bone from the proximal aspect of the osteotomy fragment (proximal to the attachment of the patella tendon) allowing the fragment to be fixed more proximally on the tibia, thus raising the patella relative to the joint line (Figure 7-2B). At the end of the case, the osteotomy site is fixed with 2 3.5-mm cortical screws with washers (Figures 7-2C and D). When this method is employed we use a stemmed tibial component to bypass the osteotomy site. The stem is uncemented to prevent extravasation of cement into the osteotomy site, which would interfere with healing. Wiring offers a viable alternative to screw fixation for TTO, particularly if the stemmed tibial component interferes with the placement of the screws. Once adequate fixation of the osteotomy fragment is achieved, most authors feel that no changes to the standard rehabilitation protocol are necessary.

When the proximal tibial bone is compromised or poor soft tissues distally preclude the use of a TTO, a V-Y turndown can be utilized to increase exposure. This approach allows for good visualization, but commonly causes excessive scar tissue and can result in an extensor lag.[67] The turndown is accomplished by first performing a medial parapatellar arthrotomy. The capsular incision is extended 45 degrees distally and laterally from the apex of the arthrotomy toward the proximal tibia and around the lateral aspect of the patella. It is carried distally until adequate exposure is achieved. Care should be taken to avoid injury to the inferior lateral geniculate artery in order to prevent hematoma and devascularization of the patella. Closure is performed with the knee in slight flexion using nonabsorbable suture. The lateral aspect of the turndown can be left open as a lateral release if needed for patellar tracking. The knee is flexed following the repair and the angle is noted at which significant tension occurs. Postoperatively, the patient is placed in a hinged knee brace blocked 5 degrees short of this angle. Passive and active flexion to this point are allowed, as is passive extension. Active extension is prohibited, and the brace is locked in extension during ambulation for 4 to 6 weeks, at which point quadriceps strengthening and range of motion exercises are initiated.

Component Removal

Once adequate exposure is achieved, the components are removed. The modular polyethylene insert is removed first, using an osteotome or manufacturer-specific extraction device to disrupt the locking mechanism. Our preference is to then remove the femur, followed by the tibia and then the patella, if necessary. The primary goal during this process is to preserve as much bone stock as possible. After each component is removed, fibrotic tissue is débrided from the interfaces and medullary canals and is again sent for frozen section analysis and culture to rule out active infection.

If the femoral component is loose, it may be easily removed with a prosthesis-specific extraction device or bone tamp. Care should be taken to apply equal force medially and laterally, especially when removing a PS or TS component, to reduce the risk of an iatrogenic condylar fracture. Removal becomes more difficult when the component is well fixed. The implant-cement (in a cemented prosthesis) or implant-bone (with a press-fit design) interface needs to be completely disrupted to allow atraumatic removal. Several different tools can be used to accomplish this, including an oscillating saw, Gigli saw, flexible or stiff osteotomes, burr, or any combination thereof. The senior author (WKB) prefers to first disrupt the anterior aspect of the component from the anterior femur. Flexible osteotomes are used until they can be passed completely from medial to lateral. Flexible osteotomes are then used to disrupt the anterior and posterior chamfers, as well as the distal aspect of the component. An open-box PS component should be freed completely along the sides of the box. Finally, the posterior condyle interfaces are disrupted using a quarter-inch stiff osteotome. Access to this area is sometimes difficult; however, it is important to take time to perform this step to prevent the entire posterior condyle from coming off when the component is removed. Once the interfaces have been divided, an extraction device is used to tap the femur off. If resistance is encountered, osteotomes are again used to free any missed areas of cement bonding. Once the component is removed, the remaining cement is extracted in small pieces under direct visualization using a rongeur, osteotome, or burr. Extreme care should be taken to preserve bone stock during this process.

Attention is next turned to the tibial component. If the tibia is well fixed, an oscillating saw is used to cut just beneath the component at the cement-implant interface. This is done in all accessible areas, making sure to protect the patellar tendon and collateral ligaments with retractors. Flexible and stiff osteotomes are then used to free the implant in areas where the saw cannot reach. Care should be taken to ensure the posterior aspect of the tibial component is completely separated or the posterior tibia may be avulsed during implant removal, creating a difficult reconstructive problem. Implant-specific extraction devices or bone tamps are then used to tap out the component. As with the femur, the cement is removed under direct visualization.

A domed polyethylene patellar component should be left in place if it is well fixed, in good position, and has no damage or significant wear. If these conditions are not met, an oscillating saw is used to cut the component off. The remaining pegs can then be dug out using a curette or drill. Even if an uncemented metal-backed patella is well fixed (and sufficient host bone remains), it may be advisable to replace the component since these designs have higher failure rates. A diamond wheel saw can be used to divide the component from its pegs. A pencil-tip drill is then used to remove these pegs.[69]

After the implants have been removed, the surgeon must carefully evaluate the integrity of the soft tissues as well as the quantity and quality of the remaining bone. Unanticipated findings may require that the preoperative plan be changed with regard to implant selection or reconstructive management of bone loss. For this reason, multiple options should be available at the time of surgery.

Bone Preparation

Restoration of the joint line, proper component rotation, and overall limb alignment are critical to the outcome of revision TKA. A key principle during revision TKA is to preserve existing healthy bone and minimize additional bone resection. Only 1 to 2 mm of bone should be removed from the most prominent femoral and tibial surfaces to provide a unicondylar platform on which the resection guides are placed. Residual defects can be reconstructed with either bone graft or prosthetic augmentation. Stem options are discussed later in this chapter.

Tibial Component

We favor preparation of the tibia first, as the tibial cut affects both the flexion and extension gaps. The tibial canal is reamed with increasing diameter straight reamers until a tight fit is achieved in the diaphyseal medullary canal. The final reamer is left in the tibia as a resection guide. Using jigs specific to the implant system, the surface is resected perpendicular to the long axis of the tibia in both the coronal and sagittal planes. Often bone loss is unequal between the medial and lateral plateau, in which case the level of resection is referenced from the high side. The low side is then built up to create a stable platform perpendicular to the mechanical axis, using the algorithm for bone loss reconstruction described above. We frequently use block augments (Figure 7-3) to provide a foundation for the prosthesis. The size of the augment (dependent on the options available in the implant system) is determined by the height discrepancy. The augment selected is typically slightly thicker than the residual defect, and a clean-up cut is made to create a flat surface for the augment to sit. When a larger bone deficiency exists, augments can be used on both sides of the tibial plateau to decrease the necessary polyethylene thickness. In this situation, often the proximal fibular head may be visualized and can be used to help support the tibial component.

Figure 7-3. Intraoperative photograph showing the trial in place after preparation for the tibia. A 5-mm medial augment was used to correct a focal defect.

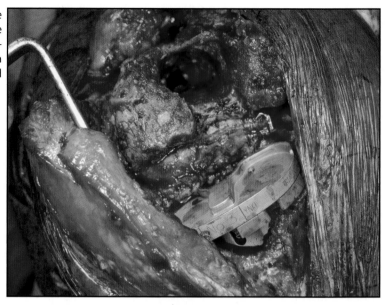

The size of the tibial component is estimated by comparing the remaining upper tibia with the available trial components. The augment and stem trials are connected, and the construct is checked for appropriate size and stability. An offset stem may be needed to avoid medial overhang and subsequent irritation of the soft tissues. To determine the proper tibial component rotation, we recommend using the junction of the medial and middle third of the tibial tubercle as a reproducible landmark. This is marked with an electrocautery to maintain accurate positioning during trialing and implantation.

When type III defects are encountered, the senior author (WKB) prefers to use trabecular metal cones for reconstruction. The cavitary defect is contoured with a high-speed burr, as guided by manufacturer-specific trials, to ensure a press-fit application. If there is a void that prohibits contact between the cone and the remaining host bone, morselized bone graft should be impacted to maximize fit. Both full and stepped cones are available and should be chosen based on which best restores the proximal tibial metaphysis to provide a scaffold for the tibial tray. The final tibial component will later be cemented onto the tibial cone with either a press-fit stem extension or cement stem extension.

Whichever techniques are used, care must be taken to ensure that the reconstructed tibial surface is perpendicular to the anatomic axis of the tibia. With the flexion gap method described below, correct alignment of the femoral component is predicated on tibial alignment, and placement of the tibia in varus can predispose the knee to internal rotation of the femoral component.

Femoral Component

Preparation of the femur begins with reaming the medullary canal to achieve a tight fit. This is of paramount importance, as the reamer position will determine the alignment of the distal cut. The distal femoral cutting jig is generally available at 5 to 7 degrees of valgus, which re-establishes the correct mechanical alignment. The angle of the cut is specific to each implant system and is determined by the angle of stem take-off from the femoral component. Some surgeons advocate that if the medial collateral ligament is incompetent, the femur should be cut in less than 5 degrees of valgus to put the mechanical axis in slight varus and thus protect the medial side. However, we believe the level of implant constraint should be increased to overcome this problem instead of altering the alignment of the distal cut. We prefer to cut the distal femur in 6 degrees of valgus

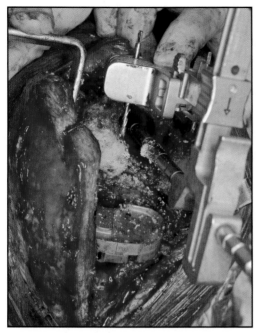

Figure 7-4. The distal femoral resection guide is referenced from the intramedullary reamer.

(secondary to the implant system used), removing only diseased bone and freshening the surface (Figure 7-4). The cut may only re-establish a flat bony surface on one of the condyles and may not remove bone from the other condyle, depending on the degree of bone loss. The cut femoral surface provides a reference line that should be parallel to the tibial cut.

The sizing of the femoral component is dependent on 2 factors. First, the dimensions of the remaining native femur dictate the size of the femoral component. The component size that best matches the remaining femur in both dimensions is chosen with the assistance of the manufacturer's sizing jig, being careful not to downsize and artificially increase the flexion gap, which is already frequently loose in the revision setting. Also, the size of the tibial component dictates the size of the femoral component in most revision knee arthroplasty systems. Hence, it is important to size the femur after the tibia has been prepared and be familiar with the properties of the chosen system.

Next, we direct our attention to re-establishing the correct height of the joint line. Accurately restoring the joint line can be difficult but is nonetheless required for optimal stability and joint kinematics. The joint line should be re-established within 8 mm of the native joint line for optimal outcomes.[70] Detailed anatomical studies have shown the joint line to be positioned at a mean distance of 3.1 cm below the medial epicondyle and 2.5 cm below the lateral epicondyle.[71] The fibular head is usually 2 cm distal to the joint line; however, this is less reliable than referencing from the epicondyles.[72] We recommend using the medial epicondyle to determine the position of the joint line (Figure 7-5). A ruler is placed on the epicondyle and the remaining bone depth is noted. Distal femoral augments are used on the lateral and/or medial sides in conjunction with the thickness of prosthesis to position the new joint line 3 cm distal to the epicondyle. If this landmark is not available due to bone loss, then the lateral epicondyle or fibular head can be used. At this point in the femoral reconstruction, the limb alignment and the joint line (ie, extension gap) have been anatomically re-established.

Next, the femoral component rotation and flexion gap are determined. It is well established that internal rotation of the femur can result in poor patellar tracking and subluxation, patellar clunk, increased component wear, and anterior knee pain.[24] As internal rotation of the femoral

Figure 7-5. The medial epicondyle is identified, and a ruler is used to estimate the location for the joint line after reconstruction.

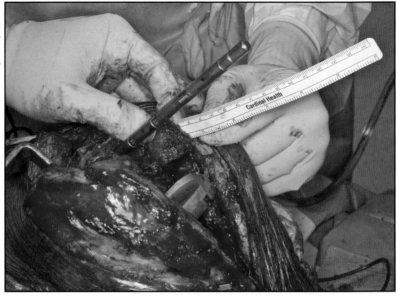

component is frequently found in the failed arthroplasty, the surgeon must be cognizant to correct any rotational abnormalities during the reconstruction. This will help ensure medial-lateral balance within the flexion gap and prevent postoperative instability due to relative laxity of the lateral ligaments. Several anatomic landmarks have been described to guide femoral component rotation including the posterior condylar axis, Whiteside's line, and the transepicondylar axis (TEA).[16,71] However, the posterior condylar axis and Whiteside's line are not useful in the revision setting due to bone loss. The TEA is a consistent landmark for recreating the femoral rotation during revision surgery and should be marked for reference during this part of the procedure.

A combined method is used to ensure proper femoral component rotation. The femoral component should be oriented parallel to the TEA, and when the collateral ligaments are equally tensioned, the anterior femoral cut is made parallel to the tibial cut, ensuring a rectangular flexion gap with the posterior condyles of the implant. First, the 4-in-1 cutting block of the previously determined size is selected and placed over the intramedullary stem. We place a saw blade through the anterior slot of the 4-in-1 block, which is positioned roughly flush to the anterior surface of the femur by using an appropriately sized femoral offset bushing. This translates the femoral component posteriorly and subsequently helps to fill the flexion gap, which is usually larger than the corresponding extension gap in the revision setting. A spacer block, tensor, or laminar spreader is placed between the tibia and the femoral cutting block and is used to distract the flexion space. This creates medial-lateral balance within the space when the collateral ligaments are equally tensioned. The cutting block is secured after double-checking the rotation against the TEA, and the anterior and chamfer clean-up cuts are made. Restoration of the posterior offset of the femur is important to improve postoperative flexion. Based on how we place our 4-in-1 cutting block to fill the flexion gap, we routinely use posterior augments as needed to fill the flexion gap. Clean-up cuts are made to the remaining posterior medial and lateral condyles through the appropriate slots of the block, which correspond to the size of the augment needed.

The trial augments are placed on the trial femoral component, and the fit with the native distal femur is assessed. We then use the previous 90/90 tibial cut as a final double check of femoral rotation. Sequentially larger spacer blocks are placed in the flexion gap and are used to ensure proper ligamentous tension (ie, a rectangular flexion gap). The block is also used to check the extension gap to preliminarily determine balance, and adjustments are made as needed based on the algorithm presented in Table 7-1. Once the flexion and extension gaps are equal and well

TABLE 7-1. INTRAOPERATIVE TREATMENT OF FLEXION AND EXTENSION GAP IMBALANCE

	EXTENSION (NORMAL)	EXTENSION (TIGHT)	EXTENSION (LOOSE)
FLEXION (NORMAL)	Nothing	Resect distal femur Release posterior capsule	Distal femoral augmentation
FLEXION (TIGHT)	Shift femoral component anterior Downsize femoral component	Downsize polyethylene Resect proximal tibia	Distal femoral augmentation with smaller or anteriorized component
FLEXION (LOOSE)	Shift femoral component posterior Posterior augmentation	Resect distal femur Larger femoral component	Larger polyethylene insert

Reprinted with permission of *The Journal of Arthroplasty*, 21(4 suppl 1). Bottros J, Gad B, Krebs V, Barsoum WK. Gap balancing in total knee arthroplasty. Pages 11-15. Copyright 2006, with permission of Elsevier.

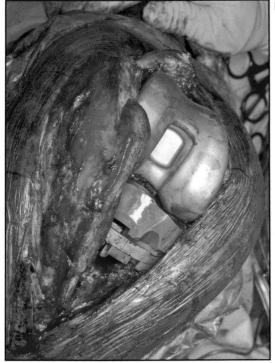

Figure 7-6. Trials in place after gap balancing.

balanced, a trial polyethylene of appropriate thickness is interposed between the femoral and tibial components (Figure 7-6).

Severe, uncontained defects that preclude the use of augments may be encountered. We encourage the use of trabecular cones for type III defects at the metaphyseal-diaphyseal junction of the femur. Again, as described for the tibia, the goal is to maximize contact with good quality host bone. The high-speed burr can be used to help contour the cavity to achieve this. Morselized bone graft mixed can be packed around the outside of the cone augment to achieve a press-fit. Fixation is achieved with cementation of the implant to the femoral cone and metaphyseal bone, along with a cemented or press-fit stem extension.

Patellar Component

As previously discussed, the patella does not always require revision. If there is sufficient bone available, a standard patellar component may be utilized. High success rates with minimal risk of patellar fracture have been reported when a domed patellar insert is used removing only 1 to 2 mm of bone.[73] The patella is prepared as in primary TKA.

If significant patellar bone deficiency is noted, then component excision is a reasonable option. This option is advocated when there is less than the 10- to 12-mm thickness required for replantation. There have been reports of up to 30% incidence of anterior knee pain with this technique. Restoring the thickness of the patella may improve strength and diminish extensor lag. Advanced strategies for reconstructing patellar thickness include bone grafting or the use of a porous tantalum metal insert. However, these have been associated with patellar pole fracture and implant migration, and thus should be used with caution.

Knee Balancing

As postoperative instability is a common mode of failure after revision TKA, careful attention must be paid during the balancing process to ensure stability. The construct balance is fine-tuned after the trials are placed. The flexion (90 degree) and extension (0 degree) gaps are assessed for symmetry as in primary TKA. It is also important to assess for stability in mid-flexion (30 and 45 degrees), because alterations in the joint line, which are frequent during revision TKA, can lead to mid-flexion instability. During trialing, the surgeon must be aware of the multiple asymmetries that influence the stability of the flexion and extension gaps. Similar to primary TKA, an algorithm is used to sequentially balance each mismatch (see Table 7-1).[74] Adjustments are made as necessary until the knee is well balanced. If a TS implant is planned, we recommend first trialing with a PS insert. This allows the surgeon to get a better assessment of the balance and stability of the construct. Finally, in revisions being done for instability, we recommend ensuring that stability with the chosen construct is adequate with the leg in the "figure 4" position.

Implant Fixation

We routinely use antibiotic-impregnated cement (Simplex-P with Tobramycin, Stryker Orthopaedics, Mahwah, NJ) during revision TKA. Antibiotic cement has been shown to reduce the risk of infection without compromising the strength of the construct.[75,76] We use modern cementation practices including pulsatile lavage, thorough drying of the bone surfaces, and finally finger impaction of the cement.[77] When stems are cemented, cement restrictors are placed and a cement gun is used to pressurize the canals (Figure 7-7).

Bone quality in revision surgery is often compromised. Thus, tibial and femoral stems are used in a majority of revision knee arthroplasties, as they provide improved fixation, bypass poor quality bone, and improve stress distribution.[78,79] Debate remains over whether cemented or cementless stems should be used, and no widely accepted guidelines or criteria exist. Some series show excellent outcomes with cemented stems,[80-82] while others show very good results with press-fit stems.[83-86]

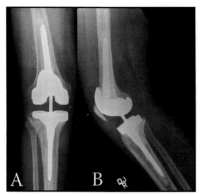

Figure 7-7. Postoperative (A) anteroposterior and (B) lateral radiographs showing the final reconstruction using total stabilized prosthesis with cemented femoral and tibial stems (Triathlon TS, Stryker Orthopaedics, Mahwah, NJ). Distal femoral augments were used to restore the joint line, with medial tibial and posterior-medial femoral augments also used to reconstruct bone defects.

In the setting of previous infection, our preference is to use uncemented stems. Uncemented stems are usually easier to revise should the prosthesis become reinfected. However, some surgeons prefer to use cemented stems in infected cases, using the cement as a local delivery system for antibiotics. We also prefer press-fit stems in situations of extreme bone loss and when highly constrained implants are used, as they help with load sharing.[84,87,88] The diameter of an uncemented stem is determined by the size of the medullary canal, as the stem must be large enough to achieve a stable press-fit. The stem should bypass any stress risers resulting from bone loss, fracture, or tibial tubercle osteotomy. Stem offsets are used to optimally position the component when the joint line is offset from the medullary canal, which may also help with gap balancing. Offset stems should not be cemented, as this greatly increases the difficulty of subsequent implant extraction and may ultimately lead to greater bone loss at rerevision.

When there is minimal bone loss and a PS design is used, the use of stems is based on surgeon preference. If stems are used in this setting, we use short (30 to 50 mm), small diameter tapered stems. The femoral component is implanted with additional cement in the metaphyseal region, but we do not cement the stem itself. On the tibial side, we prefer fully cemented stems with a cement restrictor placed in the canal to allow for a 1-cm distal plug. As discussed previously, tibial stems used in the setting of a TTO should be uncemented, preventing cement extravasation into the osteotomy site.

Closure

Soft tissue management is an integral factor in a successful outcome following revision TKA. The tourniquet is released once the cement has hardened. Care should be taken to obtain meticulous hemostasis to minimize postoperative hematoma.

Closure with the knee positioned at 90 degrees of flexion has been shown to improve range of motion at 6 months following primary TKA when compared to closure in full extension.[89] A subsequent series of 26 revision TKAs demonstrated significantly more knee flexion at 1 year postoperatively in the group closed in flexion.[90] We advocate that, when possible, closure should be undertaken in 90 degrees of knee flexion.

The extensor mechanism is meticulously closed using interrupted sutures. Details regarding the repair of enhanced exposure techniques were discussed previously. Careful attention should be given to patellar tracking, and appropriate releases should be undertaken to ensure the patella is captured in the trochlea throughout flexion. If a lateral release is done, we recommend an inside-out technique to preserve the integrity of the capsule, when possible, to prevent postoperative hematoma. The subcutaneous tissue is closed with interrupted subcutaneous sutures and the skin is closed according to the surgeon's preference. A watertight closure is necessary to minimize postoperative drainage and the risk of infection.

POSTOPERATIVE MANAGEMENT

Patients undergoing revision TKA have higher complication rates than primary TKA patients. These patients require diligent postoperative care to minimize of the risk of complications.[91]

One of the most common complications following TKA is venous thromboembolism. As a result, all patients must be initiated on a multimodal venous thromboembolism prophylaxis regimen. Pneumatic compression stockings provide a simple and low-risk method for deep venous thrombosis prophylaxis and should be worn by patients immediately following surgery. Chemoprophylaxis should be initiated within 24 hours of surgery. Our preference is to use a low-molecular-weight heparin continued for 3 to 4 weeks. However, multiple regimens are accepted.[92]

Perioperative antibiotic therapy is a critical component of infection prevention. For previously noninfected patients, we continue prophylactic antibiotics for 24 hours postoperatively. In patients who were previously infected, we prefer to continue antibiotics until the surgical cultures are finalized, often 3 to 4 days after surgery. For these patients, we use the organism-specific antibiotics with which they were previously treated.

Continuous passive motion may be used at the surgeon's discretion. In primary TKA, continuous passive motion has been shown to improve early postoperative knee flexion, but has no effect on long-term knee flexion or functional scores.[93] We do not typically use continuous passive motion after revision TKA, except in patients with preoperative arthrofibrosis.

We follow a rehabilitation protocol similar to primary TKA for most knee revisions. Patients should be mobilized as quickly as possible with assistive devices. We allow weightbearing as tolerated, unless a structural allograft was used. Range of motion is restricted when a TTO or V-Y turndown exposure was done, as previously described. Otherwise, active and passive range of motion are encouraged, and closed-chain resistance exercises can be started at 3 to 4 weeks after surgery.

REFERENCES

1. Kurtz S, Mowat F, Ong K, Chan N, Lau E, Halpern M. Prevalence of primary and revision total hip and knee arthroplasty in the United States from 1990 through 2002. *J Bone Joint Surg.* 2005;87(7):1487-1497.
2. Lavernia CJ, Drakeford MK, Tsao AK, Gittelsohn A, Krackow KA, Hungerford DS. Revision and primary hip and knee arthroplasty. A cost analysis. *Clin Orthop Relat Res.* 1995;2(311):136-141.
3. Losina E, Walensky RP, Kessler CL, et al. Cost-effectiveness of total knee arthroplasty in the United States: patient risk and hospital volume. *Arch Intern Med.* 2009;169(12):1113-1121; discussion 1121-1122.
4. Callahan CM, Drake BG, Heck DA, Dittus RS. Patient outcomes following tricompartmental total knee replacement. A meta-analysis. *JAMA.* 1994;271(17):1349-1357.
5. Bourne RB. Measuring tools for functional outcomes in total knee arthroplasty. *Clin Orthop Relat Res.* 2008;466(11):2634-2638.
6. Kurtz S, Ong K, Lau E, Mowat F, Halpern M. Projections of primary and revision hip and knee arthroplasty in the United States from 2005 to 2030. *J Bone Joint Surg.* 2007;89(4):780-785.
7. Sharkey PF, Hozack WJ, Rothman RH, Shastri S, Jacoby SM. Insall Award paper. Why are total knee arthroplasties failing today? *Clin Orthop Relat Res.* 2002;11(404):7-13.
8. Bozic KJ, Kurtz SM, Lau E, et al. The epidemiology of revision total knee arthroplasty in the United States. *Clin Orthop Relat Res.* 2010;468(1):45-51.
9. Mortazavi SM, Schwartzenberger J, Austin MS, Purtill JJ, Parvizi J. Revision total knee arthroplasty infection: incidence and predictors. *Clin Orthop Relat Res.* 2010;468(8):2052-2059.
10. Dennis DA. A stepwise approach to revision total knee arthroplasty. *J Arthroplasty.* 2007;22(4 suppl 1):32-38.
11. Mason JB, Fehring TK, Odum SM, Griffin WL, Nussman DS. The value of white blood cell counts before revision total knee arthroplasty. *J Arthroplasty.* 2003;18(8):1038-1043.
12. Trampuz A, Hanssen AD, Osmon DR, Mandrekar J, Steckelberg JM, Patel R. Synovial fluid leukocyte count and differential for the diagnosis of prosthetic knee infection. *Am J Med.* 2004;117(8):556-562.
13. Joseph TN, Mujtaba M, Chen AL, et al. Efficacy of combined technetium-99m sulfur colloid/indium-111 leukocyte scans to detect infected total hip and knee arthroplasties. *J Arthroplasty.* 2001;16(6):753-758.

14. Moon HK, Han CD, Yang IH, Cha BS. Factors affecting outcome after total knee arthroplasty in patients with diabetes mellitus. *Yonsei Med J.* 2008;49(1):129-137.

15. Parvizi J, Sullivan TA, Trousdale RT, Lewallen DG. Thirty-day mortality after total knee arthroplasty. *J Bone Joint Surg.* 2001;83-A(8):1157-1161.

16. Whiteside LA. Ligament balancing in revision total knee arthroplasty. *Clin Orthop Relat Res.* 2004;(423):178-185.

17. Krackow KA. Revision total knee replacement ligament balancing for deformity. *Clin Orthop Relat Res.* 2002;(404):152-157.

18. McAuley JP, Engh GA, Ammeen DJ. Treatment of the unstable total knee arthroplasty. *Instr Course Lect.* 2004;53:237-241.

19. Mihalko WM, Krackow KA. Flexion and extension gap balancing in revision total knee arthroplasty. *Clin Orthop Relat Res.* 2006;446:121-126.

20. Parratte S, Pagnano MW. Instability after total knee arthroplasty. *Instr Course Lect.* 2008;57:295-304.

21. Mihalko WM, Saleh KJ, Krackow KA, Whiteside LA. Soft-tissue balancing during total knee arthroplasty in the varus knee. *J Am Acad Orthop Surg.* 2009;17(12):766-774.

22. Clarke HD, Scuderi GR. Flexion instability in primary total knee replacement. *J Knee Surg.* 2003;16(2):123-128.

23. Mihalko WM, Miller C, Krackow KA. Total knee arthroplasty ligament balancing and gap kinematics with posterior cruciate ligament retention and sacrifice. *Am J Orthop (Belle Mead NJ).* 2000;29(8):610-616.

24. Hoeffel DP, Rubash HE. Revision total knee arthroplasty: current rationale and techniques for femoral component revision. *Clin Orthop Relat Res.* 2000;11(380):116-132.

25. Bush JL, Wilson JB, Vail TP. Management of bone loss in revision total knee arthroplasty. *Clin Orthop Relat Res.* 2006;452:186-192.

26. Huff TW, Sculco TP. Management of bone loss in revision total knee arthroplasty. *J Arthroplasty.* 2007;22(7 suppl 3):32-36.

27. Lucey SD, Scuderi GR, Kelly MA, Insall JN. A practical approach to dealing with bone loss in revision total knee arthroplasty. *Orthopedics.* 2000;23(10):1036-1041.

28. Engh GA, Ammeen DJ. Bone loss with revision total knee arthroplasty: defect classification and alternatives for reconstruction. *Instr Course Lect.* 1999;48:167-175.

29. Clatworthy MG, Ballance J, Brick GW, Chandler HP, Gross AE. The use of structural allograft for uncontained defects in revision total knee arthroplasty. A minimum five-year review. *J Bone Joint Surg.* 2001;83-A(3):404-411.

30. Reichel H, Hube R, Birke A, Hein W. Bone defects in revision total knee arthroplasty: classification and management. *Zentralbl Chir.* 2002;127(10):880-885.

31. Meneghini RM, Lewallen DG, Hanssen AD. Use of porous tantalum metaphyseal cones for severe tibial bone loss during revision total knee replacement. *J Bone Joint Surg Am.* 2008;90(1):78-84.

32. Radnay CS, Scuderi GR. Management of bone loss: augments, cones, offset stems. *Clin Orthop Relat Res.* 2006;446:83-92.

33. Rand JA. Modular augments in revision total knee arthroplasty. *Orthop Clin North Am.* 1998;29(2):347-353.

34. Ritter MA, Harty LD. Medial screws and cement: a possible mechanical augmentation in total knee arthroplasty. *J Arthroplasty.* 2004;19(5):587-589.

35. Ritter MA. Screw and cement fixation of large defects in total knee arthroplasty. *J Arthroplasty.* 1986;1(2):125-129.

36. Ritter MA, Keating EM, Faris PM. Screw and cement fixation of large defects in total knee arthroplasty. A sequel. *J Arthroplasty.* 1993;8(1):63-65.

37. Werle JR, Goodman SB, Imrie SN. Revision total knee arthroplasty using large distal femoral augments for severe metaphyseal bone deficiency: a preliminary study. *Orthopedics.* 2002;25(3):325-327.

38. Pagnano MW, Trousdale RT, Rand JA. Tibial wedge augmentation for bone deficiency in total knee arthroplasty. A followup study. *Clin Orthop Relat Res.* 1995;12(321):151-155.

39. Dorr LD, Ranawat CS, Sculco TA, McKaskill B, Orisek BS. Bone graft for tibial defects in total knee arthroplasty. 1986. *Clin Orthop Relat Res.* 2006;446:4-9.

40. Dennis DA. The structural allograft composite in revision total knee arthroplasty. *J Arthroplasty.* 2002;17(4 suppl 1):90-93.

41. Dennis DA, Little LR. The structural allograft composite in revision total knee arthroplasty. *Orthopedics.* 2005;28(9):1005-1007.

42. Engh GA, Herzwurm PJ, Parks NL. Treatment of major defects of bone with bulk allografts and stemmed components during total knee arthroplasty. *J Bone Joint Surg Am.* 1997;79(7):1030-1039.

43. Parks NL, Engh GA. The Ranawat Award. Histology of nine structural bone grafts used in total knee arthroplasty. *Clin Orthop Relat Res.* 1997;12(345):17-23.

44. Bobyn JD, Stackpool GJ, Hacking SA, Tanzer M, Krygier JJ. Characteristics of bone ingrowth and interface mechanics of a new porous tantalum biomaterial. *J Bone Joint Surg Br.* 1999;81(5):907-914.

45. Brooks DH, Fehring TK, Griffin WL, Mason JB, McCoy TH. Polyethylene exchange only for prosthetic knee instability. *Clin Orthop Relat Res.* 2002;12(405):182-188.

46. McAuley JP, Engh GA, Ammeen DJ. Revision of failed unicompartmental knee arthroplasty. *Clin Orthop Relat Res.* 2001;11(392):279-282.

47. Gebhard JS, Kilgus DJ. Dislocation of a posterior stabilized total knee prosthesis. A report of two cases. *Clin Orthop Relat Res.* 1990;5(254):225-229.

48. Laskin RS, Ohnsorge J. The use of standard posterior stabilized implants in revision total knee arthroplasty. *Clin Orthop Relat Res.* 2005;440:122-125.

49. Rand JA. Revision total knee arthroplasty using the total condylar III prosthesis. *J Arthroplasty.* 1991;6(3):279-284.

50. Rosenberg AG, Verner JJ, Galante JO. Clinical results of total knee revision using the Total Condylar III prosthesis. *Clin Orthop Relat Res.* 1991;12(273):83-90.

51. Donaldson WF 3rd, Sculco TP, Insall JN, Ranawat CS. Total condylar III knee prosthesis. Long-term follow-up study. *Clin Orthop Relat Res.* 1988;1(226):21-28.

52. Karpinski MR, Grimer RJ. Hinged knee replacement in revision arthroplasty. *Clin Orthop Relat Res.* 1987;7(220):185-191.

53. Inglis AE, Walker PS. Revision of failed knee replacements using fixed-axis hinges. *J Bone Joint Surg Br.* 1991;73(5):757-761.

54. Westrich GH, Mollano AV, Sculco TP, Buly RL, Laskin RS, Windsor R. Rotating hinge total knee arthroplasty in severly affected knees. *Clin Orthop Relat Res.* 2000;10(379):195-208.

55. Barrack RL. Evolution of the rotating hinge for complex total knee arthroplasty. *Clin Orthop Relat Res.* 2001;11(392):292-299.

56. Pour AE, Parvizi J, Slenker N, Purtill JJ, Sharkey PF. Rotating hinged total knee replacement: use with caution. *J Bone Joint Surg Am.* 2007;89(8):1735-1741.

57. Burnett RS, Aggarwal A, Givens SA, McClure JT, Morgan PM, Barrack RL. Prophylactic antibiotics do not affect cultures in the treatment of an infected TKA: a prospective trial. *Clin Orthop Relat Res.* 2010;468(1):127-134.

58. Colombel M, Mariz Y, Dahhan P, Kenesi C. Arterial and lymphatic supply of the knee integuments. *Surg Radiol Anat.* 1998;20(1):35-40.

59. Haertsch PA. The blood supply to the skin of the leg: a post-mortem investigation. *Br J Plast Surg.* 1981;34(4):470-477.

60. Adam RF, Watson SB, Jarratt JW, Noble J, Watson JS. Outcome after flap cover for exposed total knee arthroplasties. A report of 25 cases. *J Bone Joint Surg Br.* 1994;76(5):750-753.

61. Hierner R, Reynders-Frederix P, Bellemans J, Stuyck J, Peeters W. Free myocutaneous latissimus dorsi flap transfer in total knee arthroplasty. *J Plast Reconstr Aesthet Surg.* 2009;62(12):1692-1700.

62. Gold DA, Scott SC, Scott WN. Soft tissue expansion prior to arthroplasty in the multiply-operated knee. A new method of preventing catastrophic skin problems. *J Arthroplasty.* 1996;11(5):512-521.

63. Lonner JH, Desai P, Dicesare PE, Steiner G, Zuckerman JD. The reliability of analysis of intraoperative frozen sections for identifying active infection during revision hip or knee arthroplasty. *J Bone Joint Surg.* 1996;78(10):1553-1558.

64. Bauer TW, Parvizi J, Kobayashi N, Krebs V. Diagnosis of periprosthetic infection. *J Bone Joint Surg.* 2006;88(4):869-882.

65. Garvin KL, Scuderi G, Insall JN. Evolution of the quadriceps snip. *Clin Orthop Relat Res.* 1995;(321):131-137.

66. Barrack RL, Smith P, Munn B, Engh G, Rorabeck C. The Ranawat Award. Comparison of surgical approaches in total knee arthroplasty. *Clin Orthop Relat Res.* 1998;11(356):16-21.

67. Trousdale RT, Hanssen AD, Rand JA, Cahalan TD. V-Y quadricepsplasty in total knee arthroplasty. *Clin Orthop Relat Res.* 1993;1(286):48-55.

68. Whiteside LA, Ohl MD. Tibial tubercle osteotomy for exposure of the difficult total knee arthroplasty. *Clin Orthop Relat Res.* 1990;11(260):6-9.

69. Dennis DA. Removal of well-fixed cementless metal-backed patellar components. *J Arthroplasty.* 1992;7(2):217-220.

70. Partington PF, Sawhney J, Rorabeck CH, Barrack RL, Moore J. Joint line restoration after revision total knee arthroplasty. *Clin Orthop Relat Res.* 1999;10(367):165-171.

71. Stiehl JB, Abbott BD. Morphology of the transepicondylar axis and its application in primary and revision total knee arthroplasty. *J Arthroplasty.* 1995;10(6):785-789.

72. Servien E, Viskontas D, Giuffre BM, Coolican MR, Parker DA. Reliability of bony landmarks for restoration of the joint line in revision knee arthroplasty. *Knee Surg Sports Traumatol Arthrosc.* 2008;16(3):263-269.

73. Laskin RS. Management of the patella during revision total knee replacement arthroplasty. *Orthop Clin North Am.* 1998;29(2):355-360.

74. Bottros J, Gad B, Krebs V, Barsoum WK. Gap balancing in total knee arthroplasty. *J Arthroplasty.* 2006;21(4 suppl 1):11-15.

75. Jiranek WA, Hanssen AD, Greenwald AS. Antibiotic-loaded bone cement for infection prophylaxis in total joint replacement. *J Bone Joint Surg Am.* 2006;88(11):2487-2500.

76. Chiu FY, Lin CF. Antibiotic-impregnated cement in revision total knee arthroplasty. A prospective cohort study of one hundred and eighty-three knees. *J Bone Joint Surg Am.* 2009;91(3):628-633.

77. Ritter MA, Herbst SA, Keating EM, Faris PM. Radiolucency at the bone-cement interface in total knee replacement. The effects of bone-surface preparation and cement technique. *J Bone Joint Surg Am.* 1994;76(1):60-65.

78. Bugbee WD, Ammeen DJ, Engh GA. Does implant selection affect outcome of revision knee arthroplasty? *J Arthroplasty.* 2001;16(5):581-585.

79. Brooks PJ, Walker PS, Scott RD. Tibial component fixation in deficient tibial bone stock. *Clin Orthop Relat Res.* 1984;4(184):302-308.

80. Mabry TM, Vessely MB, Schleck CD, Harmsen WS, Berry DJ. Revision total knee arthroplasty with modular cemented stems: long-term follow-up. *J Arthroplasty.* 2007;22(6 suppl 2):100-105.

81. Whaley AL, Trousdale RT, Rand JA, Hanssen AD. Cemented long-stem revision total knee arthroplasty. *J Arthroplasty.* 2003;18(5):592-599.

82. Fehring TK, Odum S, Olekson C, Griffin WL, Mason JB, McCoy TH. Stem fixation in revision total knee arthroplasty: a comparative analysis. *Clin Orthop Relat Res.* 2003;11(416):217-224.

83. Wood GC, Naudie DD, MacDonald SJ, McCalden RW, Bourne RB. Results of press-fit stems in revision knee arthroplasties. *Clin Orthop Relat Res.* 2009;467(3):810-817.

84. Bertin KC, Freeman MA, Samuelson KM, Ratcliffe SS, Todd RC. Stemmed revision arthroplasty for aseptic loosening of total knee replacement. *J Bone Joint Surg Br.* 1985;67(2):242-248.

85. Gofton WT, Tsigaras H, Butler RA, Patterson JJ, Barrack RL, Rorabeck CH. Revision total knee arthroplasty: fixation with modular stems. *Clin Orthop Relat Res.* 2002;11(404):158-168.

86. Haas SB, Insall JN, Montgomery W 3rd, Windsor RE. Revision total knee arthroplasty with use of modular components with stems inserted without cement. *J Bone Joint Surg.* 1995;77(11):1700-1707.

87. Completo A, Simoes JA, Fonseca F. Revision total knee arthroplasty: the influence of femoral stems in load sharing and stability. *Knee.* 2009;16(4):275-279.

88. Bourne RB, Finlay JB. The influence of tibial component intramedullary stems and implant-cortex contact on the strain distribution of the proximal tibia following total knee arthroplasty. An in vitro study. *Clin Orthop Relat Res.* 1986;(208):95-99.

89. Emerson RH Jr, Ayers C, Head WC, Higgins LL. Surgical closing in primary total knee arthroplasties: flexion versus extension. *Clin Orthop Relat Res.* 1996;10(331):74-80.

90. Emerson RH Jr, Ayers C, Higgins LL. Surgical closing in total knee arthroplasty. A series followup. *Clin Orthop Relat Res.* 1999;11(368):176-181.

91. Pulido L, Parvizi J, Macgibeny M, et al. In hospital complications after total joint arthroplasty. *J Arthroplasty.* 2008;23(6 suppl 1):139-145.

92. Kearon C, Kahn SR, Agnelli G, Goldhaber S, Raskob GE, Comerota AJ. Antithrombotic therapy for venous thromboembolic disease: American College of Chest Physicians Evidence-Based Clinical Practice Guidelines. 8th ed. *Chest.* 2008;133(6 suppl):454S-545S.

93. Lenssen TA, van Steyn MJ, Crijns YH, et al. Effectiveness of prolonged use of continuous passive motion, as an adjunct to physiotherapy, after total knee arthroplasty. *BMC Musculoskeletal Disorders.* 2008;9:60.

Joint Line Position in Revision Total Knee Arthroplasty

Kirby D. Hitt, MD

The principles of revision knee replacement are to correct limb and patellar alignment, correct implant rotation, restore flexion-extension stability, and restore the anatomic joint line. Projected increases in the number of knee revisions by 601% between 2005 and 2030[1] will result in more surgeons facing the daunting challenge of achieving these goals. Reported outcomes for revision total knee arthroplasty (TKA) have not equaled primary replacements.[2] Simplified, reproducible revision surgical techniques should result in improved survival and function and close the gap between primary and revision knee outcomes. Anatomic reproduction of the joint line in revision surgery is complicated by the loss of normal bony landmarks and scarred or deficient ligaments. Clinical results following revision TKA have been shown to have a direct correlation with accurate reproduction of the joint line.[3-18]

WHY SHOULD WE RESTORE THE JOINT LINE?

Failure to adequately restore the joint line at revision surgery has been shown to result in midflexion instability, decreased extensor strength, anterior knee pain, patellar clunk and crepitus, patellar instability, decreased motion, and decreased clinical results.

Figgie et al[7] have shown inferior clinical results associated with elevation of the joint line more than 8 mm. Functional knee scores, range of motion, patellofemoral pain, mechanical problems, revision rates, and need for manipulations were all correlated with joint line elevation. Ryu et al[14] reported on range of motion related to joint line position. Patients with a higher range of motion had a mean shift of the joint line of 2.1 mm, whereas patients with decreasing range of motion had up to 5.7 mm of shift or nearly 3 times higher.[14] Joint line shifts of 2 mm or more have been associated with decreased knee flexion.[19]

Similarly, Partington et al[12] showed elevation of the joint line by 8 mm resulted in Knee Society clinical rating scores to be on average 15 points worse compared with a 10-point improvement when the joint line was restored within 8 mm. In that study, the joint line was found to be elevated in 79% of the revision cases.

Jacofsky DJ, Hedley AK, eds.
Fundamentals of Revision Knee Arthroplasty:
Diagnosis, Evaluation, and Treatment (pp 121-132).
© 2013 SLACK Incorporated.

Altered transmission of quadriceps forces and increased patellofemoral pressures have been shown with elevation of the joint line by 2 mm.[6] Increased patellofemoral and tibiofemoral joint contact forces in normal walking and stairclimbing have been shown to have a direct correlation with elevation of the joint line in revision TKA.[20] Clinical consequences of these increased forces can result in increased wear of the tibial and patellar bearings, anterior knee pain, patellar component loosening, instability, and limited function. Singerman et al[17] similarly have shown an increase in the patellofemoral contact forces by as much as 3% per millimeter of joint line elevation.

Porteous et al[21] in a study of 114 revision patients reported restoration of the joint line in 73 patients (64%) with elevation of the joint line in 41 (36%) knees. Restoration of the joint line to within 5 mm improved the Bristol knee and functional scores and overall clinical outcome. In a cadaveric study, Martin and Whiteside[10] showed anterior displacement of the flexion joint space by 5 mm resulted in midflexion instability.

Restoration of the joint line position to within 5 mm has resulted in the need for reduced implant constraint which could result in improved long-term durability.[22] While joint line elevation is more commonly seen, depression of the joint line has been shown to result in increased risk of a patellar subluxation and retropatellar pain.[5]

In a radiographic and clinical analysis of 89 consecutive revision TKAs, Hofmann et al[23] showed that clinical outcomes are correlated to joint line position. Patients in whom the joint line was recreated within ± 4 mm of the prearthroplasty value had improved Knee Society scores, flexion and extension, and total range of motion.[23]

WHERE IS THE JOINT LINE?

Multiple studies have reported elevation of the joint line associated with revision knee arthroplasty. The tendency to raise the joint line relates to distal femoral bone loss at the time of revision and the placement of the revision femoral component on the remaining distal bone instead of appropriately restoring the joint line to a more anatomical position. In revision cases where the flexion space is wider than the extension space, attempts to balance the gaps could result in inappropriately removing distal femoral bone to balance the flexion-extension gaps. Accurately restoring the anteroposterior (AP) dimension of the femur should fill the flexion space, thus avoiding the need to resect bone from the distal femur, which is already deficient and would result in further elevation of the joint line.

In revision surgery, restoration of the joint line can be determined by 2 intraoperative methods. Prior to removal of the failed implant, marks can be made on the bone proximal and distal and measurements made to the joint line based on the existing implant. This technique assumes that the previous implant restored the joint line accurately.

Surgeons must avoid utilizing the existing implant joint line position from the primary replacement as the sole determinant to accurate joint line reconstruction at revision, as multiple studies have shown deviation of the normal joint line utilizing various implant designs.[5,7,13,15,24]

An easily accessible, identifiable intraoperative anatomic landmark is required to adequately determine the joint line. Anatomic landmarks previously studied include the medial or lateral femoral epicondyle, the meniscal scar, the inferior pole of the patella, the tibial tubercle, the fibular head, the adductor tubercle, and the epicondylar axis. Soft tissue landmarks are inaccurate due to anatomic alterations resulting from the previous surgery. Bony landmarks provide a more reliable guide to restoring joint line position.

The patella is not a good landmark for restoring the joint line in revision surgery. Scarring and pathologic changes of the patellar tendon and quadriceps mechanism can result in abnormal patellar position. The joint line should be restored at revision surgery and ligament balancing performed to achieve stability in flexion and extension, and the patellar position should be dictated by placement of the joint line based on predictable anatomic landmarks.

While the distance from the fibular head has been suggested as a reliable indicator of joint line position, large variations in measurements indicate it is a poor landmark for predictable joint line restoration.[25-27] Preoperative radiographic assessment of fibular head to joint line distance of the contralateral knee may decrease this deviation, but the difficulty in localizing the fibular head intraoperatively makes it an unreliable guide for joint line position in revision surgery.

In a cadaveric study, Mason et al[26] evaluated 4 anatomic landmarks as references for locating the joint line in revision knee surgery. The medial femoral epicondyle, the fibular head, the tibial tubercle, and inferior pole of the patella to the joint line were evaluated and validated on 94 revision cases. The most reproducible landmark was found to be the medial femoral epicondyle, which was on average 28 mm to the joint line. Stiehl and Abbott[28] reported similar findings. The average distance from the joint line in their study was 30.8 mm from the medial epicondyle and 25.3 mm from the lateral epicondyle. Similar findings have also been reported by Griffin et al.[29] In a magnetic resonance imaging (MRI) assessment of the reliability of anatomic landmarks to restore the joint line in revision surgery, the average distance from the epicondyles to the joint line was 23 mm on the lateral side and 28 mm on the medial side. Variations in distance from the epicondyles related to gender and size differences led the authors to suggest that the joint line should be calculated from the femoral width as a measured distance between the lateral and medial epicondyles. The distance from the lateral epicondyle to the distal joint line was 28% of the measured femoral width while the distance to the posterior joint line was 29%. The medial epicondyle was found to be less reliable than the lateral epicondyle, partly owing to the difficulty of determining the medial epicondylar sulcus on MRI.[25] A radiologic and computer-based study confirmed these findings, reporting that the relationship between the transepicondylar axis and the joint line is a constant relationship and can be utilized intraoperatively.[30] The authors concluded that the joint line could be derived by measuring the distance between the epicondyles and dividing by 3.4. The distance from the epicondyles to the joint line were on average 28.6 mm on the medial side and 25.7 mm laterally. Romero and associates[31] found a 59% incidence of joint line elevation in revision total knee replacements. They proposed a preoperative radiologic method to reliably determine joint line position on radiographs prior to the revision procedure. A nongender-specific coefficient of 0.4 (medial) and 0.3 (lateral), multiplied by the transepicondylar axis width, facilitates estimation of the joint line. The mean perpendicular distance from the medial epicondyle to the joint line was 31.6 ± 2.5 mm and the mean distance from the lateral epicondyle to the joint line was 25.1 ± 2.7 mm. The proximal aspect of the tibial tubercle has also been utilized as a possible bony landmark for determining joint line position.[7,25] On sagittal x-rays, the distance from the anterior aspect of the tubercle to the tibial insert assumes that the joint line was adequately restored at the time of the primary procedure. When working distal to the joint, the tibial tubercle is the most reliable indicator for determining joint line positioning.

While the joint line in extension has been studied extensively, a paucity of literature exists related to the joint line in flexion. Improved postoperative range of motion associated with preservation of the posterior condylar offset has been shown.[32,33] Seventeen (85%) of 20 knees in a study by Sato et al[34] showed anterior movement of the posterior joint line following primary knee replacement. To maximize our revision knee results, the surgeon needs to consider the flexion joint line as well. The distance from the lateral epicondyle to the posterior lateral condyle has been shown to be approximately 24 mm. Likewise, the distance from the medial epicondyle to the posterior medial condyle and distal medial condyle averaged 28 mm.

Bottom Line

The most consistent identifiable bony landmark for determining intraoperative joint line position that results in the least variability is the medial epicondyle. Multiple studies suggest placing the joint line 28 mm from the medial epicondyle will allow for size and gender differences and allow restoration of the joint line to within 3 to 5 mm.[26,28-30,35] Alternatively the joint line can be adequately restored by placing the femoral component 25 mm from the lateral epicondyle.[26,28-30] Newer instrumentation to assist in measuring the transepicondylar axis width and multiplying this by an established coefficient could be utilized to determine joint line position and eliminate potential gender bias. If the distal femoral bone does not allow anatomic landmarks for intraoperative assessment, the surgeon must work distal to the joint, and the tibial tubercle is the most reliable indicator for determining joint line positioning.

AVOIDING JOINT LINE ELEVATION

Elevation of the joint line in revision TKAs occur up to 79% of the time.[12] Only when surgeons understand the causes of the elevation can it be avoided. Removal of a loose or well-fixed femoral implant often results in distal femoral bone loss. Routine use of distal femoral augments in revision cases should be considered and if none appear to be indicated, then the surgeon should question whether the reconstructed joint line is correct. Likewise, surgeons have a tendency to undersize the femoral component due to posterior bone loss. By placing a smaller femoral component, direct contact is achieved on the remaining bone at the risk of elevating the joint line both in flexion and extension. Thicker tibial inserts will be required to fill the flexion and extension space. It is imperative that a femoral component be chosen that restores the original AP diameter prearthroplasty to avoid introducing gap mismatch. After component removal and débridement it is not uncommon to be faced with a flexion gap that is much larger than the extension gap. This occurs because the capsuloligamentous structures in revision surgery, when compromised, affect the flexion gap more than the extension gap. Filling up the flexion gap with a larger tibial insert will result in a tighter extension gap and could lead the surgeon to inappropriately remove more distal femoral bone to balance the gaps. To avoid flexion-extension gap balancing issues, the femoral component should reproduce the original AP dimension of the knee, and the surgeon needs to ensure that the scarred posterior capsule has been adequately released off the condyles, as failure to address this could result in the inadvertent distal femoral resection.

SURGICAL TECHNIQUE

Various techniques have been reported for knee revision and balancing the flexion and extension gaps.[36-43] While some authors advocate balancing the revision knee in extension first, a more simplified approach is to balance the knee in flexion first. Once the flexion gap is stabilized, the surgeon has only to determine whether the extension gap is loose, tight, or just right.

Attempts should be made during exposure in revision cases to avoid releasing or damaging the anterior longitudinal portion of the medial collateral ligament, as this could result in an increase in the flexion space, making balancing efforts more difficult.

Correct femoral component size should not be based on the remaining AP dimension after component removal and débridement. To maximize stability in flexion when between sizes, the larger size should be chosen to avoid decreasing the posterior condylar offset by resection of posterior bone stock. The femoral component should be placed flush with the anterior cortex to maximize filling of flexion space.

Placement of a long diaphyseal fitting stem can result in extension of the femoral component and an increase in the flexion gap. Anterior displacement of the femoral component in these situations with resultant overstuffing of the anterior compartment can be avoided by the use of offset stems, allowing anterior seating of the femoral component and the inadvertent increase in the flexion space. Bone loss and compromised medial and lateral ligaments can lead to rotational errors in femoral component placement, resulting in a compromised functional result.

Surgeons should not assume that the joint line was appropriately established at the time of the index operation, as this may have been a contributing factor to the subsequent need for revision.

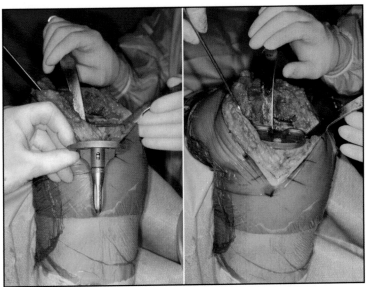

Figure 8-1. Trial base plate with planned augments and stems is inserted.

Two methods have been utilized to adequately restore joint line position intraoperatively. The flexion-extension gap balancing technique addresses the flexion gap, whereas the medial epicondylar referencing technique initially addresses the extension gap. The authors advocate a revision method that combines these approaches, but prefer to balance the knee in flexion first.

While the literature suggests that the results of revision total knee replacement are inferior to primary cases, a simplified, reproducible, stepwise surgical technique to revision cases should improve on existing results. After the initial approach, component removal, and débridement, the first step in the reconstruction plan is to prepare the tibia.

TIBIAL PREPARATION

Either intramedullary or extramedullary instrumentation can be used to make a clean-up cut of the proximal tibia. The goal is to produce a flat tibial surface with a neutral posterior slope and neutral mechanical alignment. The tibial surface can be reconstructed with bone graft or augments as necessary to restore a flat surface. Surgeons should avoid overresecting tibial bone, which could create compatibility sizing problems with the femur. Preparation of the proximal keel and stem augments are done at this time, and a trial tibial baseplate with planned augments inserted (Figure 8-1). To save operating room time, stem preparation can be done for both the tibial and femur as indicated. There is no need to consider joint line position at this step, and the surgeon should not have to ever return to the tibial side, as the flexion and extension gaps are equally affected by tibial inserts. Surgeons need to understand that soft tissue balancing and joint line placement are controlled by the position of the femoral component and not related to the tibial reconstruction.

FEMORAL PREPARATION IN FLEXION: SIZING, ROTATION, JOINT LINE, AND STABILIZATION

The surgeon should attempt to restore the original AP dimension of the femur prior to the index operation. While the original lateral x-rays could prove helpful in determining the original AP dimension, they are often not available to the revision surgeon. Utilizing the removed implant

Figure 8-2. Utilizing the removed implant to determine size is often times inaccurate.

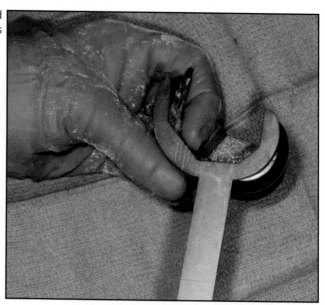

Figure 8-3. The most accurate determination of original anteroposterior dimension should be determined by the intact mediolateral dimension.

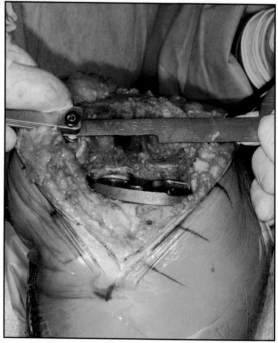

to determine sizing suggests that the appropriate size was placed at the index operation, which is not always the case and may have been a contributing factor to the need for revision (Figure 8-2). While distal and posterior bone loss is not unusual in a revision knee, the medial/lateral bone is usually preserved. As anthropometric data have been used to design current implants with improved AP/mediolateral sizing, instrumentation has been designed to allow measuring of the mediolateral femoral width to help determine the appropriate AP dimension (Figure 8-3). A secondary check to ensure that the appropriate femoral size has been chosen can be accomplished by measuring the distance from the medial epicondyle to the posterior medial condyle, which should be approximately 28 mm (Figure 8-4). When between sizes, the largest femoral component that

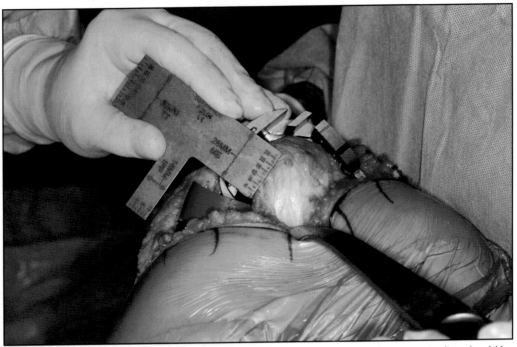

Figure 8-4. To confirm that the anteroposterior dimension is restored, the posterior joint line should be approximately 28 mm from the medial epicondyle.

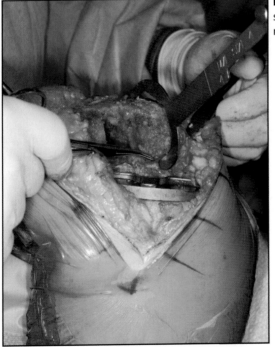

Figure 8-5. Anteroposterior sizing templating showing posterior bone loss and need for posterior augmentation.

does not result in mediolateral overhang should be utilized to avoid resection of posterior condylar bone and to maximize stability in flexion. Due to posterior bone loss from loosening of the implant or during implant removal, the need for augmentation posteriorly is common (Figure 8-5).

Figure 8-6. Trial cutting guide with balancing of the flexion space and setting rotation of the femoral component.

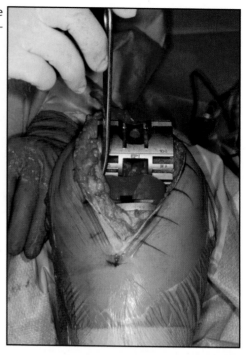

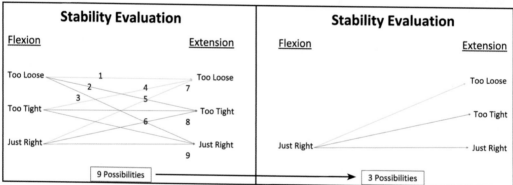

Figure 8-7. By balancing the flexion gap first, the decision making is simplified.

Normal anatomic landmarks such as Whiteside's line and the transepicondylar axis used to determine femoral rotation in the primary setting are difficult in the revision case because of bone loss and scarring. Femoral rotation is established parallel to the tibial component at 90 degrees of flexion with the medial and lateral structures under tension. This can be accomplished utilizing laminar spreaders, tibial inserts, tensor/balancers, or trial cutting guides, which allows balancing to be done prior to any bone cuts (Figure 8-6). The flexion gap is then filled with trial inserts until stability is achieved. By balancing the flexion gap first, the reconstructive balancing is simplified (Figure 8-7). The knee is then brought out in extension and because of the balanced flexion space, 3 possibilities in extension will occur: too loose, too tight, or just right. If the extension gap is too loose relative to the flexion gap, distal femoral augments should be utilized. In cases where the extension gap is too tight, options include placing a smaller distal femoral augment or resection of distal femoral bone. Because bone loss is common from the distal femur, if faced with the need to resect more distal femoral bone, the surgeon should be sure that the posterior capsule has been released off the posterior femoral condyles, which could result in a tight extension space (Figure 8-8). By placing the prepared stem on the trial femoral component or revision cutting

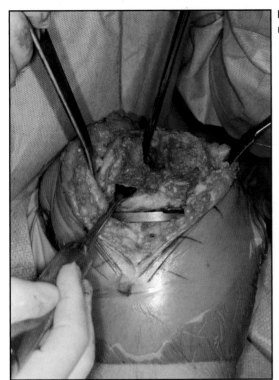

Figure 8-8. The posterior capsule should be released off the posterior condyle.

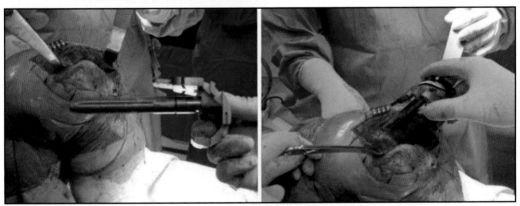

Figure 8-9. The prepared stem is attached to a trial femoral component or revision cutting guide and inserted.

guide as the knee is brought out in extension (Figure 8-9), the femoral trial will be pushed toward the femur until the knee is fully extended. With the knee balanced in extension the surgeon should assess that the extension joint line is 28 mm ± 5 mm of the medial epicondyle (Figure 8-10). In the rare situation where the extension joint line is outside the acceptable 28 mm ± 5 mm range, adjustments can be made relative to the size of the femoral component with stem offsets to maintain acceptable joint line position in flexion and extension. After completing any necessary femoral bone resections (Figure 8-11), the femoral trials are then assembled along with the previously determined tibial insert and stability is assessed. Stability assessment is best achieved with a nonconstrained insert. Once balancing efforts have been maximized, the insert constraint of choice can be placed and the knee taken through a range of motion to check for post impingement.

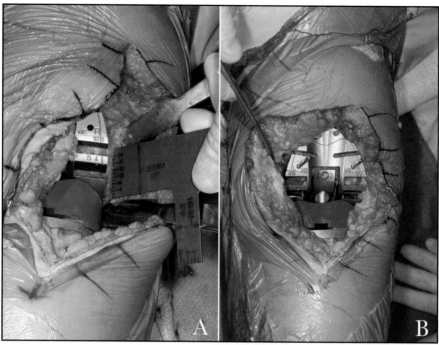

Figure 8-10. The same insert balancing the knee in flexion is utilized to balance the knee in extension, and confirming the extension joint line has been restored at approximately 28 mm from the medial epicondyle, the guide can be pinned to maintain position.

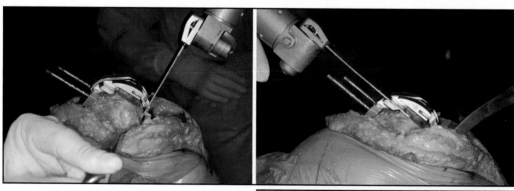

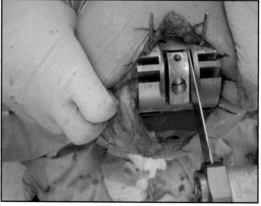

Figure 8-11. Femoral resections are performed from the trial cutting guide with need for augmentation determined and box preparation performed.

While some authors advocate re-establishing the joint line in extension first and then balancing the flexion gap utilizing different-sized femoral components,[11,40] the flexion gap first method decreases the complexity of the reconstruction.

In the majority of cases, flexion-extension balancing can be achieved utilizing these techniques. There are cases, despite maximizing balancing efforts, where flexion-extension balancing cannot be achieved and increased prosthetic constraint should be considered. Optimal stability and joint kinematics and the reduced need for prosthetic constraint can occur by re-establishing the joint line to a more anatomic level.

REFERENCES

1. Kurtz S, Ong K, Lau E, Mowat F, Halpern M. Projections of primary and revision hip and knee arthroplasty in the United States from 2005 to 2030. *J Bone Joint Surg Am.* 2007;89:780-785.
2. Ritter MA, Carr KD, Keating EM, Faris PN, Bankoff DL, Ireland PM. Revision total joint arthroplasty: does Medicare reimbursement justify time spent. *Orthopedics.* 1996;19:137-139.
3. Chao EY, Neluheni EV, Hsu RW, Paley D. Biomechanics of malalignment. *Orthop Clin North Am.* 1994;25:379-386.
4. Chiu KY, Ng TP, Tang WM, Yau WP. Review article: knee flexion after total knee arthroplasty. *J Orthop Surg (Hong Kong).* 2002;10:194-202.
5. Cope MR, O'Brien BS, Nanu AM. The influence of the posterior cruciate ligament in the maintenance of joint line in primary total knee arthroplasty: a radiologic study. *J Arthroplasty.* 2002;17:202-208.
6. Emodi GJ, Callaghan JJ, Pedersen DR, Brown TD. Posterior cruciate ligament function following total knee arthroplasty: the effect of joint line elevation. *Iowa Orthop J.* 1999;19:82-92.
7. Figgie HE 3rd, Goldberg VM, Heiple KG, Moller HS 3rd, Gordon NH. The influence of tibial-patellofemoral location on function of the knee in patients with the posterior stabilized condylar knee prosthesis. *J Bone Joint Surg Am.* 1986;68:1035-1040.
8. Goldberg VM, Figgie HE 3rd, Figgie MP. Technical considerations in total knee surgery. Management of patella problems. *Orthop Clin North Am.* 1989;20:189-199.
9. Grelsamer RP. Patella baja after total knee arthroplasty: is it really patella baja? *J Arthroplasty.* 2002;17:66-69.
10. Martin JW, Whiteside LA. The influence of joint line position on knee stability after condylar knee arthroplasty. *Clin Orthop Relat Res.* 1990;259:146-156.
11. Mihalko WM, Krackow KA. Posterior cruciate ligament effects on the flexion space in total knee arthroplasty. *Clin Orthop Relat Res.* 1999;360:243-250.
12. Partington PF, Sawhney J, Rorabeck CH, Barrack RL, Moore J. Joint line restoration after revision total knee arthroplasty. *Clin Orthop Relat Res.* 1999;367:165-171.
13. Ritter MA, Montgomery TJ, Zhou H, Keating ME, Faris PM, Meding JB. The clinical significance of proximal tibial resection level in total knee arthroplasty. *Clin Orthop Relat Res.* 1999;360:174-181.
14. Ryu J, Saito S, Yamamoto K, Sano S. Factors influencing the postoperative range of motion in total knee arthroplasty. *Bull Hosp Jt Dis.* 1993;53:35-40.
15. Scuderi GR, Insall JN. Total knee arthroplasty. Current clinical perspectives. *Clin Orthop Relat Res.* 1992;276:26-32.
16. Shoji H, Solomonow M, Yoshino S, D'Ambrosia R, Dabezies E. Factors affecting postoperative flexion in total knee arthroplasty. *Orthopedics.* 1990;13:643-649.
17. Singerman R, Heiple KG, Davy DT, Goldberg VM. Effect of tibial component position on patellar strain following total knee arthroplasty. *J Arthroplasty.* 1995;10:651-656.
18. Yoshii I, Whiteside LA, White SE, Milliano MT. Influence of prosthetic joint line position on knee kinematics and patellar position. *J Arthroplasty.* 1991;6:169-177.
19. Carpenter CW, Cummings JF, Grood ES, Leach D, Paganelli JV, Manley MT. The influence of joint line elevation in total knee arthroplasty. *Am J Knee Surg.* 1994;4:164-167.
20. Konig C, Sharenkov A, Matziolis G, et al. Joint line elevation in revision TKA leads to increased patellofemoral contact forces. *J Orthop Res.* 2010;28:1-5.
21. Porteous AJ, Hassaballa MA, Newman JH. Does the joint line matter in revision total knee replacement? *J Bone Joint Surg.* 2008;90:879-884.

22. Mahoney OM, Kinsey TL. Modular femoral offset stems facilitate joint line restoration in revision knee arthroplasty. *Clin Orthop Relat Res.* 2006;446:93-98.

23. Hofmann AA, Kurtin SM, Lyons S, Tanner AM, Bolognesi MP. Clinical and radiographic analysis of accurate restoration of the joint line in revision total knee arthroplasty. *J Arthroplasty.* 2006;21:1154-1162.

24. Kawamura H, Bourne RB. Factors affecting range of flexion after total knee arthroplasty. *J Orthop Sci.* 2001;6:248-252.

25. Servien E, Viskontas D, Giuffre BM, Coolican MR, Parker DA. Reliability of boney landmarks for restoration of the joint line in revision knee arthroplasty. *Knee Surg Sports Traumatol Arthrosc.* 2008;16:263-269.

26. Mason M, Belisle A, Bonutti P, Kolisek FR, Malkani A, Masini M. An accurate and reproducible method for locating the joint line during a revision total knee arthroplasty. *J Arthroplasty.* 2006;21:1147-1153.

27. Havet E, Gabrion A, Leiber-Wackenheim F, Vernois J, Olory B, Mertl P. Radiological study of the knee joint line position measured from the fibular head and proximal tibial landmarks. *Surg Radiol Anat.* 2007;29:285-289.

28. Stiehl JB, Abbott BD. Morphology of the transepicondylar axis and its application in primary and revision total knee arthroplasty. *J Arthroplasty.* 1995;10:785.

29. Griffin FM, Math K, Scuderi GR, Insall JN, Poilvache PL. Anatomy of the epicondyles of the distal femur: MRI analysis of normal knees. *J Arthroplasty.* 2000;15:354-359.

30. Mountney J, Karamfiles R, Breidahl W, Farrugia M, Sikorski JM. The position of the joint line in relation to the trans-epicondylar axis of the knee: complementary radiologic and computer-based studies. *J Arthroplasty.* 2007;22:1201-1207.

31. Romero J, Seifert B, Reinhardt O, Ziegler O, Kessler O. A useful radiologic method for preoperative joint-line determination in revision total knee arthroplasty. *Clin Orthop Relat Res.* 2009;463:97-120.

32. Bellemans J, Banks S, Victor J, et al. Fluoroscopic analysis of the kinematics of deep flexion in total knee arthroplasty. Influence of posterior condylar offset. *J Bone Joint Surg Br.* 2002;84:50.

33. Banks S, Bellemans J, Nozaki H, et al. Knee motion during maximum flexion in fixed and mobile-bearing arthroplasties. *Clin Orthop Relat Res.* 2003;410:131.

34. Sato T, Koga Y, Dobue T, Omori G, Tanabe Y, Sakamoto M. Quantitative 3-dimensional analysis of preoperative and postoperative joint lines in total knee arthroplasty: a new concept for evaluation of component alignment. *J Arthroplasty.* 2007;22:560-568.

35. Laskin RS. Joint line position restoration during revision total knee replacement. *Clin Orthop Relat Res.* 2002;(404):169-171.

36. Mihalko WM, Krackow KA. Flexion and extension gap balancing in revision total knee arthroplasty. *Clin Orthop Relat Res.* 2006;446:121-126.

37. Vince KG, Droll KP, Chivas D. Your next revision total knee arthroplasty: why start in flexion? *Orthopedics.* 2007;30:791-792.

38. Vince KG. A step-wise approach to revision TKA. *Orthopedics.* 2005;28:999-1001.

39. Vince K, Droll K, Chivas D. New concepts in revision total knee arthroplasty. *J Surg Orthop Adv.* 2008;17:165-172.

40. Masini MA, Kester MA. The joint reduction method of revision total knee arthroplasty. *Orthopedics.* 2004;27:813-816.

41. Whiteside LA. Ligament balancing in revision total knee arthroplasty. *Clin Orthop Relat Res.* 2004;(423):178-185.

42. Dennis DA. A stepwise approach to revision total knee arthroplasty. *J Arthroplasty.* 2007;22(4 suppl 1):32-38.

43. Fehring TK, Christie MJ, Lavernia C, et al. Revision total knee arthroplasty: planning, management, and controversies. *Instr Cours Lect.* 2008;57:341-363.

Deciding on Constraint and Hinges in Revision Total Knee Arthroplasty

Dermot Collopy, MBBS, FRACS

The world over, primary and revision total knee replacement (TKR) has become an increasingly common surgical procedure. Continual refinement of surgical technique, together with advances in prosthetic design, has allowed surgeons to achieve predictably good outcomes in the majority of cases.[1,2] TKR function is determined by implant design features, but longevity and performance have been repeatedly shown to be dependent on implant alignment, joint line preservation, mechanical axis restoration, and ligamentous balance.[3-5] Maximal range of motion and predictable kinematics rely on accurate component positioning and correct ligament tensioning.

In primary TKR, these goals are achieved by established surgical technique utilizing precise instrumentation and applying the principles of measured bone resection and gap balancing. However, in the setting of revision TKR, with the challenges posed by altered bony landmarks, deficient ligamentous support, asymmetric bone loss, and perhaps in the aftermath of infection, it is frequently impossible to recreate a stable knee (Figure 9-1). In the presence of poorly balanced or attenuated biological restraints, the surgeon is forced to choose prosthetic components with some degree of "in built" mechanical stability, or constraint, to restore stability and provide predictable kinematics.

Arguments exist as to the relative merits of unconstrained, semiconstrained, and highly constrained devices. History has shown us excessive constraint may result in restricted range of motion, polyethylene wear, and component loosening. Alternatively, insufficient constraint—especially in the setting of compromised soft tissue support—may lead to instability with resultant pain, accelerated wear, and even tibiofemoral dislocation. This chapter attempts to outline the various constraint options available to surgeons and offer some insight into their appropriate use.

Jacofsky DJ, Hedley AK, eds.
Fundamentals of Revision Knee Arthroplasty:
Diagnosis, Evaluation, and Treatment (pp 133-156).
© 2013 SLACK Incorporated.

Figure 9-1. Loosening with subsidence and varus deformity in a cemented unicompartmental tibial component.

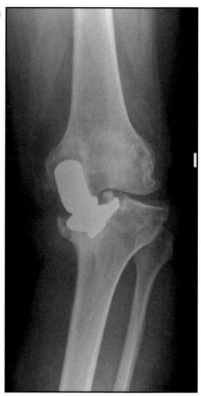

INSTABILITY

Over the past 4 decades, as prosthetic design and surgical techniques have evolved, TKR has become a highly successful procedure with survivorship rates approaching 95% at 10 years.[1,2] Surgeons have long been aware of the potential for patient dissatisfaction if the knee replacement is unstable. However, several recent articles have suggested tibiofemoral instability after total knee arthroplasty (TKA) is becoming an increasingly common entity, accounting for between 22% and 27% of early revision.[6,7]

Stability of the replaced knee is the result of complex interaction between the geometries of the contacting surfaces of the femoral and tibial components, the quality of the existing soft tissue restraints, and the mechanical alignment of the limb. In certain circumstances, if the surface geometries are nonconforming, or when important soft tissue stabilizers are deficient, clinical instability of the arthroplasty may result.[8,9] This can be exacerbated by limb malalignment.[10] Generally speaking, instability patterns are similar for most implant designs, but occasionally, implant-specific instability patterns exist, such as mid-flexion instability with cruciate-retaining (CR) designs, posterior dislocation in cam-and-post posterior stabilized (PS) or varus-valgus constrained designs, and bearing spin out in mobile bearing designs.

Soft Tissue Restraints

In the natural knee, stability is largely afforded not by the contacting joint surfaces but by the soft tissue stabilizers—the ligaments, musculotendinous units, and joint capsule—that connect the femur and tibia. Anatomic variation determines the relative contribution of each structure to the overall stability of the individual knee, but all play a role in providing resistance to angular, translational, and rotational motion.[11-13] The loss of even a single one of these supporting structures can render the knee unstable, the consequences of which may be felt immediately with functional instability, but also longer term, with premature arthritis. Perhaps the best example of this is rupture of the anterior cruciate ligament which results in abnormal tibiofemoral motion, creating excessive shearing forces on the articular surfaces, which over time, leads to meniscal attrition, accelerated articular cartilage breakdown, and ultimately to secondary osteoarthritis. Not surprisingly, in the presence of instability, these same abnormal motion patterns in an artificial knee will produce similar shear forces that are equally destructive to the tibial polyethylene surface.

Numerous anatomic, cadaveric, and clinical studies have attempted to define the exact contribution of each of these supporting structures to the overall stability and alignment of the replaced knee.[13-20] The shared goal of these studies has been to attempt to define a predictable sequence of selective release of these soft tissue restraints to achieve a balanced, well-aligned knee replacement. These studies also give some insight into the potential instability patterns surgeons may actually create in the process of "balancing the knee."

Medial collateral ligament: This is the primary stabilizer of the medial knee and has its stabilizing affect throughout the range of flexion. As it has a broad bony attachment on the medial surface of the proximal tibia, some authors have proposed a functional difference between the anterior and posterior portions of the medial collateral ligament.[19] In the flexed position, because of femoral roll-back, the tibial attachment of the anterior medial collateral ligament fibers lies further from the medial collateral ligament origin on the medial femoral epicondyle, and hence the fibers are more taut and may contribute relatively greater resistance to valgus stress in the flexed position (60 to 90 degrees). The posterior fibers are said to have more of an effect in the extended position (0 to 30 degrees).

Posterior oblique ligament: Similarly, as these posterior fibers of the medial collateral ligament attach more posteriorly on the tibia, they too tighten relatively more in extension (0 to 30 degrees).

Lateral collateral ligament: The primary lateral stabilizer of the knee, the lateral collateral ligament resists varus stress throughout the range of flexion (0 to 90 degrees). It also provides resistance to tibial internal and external rotation, especially in the flexed position.

Iliotibial band: This is taut in extension only and is an important secondary varus stabilizer of the lateral side of the knee in extension (0 to 30 degrees). In the flexed knee, it resists tibial internal rotation but has no varus stabilizing effect.

Popliteus: Provides varus resistance throughout the range of flexion (0 to 90 degrees) and is also an important stabilizer against tibial external rotation.

Posterolateral corner capsule: This is a localized thickening of the posterolateral capsule and attaches immediately behind the lateral collateral ligament, onto the lateral femoral epicondyle. It provides lateral stability throughout the range of flexion, but particularly in extension (0 to 30 degrees).

Posterior joint capsule: Both the medial and lateral posterior capsule provide some medial and lateral restraint, respectively, in extension particularly, but also in flexion.

Etiology of Instability

Instability after TKA may be caused by many factors, including late ligamentous insufficiency, flexion and extension gap mismatch, improper component sizing or positioning, component loosening, bone loss, generalized soft tissue laxity, collateral ligament imbalance, and limb malalignment.[10]

Ligament Attenuation

With increasing age, some individuals experience progressive microstructural changes in elastin, collagen, and other connective tissue elements which may lead to loss of functional integrity of ligamentous and capsular supporting structures. Conditions such as rheumatoid arthritis, collagen

Figure 9-2. Sagittal instability due to late posterior cruciate ligament failure in a cruciate-retaining design.

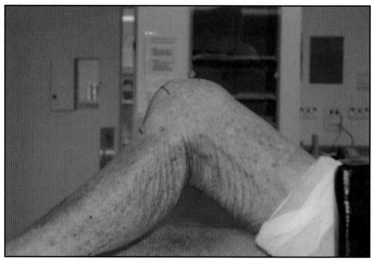

vascular disorders, and long-term steroid usage may produce similar changes. As a result, tissues generally become less supportive, and in the presence of an artificial knee, late ligamentous laxity and joint instability may ensue. This pattern is frequently seen in patients who received relatively unconstrained flat-on-flat or round-on-flat designs from the late 1980s and early 1990s. These patients may present after 10 to 12 years with generalized laxity of the replaced knee, polyethylene wear, and clinical instability. Limited revision with simple upsizing of the polyethylene insert, with the intent of retensioning the soft tissue sleeve, will temporarily improve the situation, but the soft tissue attenuation will recur and further surgery will likely be required.[21] Rather than thicker polyethylene inserts, these cases require the use of a more constrained implant to absorb the forces leading to soft tissue attenuation.

Also, designs that preserve the posterior cruciate ligament theoretically rely on the ligament's continued integrity throughout the life of the prosthesis. Histological studies have suggested this ligament is often damaged by the arthritic disease process,[22,23] and hence late insufficiency, or attrition rupture, may render the knee unstable in the sagittal plane (Figure 9-2).

Flexion-Extension Gap Balance

The concept of flexion-extension gap balance was first introduced by Freeman et al[24] and Insall et al[25] in the late 1960s and early 1970s, and still remains the cornerstone of TKA technique today. Precise bone resections from the posterior and distal femoral condyles, and from the proximal tibial plateau, create cut bone surfaces that are perpendicular to the neutral mechanical axis of the limb. The "gap" thus created will be later filled by the prosthetic components, thereby retensioning the soft tissue sleeve. Even tension in the respective collateral ligaments will only be created if this gap is of equal dimension on the medial and lateral side of the knee (ie, is rectangular in shape). If instead this gap is asymmetrical and trapezoidal in shape, then the ligaments will not be evenly tensioned, and the gap is said to be unbalanced (Figure 9-3). To achieve equal ligament tension throughout the range of motion, this gap must remain rectangular and of equal dimension in both extension and 90 degrees of flexion (and theoretically at every angle in between). If this is not the case, then the flexion or extension gap (or both) will be lax, and instability may ensue.

Component Size and Positioning

Accurate component sizing is required to restore the joint articular profile, to allow adequate bony support for reliable component fixation, and to reestablish correct posterior femoral condylar

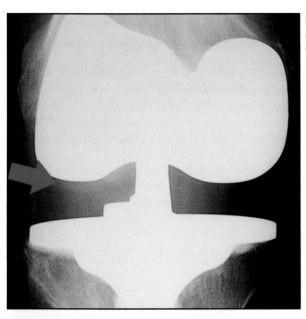

Figure 9-3. Lateral condylar lift-off due to an asymmetric extension gap from inadequate medial release in a varus knee.

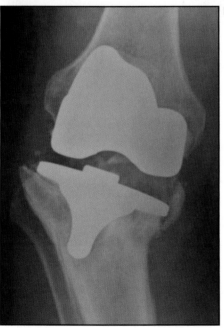

Figure 9-4. Varus subsidence of a loose tibial component.

offset, which is necessary to achieve a balanced flexion gap. In the revision scenario, femoral component undersizing may lead to underfilling of the flexion gap, with resultant sagittal instability. Similarly, under- or overresection of bone from the posterior or distal femur may create an unequal flexion or extension gap.

Loosening and Bone Loss

With septic or aseptic loosening, component subsidence may occur, which can contribute to instability. This is typically seen in asymmetric (usually varus) subsidence of a loose tibial component or proximal migration of a loose femoral component (Figure 9-4).

Gap Imbalance: The Final Common Pathway to Instability

With all these concepts in mind, Krackow[10] outlined a very practical approach to the diagnosis and management of instability in TKA. He characterized all instability as being due either to collateral ligament imbalance (so-called *gap asymmetry*) or to flexion-extension gap mismatch (so-called *gap inequality*). Hence, by paying close attention to gap symmetry and flexion-extension gap parity, surgeons should be able to recognize intraoperative factors that may contribute to postoperative instability. In cases of mild deformity, sequential soft tissue releases allow a variable but usually predictable approximation of flexion-extension gap balance and mediolateral gap symmetry, at both 0 and 90 degrees flexion. However, this becomes less predictable in cases of increased angular deformity or in post-traumatic situations, such as following high tibial osteotomy (HTO) or peri-articular malunions. And gap balance and gap symmetry at 30 and 60 degrees can be quite different to 0 and 90 degrees. Many of us have learned the hard way that "sequential release" can quickly turn into "complete instability," particularly in the tight valgus knee, when that last little nick in the posterolateral corner suddenly releases everything remaining, and the lateral flexion gap springs open and the knee becomes highly unstable to varus stress, particularly at 90 degrees flexion.

Classification

Most surgeons like to think of instability according to the knee position in which the instability pattern is manifest. Hence, 4 four main instability patterns are as follows:
1. Extension instability
2. Flexion instability
3. Recurvatum
4. Global instability

Extension Instability

Varus-valgus instability is usually manifest in the extended position, and this pattern is easily recognized on clinical examination. Collateral ligament insufficiency or imbalance is the main cause, and commonly results from the incomplete release of contracted structures on the concave side of the deformity (see Figure 9-3). Occasionally, overly aggressive release of these same tight structures may result in the opposite problem—iatrogenic laxity. Slow attenuation of the collateral ligaments can occur over time, especially if the mechanical axis was not corrected at the time of the index procedure. Very occasionally, trauma may result in a complete rupture of a collateral ligament.

Flexion Instability

Sagittal plane laxity is best demonstrated at 90 degrees of flexion and is manifest as excessive posterior tibial subluxation (see Figure 9-2). This instability may be well tolerated in low-demand patients but will cause symptoms in modest and high-demand patients, especially with activities such as stair descent or when arising from a seated position.[8] It is often the result of an unbalanced flexion gap or posterior cruciate ligament insufficiency in a CR knee. This can be compounded by an excessively sloped tibial cut or an undersized femoral component with inadequate posterior condylar offset.

Recurvatum

Excessive knee hyperextension is usually the result of extensor mechanism insufficiency due to quadriceps weakness (from neuromuscular conditions such as polio and spinal stenosis) or to infrapatellar tendon rupture. It can also be iatrogenic from excessive resection of bone from the distal femur. Recurvatum is often progressive and may lead to more generalized laxity and instability.

Global Instability

Instability in more than one plane usually leads to gradual attenuation of the entire soft tissue envelope of the knee with resultant complex, multidirectional instability. Global laxity is typically a combination of recurvatum, varus-valgus extension instability, and sagittal plane flexion instability.

PROSTHETIC CONSTRAINT

Instability occurs when the available ligaments and soft tissues, in combination with prosthetic articular design and limb alignment, are unable to provide the stability necessary for adequate function in the presence of physiological stresses across the knee joint.[26] To address deficient biological soft tissue restraint, implants with varying degrees of inherent mechanical constraint have been developed. These designs achieve stability by complex interaction of the surface topography of the contacting femoral condylar and intercondylar regions with the matching tibial polyethylene surfaces.

Three basic mechanisms are employed by design engineers to enhance inherent mechanical prosthetic constraint:

1. Increased conformity between contacting curved femoral and tibial condylar surfaces.
2. Addition of a vertical polyethylene extension from the central tibia, which engages within a modified intercondylar section of the femoral component.
3. Formal linkage of the femoral and tibial components via an axial hinge connection.

Conforming Surface Geometries

By altering the degree of conformity between the curved profiles of femoral and tibial prosthetic surfaces, design engineers can influence the intrinsic mechanical stability (constraint) of the knee design.

For many years now, the femoral component sagittal profile has been near-anatomic, and despite marketing hype to the contrary, little difference exists between many designs. Instead, it has been the concave sagittal geometry of the tibial polyethylene insert that has seen most variation in design philosophy. Early-generation posterior cruciate ligament-retaining tibial designs were quite flat in the sagittal plane, working under the assumption the retained posterior cruciate ligament would consistently induce rollback, and the flattened insert would permit physiologic rotation during flexion. Relying solely on soft tissue stabilizers to restrain motion, these round-on-flat and flat-on-flat designs offered little resistance to rotational and translational forces and often suffered from markedly abnormal kinematics, which contributed to disappointing failure rates as a result of wear and instability.

More contemporary tibial insert designs have seen a subtle reintroduction of increased sagittal curvature to enhance conformity with the femoral component. Some knee systems have gone one step further and offer inserts with additional height of polyethylene material anteriorly and posteriorly (conforming or deep-dish inserts) to better resist paradoxical anterior femoral translation. This greater conformity is beneficial for increased anteroposterior and rotational stability, but may come at the cost of reduced motion and increased shear stress transmission to the prosthetic-cement-bone interfaces. To counter the kinematic conflict inherent in these highly conforming designs, companies have developed patented design features to permit physiologic rotation. Femoral components with a single coronal plane mediolateral curvature or tibial polyethylene inserts with an elliptical rotary arc are 2 examples of design innovations that permit tibiofemoral rotation in the presence of enhanced sagittal constraint. Other designs have gone to mobile-bearing tibial components to achieve this.

Figure 9-5. Intercondylar stabilized designs, showing (A) a box-and-cam design and (B) a post-and-box housing design.

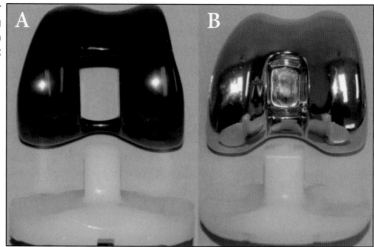

Intercondylar Stabilization

An alternate technique to achieve enhanced mechanical constraint in total knee design is by the creation of additional surfaces of contact between the articulating femoral and tibial components with the goal of guiding or resisting motion in one or more directions. This is achieved through a vertical tibial polyethylene post or spine articulating against a transverse intercondylar femoral cam or engaging within an intercondylar box housing (Figure 9-5).

Early condylar knee designs were plagued by posterior instability with a tendency for progressive posterior tibial subluxation and reduced range of motion due to posterior impingement.[27] To counter this, engineers developed a post-and-cam mechanism to act as a physical stop to posterior tibial translation, with resultant increased motion and improved stability.[27] In its first iteration, as the Total Condylar II design, this posterior femoral cam was part of an intercondylar box housing. However, it was soon recognized that uncontrolled contact of the tibial post with the roof and anterior cam of the femoral box housing sometimes occurred. This undesirable contact was eliminated by converting the intercondylar box housing to a single transverse intercondylar cam, and thus the Posterior-Stabilized Total Condylar Prosthesis was born (later to evolve into the highly successful Insall-Burstein knee). Many iterations of this original post-and-cam mechanism now exist, and all have subtle differences in design and kinematics. Most devices aim for cam-post contact somewhere between 60 and 90 degrees of flexion, after which the femur will be guided posteriorly through further flexion. Design variables such as relative anteroposterior location of the post, post height, post angulation, cam location, cam profile, and anterior femoral flange location have all been shown to potentially adversely influence knee function and longevity.

Despite problems, the original concept of a tibial post engaging within a femoral intercondylar box housing was not completely abandoned, once it was appreciated that additional contact between the post and the box sidewalls may be beneficial in patients with varus-valgus instability.[27] Thus the Total Condylar III was born, with a taller, more robust tibial post that conformed tightly to the internal dimensions of the femoral box housing. Later iterations included the constrained condylar knees, the varus-valgus constrained, and total stabilized designs. All permit only very limited varus-valgus and rotational play, yet allow unrestricted flexion. While successful in limiting varus-valgus, sagittal, and rotational instability in many situations, these intercondylar-stabilized designs have inherent problems due to their increased constraint. Component loosening, tibial post wear and breakage, locking mechanism failure, and tibiofemoral dislocations have all been reported.

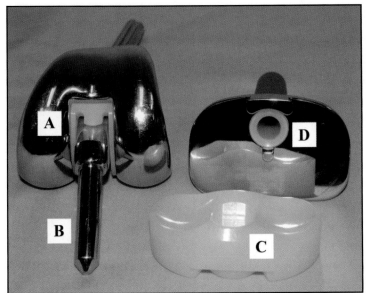

Figure 9-6. An example of a modern rotating hinge design showing an (A) intercondylar linkage, (B) vertical hinge extension arm, (C) mobile polyethylene bearing with conforming surface geometry, and (D) central tibial well within a tibial tray.

Prosthetic Linkage (Hinge Designs)

The last engineering method of introducing additional constraint and conferring stability is to formally link the femoral and tibial components, usually via an axial hinge mechanism through the condylar body of the femoral component. Depending on the designed rigidity of the linkage, these hinged designs can be rigid and permit virtually no varus-valgus or rotational play, or they can be sloppy and permit 2 to 5 degrees of varus-valgus and rotation motion. Hinged knees have been available since the 1950s, but the first- and second-generation designs had disappointingly high failure rates as a consequence of their excessive rigidity, primarily from loosening and infection. With the introduction of the sloppy hinge and more recently the rotating hinge, improved results have been obtained (Figure 9-6).

ADVANTAGES OF CONSTRAINT

Early generation knee arthroplasty designs of the 1950s and 1960s often failed as a result of excessive constraint, with high rates of tibial loosening and poor range of motion reported. Designs then moved away from significant constraint and an era of low conformity ensued, with flat-on-flat and curved-on-flat designs emerging in the 1980s and early 1990s. Although they delivered improved range of motion, these unconstrained designs frequently demonstrated markedly abnormal kinematics.

Improved Kinematics

Despite the best efforts of design engineers for more than 4 decades, TKAs still fail to replicate normal knee kinematics. With the introduction of increased sagittal curvature and conformity and by the use of intercondylar post-cam contacts, designers have attempted to improve triplanar stability and diminish abnormal motion in these partially constrained designs. Multiple studies using in vivo fluoroscopic analysis of well-functioning TKR have repeatedly demonstrated markedly abnormal kinematics including reduced posterior femoral rollback, paradoxical anterior femoral translation, reverse axial rotation patterns, and femoral condylar lift-off.[28-31] CR designs performed worst of all. Inserts with additional constraint, while by no means perfect, did show less

Figure 9-7. Gross loosening with osteolysis in a fixed-hinge device.

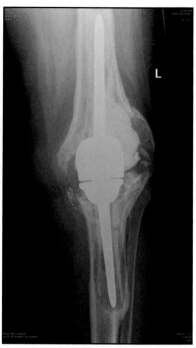

variability in motion paths and less variation between different surgeons. Ultracongruent mobile-bearing designs proved more predictable than either PS or CR designs.

Lower Failure Rate

Several papers have looked at survivorship and reoperation rates for revision knee arthroplasty patients and have shown variable survivorship of different constraint groups.[32,33] All have shown better results with revision undertaken with more constrained inserts. Numerous series have shown revision with CR (unconstrained) inserts have a higher failure rate.[34,35]

DISADVANTAGES OF CONSTRAINT

As a direct result of the intentional increased contact between articulating surfaces in constrained inserts, the components experience greatly increased shear and rotational torque forces. In the normal knee, soft tissue restraints would modulate and dissipate these forces, but in the revision arthroplasty with deficient soft tissue supports, these forces are born directly by the constraining mechanisms—the conforming tibial polyethylene surface, the post of the cam-post mechanism, or the axial hinge of the linked components. Not surprisingly, we have seen failure scenarios as a consequence of these increased forces.

Loosening

Constrained implants experience high torsional and shear loads, which are transferred by the prosthetic linkages, or condylar surfaces, to the implant fixation interfaces, either the prosthesis-bone interface in uncemented knee or the cement-bone interface in cemented implants. If this cyclical loading exceeds a certain threshold, it will lead to premature loosening of the implant.[36] The greater the degree of constraint, the more likely this loosening will develop. This was the case with early hinged knee implants of the 1950s and 1960s, which were rigid uniaxial hinge designs with no rotation nor varus-valgus laxity. Loosening was common (Figure 9-7). Complication rates

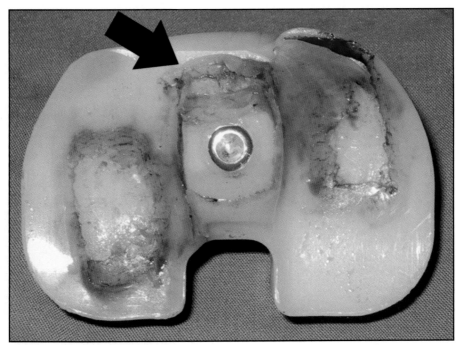

Figure 9-8. Significant post wear, especially on its anterior surface, from adverse contact against anterior femoral flange in extension.

of between 23%[37] and 70%,[38] loosening rates of 27% at 1 to 3 years,[39] and implant breakage rates of up to 10%[40] have been reported. Contemporary design hinged devices now permit axial rotation and have demonstrated improved results.[41,42] Even in nonlinked constrained devices, numerous reports cite a significant incidence of progressive radiolucent lines and aseptic loosening of both cemented and uncemented femoral and tibial components, with a quoted incidence of between 30% and 70%.[36,43-45]

Post Wear

Intentional contact between the tibial polyethylene post and the cam or box housing confers increased mechanical stability in situations with compromised soft tissue support. However, it is recognized that certain circumstances may lead to excessive post-cam or post-box contact, with deleterious results. This was first reported soon after the PS design was introduced by Insall and coworkers in the mid 1970s.[25] Many articles have appeared over the past decade documenting the adverse sequelae of unintentional post contact against the surfaces of the intercondylar box, and significant polyethylene wear and post deformation have been consistently observed[46] (Figure 9-8). Repetitive contact of the distal edge of the femoral component anterior flange against the base of the tibial spine (at heel strike and with knee hyperextension) leads to polyethylene scoring, fatigue failure, and post breakage in both PS[47,48] and constrained condylar designs.[49,50] Factors that predispose implants to this are design and technique dependent[51,52] and include flexed femoral component orientation, excessive posterior tibial slope, relative anterior location of tibial spine, or excessive extension gap with resultant recurvatum.

Backside Wear

Contemporary revision knee systems all offer modular tibial polyethylene inserts to allow surgeons flexibility in addressing variable flexion-extension gap dimensions, as well as provide

Figure 9-9. Locking mechanism failure with tibial insert dislodgement.

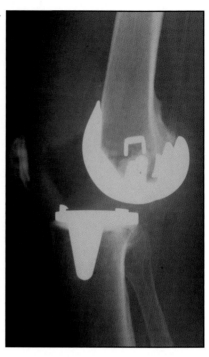

inserts with a choice of constraint. These inserts engage into the metal tibial baseplate by a variety of locking mechanisms. While effective in the broad sense, no current locking mechanism design is infallible, and varying degrees of motion occur between the baseplate and the polyethylene insert,[53] with the potential for abrasive wear of the undersurface of the tibial insert (also known as backside wear) and osteolysis. Wasielewski[54] showed in a laboratory study that inserts with increasing levels of constraint exhibit greater shear motion.

Locking Mechanism Failure

In a similar manner, the locking mechanism is required to absorb the increased anteroposterior, varus-valgus, and rotational forces imparted to it by the contacting femorotibial surfaces. Despite recent improvements in rigidity of locking mechanisms, reports of cases of locking mechanism failure, with or without tibial insert dislodgement, have appeared in the literature (Figure 9-9). As a result, some designs incorporate vertical metal rods and/or locking screws within the tibial post to act both as a secondary locking mechanism and also to reinforce the tibial post and provide resistance to polyethylene deformation. Numerous reports of loosening and dislodgement of these locking screws have appeared in the literature, both in PS designs[55] and constrained condylar designs.[56]

Dislocation

In both PS and constrained condylar designs, the tibial post serves a dual purpose. It provides a rigid stop against unwanted posterior tibial subluxation and also guides femoral rollback through its interaction with the transverse intercondylar cam. In many implant designs, as the femur moves into deeper flexion (90 degrees and beyond), the cam rides superiorly along the posterior surface of the tibial spine. It is possible for the cam to ride up and over the spine, resulting in a posterior dislocation of the tibia on the femur.[57] This usually only occurs in cases of excessive, unbalanced flexion gap or combined flexion-rotation laxity. The cam jump height varies between designs[58] and is influenced by the post height, cam position, the post anteroposterior placement, the radius of curvature of the posterior femoral condyles, and the cam geometry. Increased knee flexion angles beyond 90 degrees usually result in decreasing jump height and the risk of posterior dislocation increases with deep flexion.

CONSTRAINT OPTIONS IN MODULAR INSERTS

Since the advent of modular tibial trays, most manufacturers have offered surgeons some choice of tibial articular surface geometry. Recent times have seen a move to offer a choice for the level of constraint as well.

Unconstrained

Cruciate-Retaining Insert

CR inserts are minimally conforming in the sagittal plane, with at most a modest anterior lip and frequently a very minimally dished mid and posterior plateau. Newer high-flex designs often have even less posterior sagittal profile (also known as *posterior relief*) to permit greater bicondylar rollback and tibial rotation in deep flexion.

By convention, all CR inserts are designed for primary TKR situations, and their success is predicated on the presence of competent, functional collateral and posterior cruciate ligament structures together with a balanced flexion and extension gap. As outlined earlier in this chapter, even in ideal circumstances, CR designs may exhibit unpredictable kinematics. The place for the use of CR inserts in revision TKR—either as an isolated polyethylene exchange or as part of a full revision—is therefore limited. Published results of isolated polyethylene exchange for the treatment of instability is reasonably damning. Pagnano et al[8] reported a series of patients with flexion instability, 3 of whom were managed by isolated tibial poly exchange, and 2 of the 3 inserts failed and were rerevised. In a similar series, Engh et al[34] performed isolated exchange on 8 patients with flexion instability, and only stabilized 4. Babis et al,[35] in a larger series from the Mayo Clinic, reported on 27 patients treated for instability with isolated polyethylene exchange and showed an overall failure rate of 44% and a rerevision rate of 30% at average 3-year follow-up.

Indication

The indications for use of a CR insert in revision TKR remains the same as for a primary TKR: competent, functional collateral and posterior cruciate ligament structures together with balanced flexion and extension gaps. The definition of balanced flexion-extension gaps is a little vague, as surgeons may differ in the degree of ligament tension and mild gap asymmetry they will accept. However, as a useful figure, most surgeons would ideally accept only 2 to 3 mm of gap asymmetry and 2 to 3 mm of flexion-extension gap inequality when choosing CR inserts. In elderly or low-demand patients, having revision for polyethylene wear with minimal instability—or in cases of revision of a failed unicompartmental knee—these criteria may be met. However, in most other scenarios, the author would advise revision to a design with an increased level of constraint.

Semiconstrained

Posterior Stabilized Insert

These inserts were also designed for primary TKR, and again require intact collateral ligaments and balanced flexion-extension gaps.[59] These inserts typically have a slightly more dished design when compared to CR inserts, as the cam-post mechanism will drive rollback even in the presence

Figure 9-10. Posterior stabilized designs do not provide any varus-valgus nor rotational constraint, and post dislocation may occur in the presence of poor flexion gap balance.

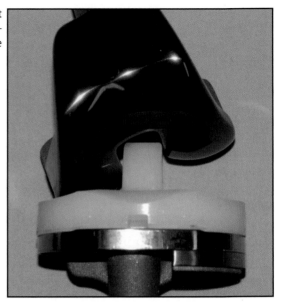

of a small posterior lip. The relative location of the tibial post and femoral cam dictate the flexion angle of cam engagement as well as the motion path of the cam against the post. In many designs, as the knee goes into deeper flexion, the cam unavoidably travels superiorly on the post, and the threshold for dislocation reduces.[57] Hence, many newer designs attempt to maintain cam-post contact near the base of the post.

Although differences in cam-and-post mechanics exist, most PS designs address moderate sagittal plane instability when due to functional incompetence or surgical excision of the posterior cruciate ligament (hence the alternate name, posterior cruciate-substituting design). These PS designs will not be sufficient to address sagittal plane instability due to an unbalanced or asymmetric flexion gap, and it is vital this fact is understood. Most complications of PS design knees occur as a direct result of inadequate flexion gap balance, where significant varus-valgus and rotational motion can occur in mid and late flexion and the tibial post is exposed to uncontrolled contact within the femoral box housing (Figure 9-10). As a result, post wear, locking mechanism failure, and cam-post dislocation may occur.

Indication

For a PS insert to be used in a revision, it is the author's preference for well-balanced flexion-extension gaps to be present, with less than 2 to 3 mm of gap asymmetry and 2 to 3 mm of flexion-extension gap inequality. Any gap asymmetry greater than that risks recurrence of varus-valgus instability, and more than 2 to 3 mm of flexion laxity risks post wear and dislocation. This is supported by other authors.[59]

Deep-Dish Inserts

An alternate bearing available in cases of moderate sagittal instability is the ultracongruent or deep-dish insert. As the name implies, these inserts have augmented anterior and posterior sagittal profiles (Figure 9-11) to provide increased resistance to anterior femoral translation in early and mid-flexion and posterior tibial subluxation at 90 degrees. Because of their increased conformity, they provide some limited resistance to rotation as well. Conceptually, these inserts represent a hybrid of cruciate-preserving and cruciate-sacrificing design philosophies. They have recently become more popular and may provide a similar PS effect without the need for a cam-and-post mechanism.[60]

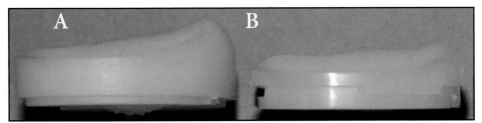

Figure 9-11. Example of (A) a deep-dish insert compared to (B) a cruciate-retaining insert. Note the additional 4 to 7 mm of polyethylene material anteriorly to resist anterior femoral translation.

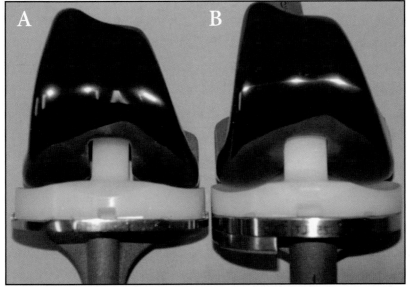

Figure 9-12. Comparison of tibial post dimensions and relative "fill" of intercondylar housing in (A) a posterior stabilized design and (B) a constrained condylar insert.

Indication

These inserts are typically used when a CR knee has developed posterior instability, due either to posterior cruciate ligament incompetence at the time of primary surgery or as a result of late posterior cruciate ligament attrition failure. As with their semiconstrained cousin, the PS insert, these deep-dish conforming inserts require a well-balanced flexion gap.

Highly Constrained

Constrained Condylar Insert

By increasing the height and width of the tibial polyethylene post and making it conform tightly to the internal dimensions of the femoral intercondylar box housing, design engineers have produced modular inserts with enhanced mechanical stability (Figure 9-12). Variously known as constrained condylar or varus-valgus constrained designs, these inserts provide significant resistance to angular, rotational, and translational forces and are the most highly constrained modular inserts available. They are sometimes incorrectly referred to as *nonlinked hinges*.

Although some variation exists between designs, the majority of these constrained condylar implants permit only 2 to 5 degrees of varus-valgus angulation and a similar amount of rotational constraint. Surgeons should be aware that the degree of tibial post engagement within the femoral box housing may vary, and with increasing flexion, the post may become uncovered and no longer fully captured by the box housing. This is especially true in designs where the tibial post is relatively anteriorly positioned or is rounded or beveled. Some variation in post height exists between different designs, but post height alone does not dictate varus-valgus constraint, nor resistance to dislocation. Also, many modern constrained condylar designs have additional topographical features to further enhance rotational constraint, with significantly greater sagittal and coronal conformity in both the flexed and extended positions when compared to the less-constrained CR and PS insert designs. These features have been added in an attempt to load-share and reduce forces on the tibial post.

Constrained condylar designs provide sufficient mechanical stability to be used in situations where the normal soft tissue stabilizers are significantly compromised, such as in cases with attenuation of either or both collateral ligaments, cases where major bone loss has compromised soft tissue attachments, or cases requiring extensive release to correct major angular deformities. Constrained condylar designs are also useful in situations where it is difficult or impossible to balance flexion and extension gaps, such as the multiply-operated knee or the globally unstable knee.

In some revision scenarios, the requirement for absolute intrinsic mechanical prosthetic constraint is only short lived, existing for the first few months after surgery, and here the post acts as an internal brace, neutralizing varus-valgus and rotational forces while healing of the soft tissue envelope occurs. In other situations, the soft tissue restraints will never repair themselves and the implants are required to provide intrinsic mechanical constraint for the life of the prosthesis. It is in these cases that we sometimes see failure of these devices. Complete loss of the functional integrity of the medial collateral ligament—either through attrition, trauma, or iatrogenic injury—induces a complex multidirectional instability pattern, with varus-valgus instability in extension and flexion coupled with rotational laxity. In this setting, a constrained condylar implant will provide adequate initial stability, but with the passage of time, recurrent instability invariably develops, often with catastrophic consequences.[41]

Indication

Constrained condylar devices are indicated in cases with major collateral ligament insufficiency, in situations when moderate flexion-extension imbalance exists, and in cases requiring correction of major angular deformity. Once again, individual surgeons' criteria may differ, but flexion gap laxity greater than 4 to 5 mm, but less than 10 mm, and angular deformity greater than 15 degrees valgus or 20 degrees varus are best treated with a constrained condylar device.

HINGE DESIGNS

It is interesting to note that hinge-style designs were in fact the very first TKRs to enjoy commercial success, and Walldius[61] is credited with introducing one of the first of these in 1951. They have remained popular in Europe, but surgeons in North America and elsewhere quickly became disillusioned with the hinge concept because of high rates of early and midterm failure (see Figure 9-7). They instead embraced the more anatomic condylar-style total knee designs that were emerging in the mid-1970s and were showing favorable results. Over the past 15 years, however, hinge designs have enjoyed somewhat of a resurgence in popularity, as arthroplasty surgeons are faced with an ever-increasing number and complexity of revision cases, often with greater and greater degrees of instability.

Hinge Concept

The basic concept of all hinge designs is that the implants are inherently stable to varus-valgus and translational forces, requiring none of the collateral ligament or joint capsular support so vital

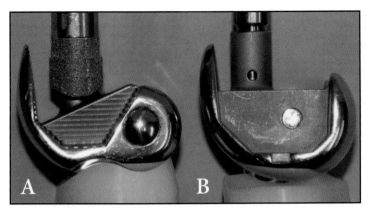

Figure 9-13. (A) Transcondylar hinge designs require considerably greater posterior bone resection than (B) intercondylar hinge designs.

to the stability of less constrained devices. Instead, these implants achieve their mechanical stability by direct linkage of the femoral and tibial components, usually by some form of axial hinge mechanism.[62]

In fixed hinge (or rigid hinge) designs, this linkage is via a simple uniaxial hinge mechanism, allowing unrestricted flexion and extension on this axis but permitting no rotation. Alternatively, in rotating hinge designs, this horizontal uniaxial hinge is coupled with a secondary articulation that permits rotation, usually via a vertical hinge extension fitting into a hollow recess within the tibial component (see Figure 9-6). By allowing axial rotation, these rotating hinge designs reduce torsional force transmission to the hinge mechanism and to the implant-bone fixation interfaces, thereby reducing wear and loosening. The linkage mechanism may span the full width of the femoral component, termed a *transcondylar linkage*, or it may be a less cumbersome hinge mechanism completely contained within the intercondylar region, also called an *intercondylar linkage* (Figure 9-13).

Historical Perspective

Traditionally, we recognize 3 distinct eras in the evolution of hinge knee design. The first-generation designs included Walldius (1951), Shiers (1953), Young (1958), Stanmore (1969), and GUEPAR (1969), and these were all highly constrained rigid hinges with metal-on-metal hinge articulations. Unfortunately, to varying degrees, all were characterized by high failure rates as a result of loosening (see Figure 9-7), implant failure, or infection (the last almost certainly a result of chronic effusions from metal particulate debris caused by fretting at the metal hinge). It soon became apparent the rigid hinge concept was problematic, and so second-generation designs gradually appeared with improved materials that avoided metal-on-metal bearings wherever possible. All had an allowance for some rotational freedom, and the Sheehan (1971), Sphereocentric (1973), and Attenborough (1974) knees were later joined by the Noiles and Kinematic knees (both in the late 1970s). These designs enjoyed improved success but were still plagued by higher than desired complications, especially loosening and patellofemoral problems.[63,64] So current third-generation devices, such as the S-ROM hinge, the Finn knee, and the NextGen RH knee, have moved further and further away from the old fixed hinge design, and now have multiple size options, load-sharing highly conforming condylar profiles, modular augments and stem extensions, and even metaphyseal-filling sleeves (Figure 9-14).

Design Features of the Modern Hinge Knee

It is useful to briefly review several design features inherent to all modern hinge designs, as they each have a bearing on ultimate knee function.[62]

Figure 9-14. Examples of different rotating hinge designs: (A) Kinematic Rotating Hinge, (B) S-ROM, and (C) NextGen RH Knee.

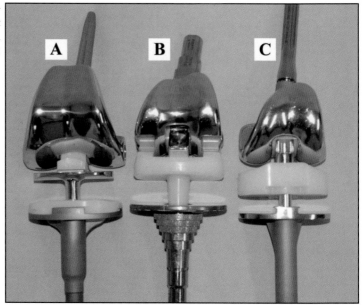

Linkage Mechanism

As outlined previously, the femoral and tibial components are linked directly via some form of axial hinge mechanism. In transcondylar linkages, this usually constitutes a robust axle that passes from the medial to the lateral condylar bodies and transfixes a vertical tibial post. These bulky metal condylar replacements require considerable distal and posterior bone removal (see Figure 9-13), especially if the axis of flexion approximates the epicondylar axis. The intercondylar linkage is an alternative design that is less bulky, but some authors have expressed concern that these linkages may not be sufficiently robust in certain situations.[62]

Location of Flexion Axis

If the anatomic axis of flexion is maintained close to the epicondylar axis, tibiofemoral and patellofemoral kinematics are optimal. However, some transcondylar linkage designs have shifted this flexion axis distally and posteriorly in an attempt to limit excessive bone resection. This may introduce adverse kinematics, with "booking" and patellofemoral tracking issues.

Mechanism of Rotation and Rotation Limits

Tibial internal and external rotation usually occurs around a vertical hinge extension post passing out of the intercondylar region and fitting within a well in the tibial baseplate. This is usually a post-in-cylinder mechanism (see Figure 9-6), and considerable variation exists among different designs in the shape and relative material of each element (see Figure 9-14). The length and cylindrical conformity of this post has been shown to have a bearing on the resistance to dislocation of the mechanism.[65] Studies have shown designs with shorter, tapered post extension, especially if made of polyethylene alone, have a greater tendency to bearing dissociation.[65] Many modern designs also incorporate some form of limit to polyethylene insert rotation, which has helped somewhat reduce the incidence of patellofemoral instability.

Load Transfer

Virtually all early hinge designs saw 100% of the tibiofemoral load transmission borne by the axial hinge, and as a result, many of these devices suffered from hinge wear or condylar breakage. Newer designs have incorporated features of the ultraconforming constrained condylar designs

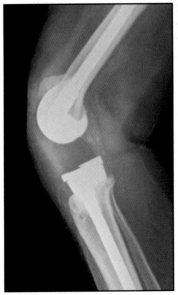

Figure 9-15. An example of a situation requiring use of a hinged device to compensate for extreme soft tissue attenuation and chronic extensor mechanism disruption.

discussed previously, with full contact between the highly conforming femoral and tibial condyles throughout the range of motion (see Figures 9-13 and 9-14).

Bone Preservation

Depending on the type and location of the component linkage and the position of the flexion axis, a variable amount of femoral bone will need to be resected to allow implant seating (see Figure 9-14). Early transcondylar hinge designs require considerable distal and posterior femoral bone removal. While the newer intercondylar linkages avoid this, the size of the intercondylar bone cut-out required for their implantation may also be problematic, especially in smaller patients.

Advantages

Because of the high degree of intrinsic mechanical stability, these modern hinge designs are ideal in revision cases with severely compromised soft tissues. Surgeons are able to accept incompletely balanced flexion and extension gaps, and disregard collateral ligament insufficiency and recurvatum. These devices provide reliable varus-valgus and rotational stability, even in the complete absence of the medial collateral ligament.

Disadvantages

Loosening, implant dissociation, and patellofemoral disorders are the most common complications seen when employing these devices. As with the constrained condylar devices discussed earlier, the additional forces absorbed by the component linkage are necessarily transferred to the component bone fixation interfaces, with the potential for loosening. Most authors advise these devices be used with at least mid-length cemented stems or long diaphyseal engaging press-fit stems.[36] While these devices are ideal for use in patients with unbalanced flexion gaps, it is possible for even hinged devices to dissociate or dislocate; however, this usually only occurs in cases with extreme global soft tissue attenuation, gross extensor mechanism deficiency (Figure 9-15), or following tumor resection.

CONSTRAINT TIPS

POSTERIOR CRUCIATE LIGAMENT DEFICIENCY	This is adequately compensated for by use of either a PS (post-and-cam) device or a deep-dish highly conforming device. Very important to distinguish sagittal instability due to posterior cruciate ligament (PCL) deficiency from sagittal instability due to an unbalanced flexion gap. The latter requires use of a constrained condylar device.
LATERAL COLLATERAL LIGAMENT DEFICIENCY	Often surprisingly well tolerated with minimally constrained devices, as long as limb alignment is neutral. Otherwise requires a constrained condylar device.
LOOSE FLEXION GAP	Probably one of the most commonly unrecognized problems that leads to failure and early revision. Rule of thumb: ■ Mild laxity (3 to 5 mm) requires correction of gap imbalance and a PS device. ■ Moderate gap laxity (5 to 10 mm) requires constrained condylar device. ■ Extreme flexion gap laxity (greater than 15 to 20 mm) necessitates a hinge.
MEDIAL COLLATERAL LIGAMENT DEFICIENCY	■ Again, one of the common recurring errors of surgeon judgment. ■ An attenuated but intact medial collateral ligament requires a constrained condylar device. ■ Complete functional absence of the medial collateral ligament requires a hinge....every time!
LOOSE EXTENSION GAP	Recurvatum, if not correctable by distal femoral augmentation, requires a hinge.
EXTENSOR MECHANISM DEFICIENCY	Chronic extensor mechanism disruption is often associated with circumferential soft tissue attenuation and global instability. This requires a hinged device or knee fusion.

Indications

Hinge implants are most commonly indicated in cases with extreme flexion gap imbalance (greater than 15 to 20 mm) or where complete absence of the medial collateral ligament exists. Chronic extensor mechanism disruption or deficiency also requires a hinged device to resist the hyperextension instability that frequently develops in these cases. They are also useful in situations of massive bone loss.

SUMMARY

As the volume and complexity of revision TKR cases continue to rise, surgeons are increasingly faced with cases involving severely compromised bone and soft tissue support. To address these situations, revision implants are required with varying degrees of inherent mechanical constraint. Experienced surgeons differ in their approach to constraint: some espouse a minimalist philosophy and advocate the use of the least constraint possible; others believe more is better. The author feels the correct answer lies somewhere between these extremes. The surgeon must choose the appropriate level of constraint in any particular situation to ensure a stable knee with predictable kinematics while taking care to minimize the adverse consequences of the chosen level of constraint. This involves consideration of component size and positioning, careful attention to flexion-extension gap balancing, augmentation or reconstruction of deficient bone stock, and the use of appropriate length and fixation of stem extensions. Most importantly, the surgeon must undertake a critical assessment of the final on-table stability of the knee before the level of constraint is chosen.

REFERENCES

1. Ranawat CS, Flynn WF Jr, Saddler S, Hansraj KK, Maynard MJ. Long-term results of the total condylar knee arthroplasty. A 15-year survivorship study. *Clin Orthop Relat Res.* 1993;286:94-102.
2. Ritter MA, Berend ME, Meding JB, Keating EM, Faris PM, Crites BM. Long-term followup of anatomic graduated components posterior cruciate-retaining total knee replacement. *Clin Orthop Relat Res.* 2001;388:51-57.
3. Benjamin J. Component alignment in total knee arthroplasty. *AAOS Instr Course Lect.* 2006;55:405-412.
4. Berend M, Ritter MS, Meding J, et al. Tibial component failure mechanisms in total knee arthroplasty. *Clin Orthop Relat Res.* 2004;428:26-34.
5. Ritter MA, Faris PM, Keating M, Meding J. Postoperative alignment of total knee replacement: its effect on survival. *Clin Orthop Relat Res.* 1994;299:153-156.
6. Fehring TK, Odum S, Griffin WL, Mason JB, Nadaud M. Early failures in total knee arthroplasty. *Clin Orthop Relat Res.* 2001;392:315-318.
7. Sharkey PF, Hozack WJ, Rothman RH, Shastri S, Jacoby SM. Why are total knee arthroplasties failing today? *Clin Orthop Relat Res.* 2002;404:7-13.
8. Pagnano MW, Hanssen AD, Lewallen DG, Stuart MJ. Flexion instability after primary posterior cruciate retaining total knee arthroplasty. *Clin Orthop Relat Res.* 1998;356:39-46.
9. Schwab JH, Haidukewych GJ, Hanssen AD, Jacofsky DJ, Pagnano MW. Flexion instability without dislocation after posterior stabilized total knees. *Clin Orthop Relat Res.* 2005;440:96-100.
10. Krackow KA. Instability in total knee arthroplasty. *J Arthroplasty.* 2003;16(3 suppl 1):S45-S47.
11. Grood ES, Noyes FR, Butler DL. Ligamentous and capsular restraints preventing straight medial and lateral laxity intact human cadaver knees. *J Bone Joint Surg Am.* 1981;63A:1257-1269.
12. Grood ES, Stowers SF, Noyes FR. Limits of movement in the human knee: effect of sectioning the posterior cruciate ligament and posterolateral structures. *J Bone Joint Surg Am.* 1988;70A:88-97.
13. Whiteside LA. Selective ligament release in total knee arthroplasty of the knee in valgus. *Clin Orthop Rel Res.* 1999;367:130-140.
14. Krackow KA, Mihalko WM. Flexion-extension joint gap changes after lateral structure release for valgus deformity correction in total knee arthroplasty: a cadaver study. *J Arthroplasty.* 1999;14:994-1004.
15. Matsueda M, Gengerke TR, Murphy M, Lew WD, Gustilo RB. Soft tissue release in total knee arthroplasty: cadaver study using knees without deformities. *Clin Orthop Relat Res.* 1999;366:264-273.
16. Krackow KA, Mihalko WM. The effect of medial release on flexion and extension gaps in cadaveric knees: implications for soft tissue balancing total knee arthroplasty. *Am J Knee Surg.* 1999;12:222-228.
17. Peters CL, Mohr RA, Bachus KN. Primary total knee arthroplasty in the valgus knee: creating a balanced soft tissue envelope. *J Arthroplasty.* 2001;16:721-729.
18. Saeki K, Mihalko WM, Patel V, et al. Stability after medial collateral ligament release in total knee arthroplasty. *Clin Orthop Relat Res.* 2001;392:184-189.
19. Whiteside LA, Saeki K, Mihalko WM. Functional medial ligament balancing in total knee arthroplasty. *Clin Orthop Relat Res.* 2000;380:45-57.
20. Kanamiya T, Whiteside LA, Nakamura T, Mihalko WM, Steiger J, Naito M. Effect of selective lateral ligament release on stability in total knee arthroplasty. *Clin Orthop Relat Res.* 2002;404:24-31.
21. Babis GC, Trousdale RT, Morrey B. The effectiveness of isolated tibial insert exchange in revision total knee arthroplasty. *J Bone Joint Surg Am.* 2002;84(A):64-68.
22. Nelissen RG, Hogendoorn PC. Retain or sacrifice the posterior cruciate ligament in total knee arthroplasty? A histopathological study of the cruciate ligament in osteoarthritic and rheumatoid disease. *J Clin Pathol.* 2001;54:381-384.

23. Allain J, Goutallier D, Voisin MC. Macroscopic and histological assessments of the cruciate ligaments in arthrosis of the knee. *Acta Orthop Scand.* 2001;72:266-269.

24. Freeman MA, Todd RC, Bamert P, Day WH. ICHL arthroplasty of the knee: 1968-1977. *J Bone Joint Surg Br.* 1978;60-B:339-344.

25. Insall JN, Binazzi R, Soudry M, Mestriner LA. Total knee arthroplasty. *Clin Orthop Relat Res.* 1985;192:13-22.

26. Morgan H, Battista V, Leopold SS. Constraint in primary total knee arthroplasty. *J Am Acad Orthop Surg.* 2005;13(8):515-524.

27. Insall J, Tria AJ, Scott WN. The total condylar knee prosthesis: the first five years. *Clin Orthop Relat Res.* 1979;145:68-77.

28. Dennis D, Komistek RD, Mahfouz MR, Hass BD, Stiehl JD. Multicenter determination of in vivo kinematics after total knee arthroplasty. *Clin Orthop Relat Res.* 2003;416:37-57.

29. Banks SA, Harman MK, Bellemans J, Hodge WA. Making sense of knee arthroplasty kinematics: news you can use. *J Bone Joint Surg Am.* 2003;85-A(suppl 4):64-72.

30. Dennis DA, Komistek RD, Mahfouz MR, Walker SA, Tucker A. A multicenter analysis of axial femorotibial rotation after total knee arthroplasty. *Clin Orthop Relat Res.* 2004;428:180-189.

31. Mahoney OM, Kinsey TL, Banks AZ, Banks SA. Rotational kinematics of a modern fixed-bearing posterior stabilized total knee arthroplasty. *J Arthroplasty.* 2009;24(4):641-645.

32. Bugbee WD, Ammen DJ, Engh GA. Does implant selection affect outcome of revision knee arthroplasty? *J Arthroplasty.* 2001;16:581-585.

33. Peters CL, Hennessey R, Barden RM, Galante JO, Rosenberg AG. Revision total knee arthroplasty with a cemented posterior-stabilized or constrained condylar prosthesis. A minimum 3-year and average 5-year follow-up study. *J Arthroplasty.* 1997;12:896-903.

34. Engh GA, Koralewicz LM, Pereles TR. Clinical results of modular polyethylene insert exchange with retention of total knee arthroplasty components. *J Bone Joint Surg Am.* 2000;82-A:516-523.

35. Babis GC, Trousdale RT, Morrey BF. The effectiveness of isolated tibial insert exchange in revision total knee arthroplasty. *J Bone Joint Surg Am.* 2002;84-A:64-68.

36. Vince KG, Long W. Revision knee arthroplasty. The limits of press fit medullary fixation. *Clin Orthop Relat Res.* 1995;317:172-177.

37. Hui FC, Fitzgerald RH Jr. Hinged total knee arthroplasty. *J Bone Joint Surg Am.* 1980;62-A:513-519.

38. Hoikka V, Vankka E, Eskola A, Lindholm TS. Results and complications after arthroplasty with a totally constrained total knee prosthesis (GUEPAR). *Ann Chir Gynaecol.* 1989;78:94-96.

39. Jones EC, Insall JN, Inglis AE, Ranawat CS. GUEPAR knee arthroplasty results and late complications. *Clin Orthop Relat Res.* 1979;140:145-152.

40. Springer BD, Hanssen AD, Sim FH, Lewallen DG. The kinematic rotating hinge prosthesis for complex knee arthroplasty. *Clin Orthop Relat Res.* 2001;392:283-291.

41. McAuley JP, Engh GA. Constraint in total knee arthroplasty: when and what? *J Arthroplasty.* 2003;18(3 suppl 1):51-54.

42. Barrack RL. Evolution of the rotating hinge for complex total knee arthroplasty. *Clin Orthop Relat Res.* 2001;392:292-299.

43. Kim YH. Salvage of failed hinge knee arthroplasty with a Total Condylar III type prosthesis. *Clin Orthop Relat Res.* 1987;221:272-277.

44. Rosenberg AG, Verner JJ, Galante JO. Clinical results of total knee revision using the Total Condylar III prosthesis. *Clin Orthop Relat Res.* 1991;273:83-90.

45. Haas SB, Insall JN, Montgomery W 3rd, Windsor RE. Revision total knee arthroplasty with use of modular components with stems inserted without cement. *J Bone Joint Surg Am.* 1995;77-A:1700-1707.

46. Puloski SKT, McCalden RW, MacDonald SJ, Rorabeck CH, Bourne RB. Tibial post wear in posterior stabilized total knee arthroplasty. An unrecognized source of polyethylene debris. *J Bone Joint Surg Am.* 2001;83-A(3):390-397.

47. Mestha P, Shenava Y, D'Arcy JC. Fracture of the tibial post in posterior stabilizes (Insall Burstein II) total knee arthroplasty. *J Arthroplasty.* 2000;15(6):814-815.

48. Mariconda M, Lotti G, Milano C. Fracture of posterior-stabilized tibial insert in a Genesis knee prosthesis. *J Arthroplasty.* 2000;15(4):529-530.

49. McPherson EJ, Vince KG. Breakage of a Total Condylar III knee prosthesis. A case report. *J Arthroplasty.* 1993;8(5):561-563.

50. Lombardi AV Jr, Mallory TH, Fada RA, Adams JB, Kefauver CA. Fracture of the tibial spine of a Total Condylar III knee prosthesis secondary to malrotation of the femoral component. *Am J Knee Surg.* 2001;14(1):55-59.

51. Furman BD, Lipman J, Kligman M, Wright TM, Haas SB. Tibial post wear in posterior-stabilized knee replacements is design-dependent. *Clin Orthop Relat Res.* 2008;466:2650-2655.

52. Li G, Papannagari R, Most E, et al. Anterior tibial post impingement in a posterior stabilized total knee arthroplasty. *J Orthop Res.* 2005;23(3):536-541.

53. Bhimji S, Wang A, Schmalzried T. Tibial insert micromotion of various total knee arthroplasty devices. *J Knee Surg.* 2010;23(3):153-162.

54. Wasielewski RC, Parks N, Williams I, Suprenant H, Collier JP, Engh G. Tibial insert undersurface as a contributing source of polyethylene wear debris. *Clin Orthop Relat Res.* 1997;345:53-59.

55. Cho WS, Youm YS. Migration of polyethylene fixation screw after total knee arthroplasty. *J Arthroplasty.* 2009;24(5):825.e5-825.e9.

56. Rapuri VR, Clarke HD, Spangehl MJ, Beauchamp CP. Five cases of failure of the tibial polyethylene insert locking mechanism in one design of constrained knee arthroplasty. *J Arthroplasty.* 2011;26(6):976.e21-976.e24.

57. Kocmond JH, Delp SL, Stern SH. Stability and range of motion of Insall-Burstein condylar prostheses. A computer simulation study. *J Arthroplasty.* 1995;10:383-388.

58. Lombardi AV Jr, Mallory TH, Vaughn BK, et al. Dislocation following primary posterior-stabilized total knee arthroplasty. *J Arthroplasty.* 1993;8:633-639.

59. Dorr LD. Revision knee arthroplasty: how I do it. In: Insall JN, Scott WN, eds. *Surgery of the Knee.* 3rd ed. New York, NY: Churchill Livingstone; 2001:1925-1933.

60. Hofmann AA, Tkach KT, Evanich CJ, et al. Posterior stabilization in total knee arthroplasty with use of an ultracongruent polyethylene insert. *J Arthroplasty.* 2000;15(5):576-583.

61. Walldius B. Arthroplasty of the knee using an endoprosthesis. *Acta Orthop Scand.* 1957;(suppl 2)4:1-112.

62. Walker PS, Sathasivam S. Design forms of total knee replacement. *Proc Instn Mech Engrs.* 2000;214(H):101-109.

63. Rand JA, Chao EY, Stauffer RN. Kinematic rotating-hinge total knee arthroplasty. *J Bone Joint Surg Am.* 1987;69-A:489-497.

64. Shaw JA, Balcom W, Greer RB 3rd. Total knee arthroplasty using the kinematic rotating hinge prosthesis. *Orthopedics.* 1989;12:647-654.

65. Ward WG, Haight D, Ritchie P, Gordon S, Eckardt J. Dislocation of rotating hinge total knee protheses. *J Bone Joint Surg Am.* 2003;83-A:448-453.

10

Management of Infection in Total Knee Arthroplasty

Mark D. Campbell, MD

Periprosthetic infection is a devastating complication following total knee arthroplasty (TKA). It imposes heavy emotional and financial tolls on the patient, the physicians involved, and the society as a whole. An infected total joint replacement carries significant morbidity, and can ultimately threaten the viability of the affected limb. Most recent studies have estimated the incidence to be about 1% to 2% of primary TKAs.[1,2] Although early infection rates were high, multiple prophylactic measures have been instituted that have resulted in the current lower incidence.[3-5] Multiple risk factors predisposing patients to periprosthetic infection have been identified, allowing the surgeon to avoid higher-risk cases.

The diagnosis of periprosthetic infection can be challenging, and a high index of suspicion is critical. Classic signs of infection such as erythema, warmth, and drainage are rarely seen in patients presenting with an infected TKA.

Treatment goals include eradication of infection, decreased pain, and a functional TKA. A variety of treatment options exist to assist in management. Multiple factors direct the treatment choice. These include host factors, offending organism(s), and timing of the infection. This chapter will review pertinent issues—such as incidence and risk factors—as well as diagnosis and treatment options.

INCIDENCE

Although the incidence of infection is often quoted as between 1% and 2%, studies have shown an incidence as high as 12.4%.[6-13] At the Mayo Clinic, 1.2% of 3000 consecutive primary TKAs developed infection.[14] Bengtson and associates[6-8] reviewed data from the Swedish Knee Arthroplasty Project, which revealed an infection rate of 1.7% after TKA performed for osteoarthritis and a 4.4% infection rate for TKA performed for rheumatoid arthritis. In a series of 12,118 primary TKAs, Blom and associates reported the results of a study comparing infection in TKA patients before and after the advent of better prophylactic protocols.[15] In their earlier audit in 1986, the authors documented infection rates of 4.4% in 471 primary TKAs and 15% in 23 revision TKAs. Following the improved prophylaxis, the infection rates decreased to 1% in

Jacofsky DJ, Hedley AK, eds.
Fundamentals of Revision Knee Arthroplasty:
Diagnosis, Evaluation, and Treatment (pp 157-170).
© 2013 SLACK Incorporated.

931 primary TKAs and to 5.8% in 69 revision surgeries. The authors attributed the improvements to stringent preoperative antibiotic protocols, vertical laminar flow, use of occlusive clothing, and antimicrobial lavage prior to closure. Kurtz et al quantified the current and historical incidence of periprosthetic infection associated with hip and knee arthroplasty in the United States using the Nationwide Inpatient Sample, as well as corresponding hospitalization charges and length of stay.[16] The rate of infected knee arthroplasties was 0.92%, significantly greater than that of infected hip arthroplasties with 0.88%. Urban nonteaching hospitals experienced the highest burden of infection with 1.18% for hips and 1.26% for knees compared to rural (0.61% for hips and 0.69% for knees) and urban teaching hospitals (0.73% for hips and 0.77% for knees).

RISK FACTORS

All patients are at risk of developing infection. As the immune system is critical in preventing infection, those who are immunocompromised are at higher risk. In a study by Wilson et al, patients with rheumatoid arthritis, skin ulceration, and those having undergone previous surgical procedures showed a statistically significant increase infection rate.[13] The authors retrospectively reviewed the results of 4171 TKAs and found that deep infection had occurred in 67 (1.6%) knees. The primary diagnoses were rheumatoid arthritis (45 knees), osteoarthritis (16), hemophilic arthropathy (3), osteonecrosis (1), lupus erythematosus (1), and ankylosing spondylitis (1). The incidence of infection was significantly higher for patients with rheumatoid arthritis (2.2%) than for those with osteoarthritis (1%). Prior knee surgery was also an important risk factor, but only for those with osteoarthritis. In the osteoarthritic knees, the infection rate was 1.4% for patients who had prior knee surgery and 0.3% for those who had not. The presence of a remote skin ulcer was another highly significant risk factor for infection, being found in 20% of the infected knees compared with 3% of uninfected knees. There was also a trend toward infection in obese patients, those with recent urinary tract infections, and patients with oral corticosteroid dependency. Other studies have shown an increased incidence in those with diabetes mellitus and malnutrition. Operative technique is also an important variable that affects the possibility of deep infection. Increased operative time is associated with an increased risk of infection. Also, patients who require reoperation due to drainage, hematoma, or wound necrosis are at increased risk. Although an infection can occur at any time, the risk is highest within the first 3 months of the operation. Peersman and associates reported on a large retrospective review of 6489 knee replacements in 6120 patients.[17] Of these knee replacements, 116 knees became infected and 3 were lost to follow-up. One hundred of the infections occurred in patients undergoing primary knee replacement, whereas the remaining infections occurred in patients undergoing revision knee replacement. Ninety-seven of these infected knees (86%) had deep periprosthetic infections, and the remaining 16 knees had superficial wound infections. The overall early deep infection rate for patients undergoing a primary knee replacement was 0.39%, whereas the rate for patients undergoing a revision knee replacement was 0.97%. Factors that were statistically significant in increasing the risk of infection were prior open surgical procedures, immunosuppressive therapy, poor nutrition, hypokalemia, diabetes mellitus, obesity, revision surgery, and a history of smoking. Despite the best preventative efforts, infection inevitably will occur following TKA in a certain number of patients. Although risk factors should heighten the physician's suspicion for infection, the lack of such risks should not decrease suspicion.

Although *Staphylococcus aureus* is the most common organism noted in cultures in deep prosthetic infection,[13,18] the microorganisms that have been documented to be responsible include virtually all aerobic and anaerobic organisms, fungi, mycobacterium, and Brucella.[19] Mixed polymicrobial infections are often encountered where there is an actively draining wound allowing surface organisms to gain access to the joint. Furthermore, patients treated with antibiotic suppression may develop resistant bacterial strains.

DIAGNOSIS

The clinical diagnosis of infection after TKA often requires a high index of suspicion. Prompt and accurate diagnosis will greatly benefit the patient. A combination of patient history, physical exam, and various studies is required to diagnose a patient with an infected TKA. A patient presenting with an acute, painful, fulminate infection shortly after TKA is rarely observed. Most typically it is far less obvious. Persistence of a moderately painful or stiff TKA should always alert the surgeon to the possibility of postoperative infection. Early diagnosis of deep arthroplasty infection is imperative in order to maximize the likelihood that the prosthesis will be able to be salvaged with débridement and retention.[12] Superficial cultures of wound drainage appear to be of little diagnostic value, and such practice is discouraged. If a wound appears worrisome, joint arthrocentesis and evaluation of the aspirate with cell count and differential, gram stain, and bacterial culture should be performed to evaluate for deep infection.

Important historical factors to consider when subacute or chronic infection is a concern include persistent pain, postoperative wound complications, significant wound drainage, chronic or multiple courses of oral antibiotic treatment for wound difficulties, a history of potential hematogenous sources of infection, such as tooth extraction or urologic procedures, and persistent knee stiffness despite appropriate rehabilitation efforts. Despite the fact that the empiric use of antibiotics is unfortunately quite common, it should be avoided in patients with painful or stiff TKAs without a definitive diagnosis of infection. This practice, although at times "easier" than the acceptance of infection and/or the subsequent work-up to prove such, is an approach that complicates efforts to diagnose infection and makes treatment more difficult once it is confirmed.

In a study performed at the Hospital for Special Surgery, a series of patients who had been treated for infection after TKA were evaluated.[20] In this series, considerable pain was present in 96% of patients, swelling of the knee was present in 77% of patients, 27% were febrile, and 27% had active drainage. The average erythrocyte sedimentation rate (ESR) was 63 mm/hour (range: 4 to 125 mm/hr). A positive aspiration of the knee fluid was obtained in 51 of 52 infected knees, with a positive culture being present from samples taken at the time of revision arthroplasty in that one patient where aspiration was not performed because infection was not suspected.

Laboratory studies should routinely include a white blood cell count, ESR, and C-reactive protein (CRP). These values are useful, although often nonspecific and difficult to interpret, especially in patients with a history of rheumatoid arthritis.[21] Sanzen and Sundberg evaluated the laboratory findings in 23 nonrheumatoid patients with low-grade periprosthetic hip and knee infections.[22] False-negative rates of 35% and 22% were seen in the ESR and CRP, respectively. However, only 1 patient had normal values for both tests, supporting the use of both of these studies in conjunction. Greidanus et al have recently reported optimal ESR and CRP cut-off values of 22.5 mm/hr and 13.5 mg/L, respectively, in their review of 151 knees presenting for revision surgery. Using these values in combination produced a sensitivity of 88%, specificity of 93%, positive predictive value of 84%, and negative predictive value of 95%.[23]

Special tests such as serum interleukin-6 and polymerase chain reaction deserve mention. In a prospective, case-control study of 58 patients undergoing revision surgery of total hip and knee arthroplasties, serum interleukin-6 values greater than 10 pg/mL were reported to have a sensitivity of 100%, specificity of 95%, positive predictive value of 89%, negative predictive value of 100%, and accuracy of 97%.[24] Cost and availability limit these test for most practitioners at this time.

Underdiagnosis of joint sepsis occurs during aspiration when organisms present in the knee are unable to be grown in culture. The weaknesses in the culture process and in the laboratory diagnosis of infection have recently prompted intense interest in the use of polymerase chain reaction to more accurately diagnose periprosthetic infection. Very promising results have been reported.[25]

This method is used to detect and amplify the presence of bacterial DNA. It is thought to be a quick method since it is not affected by whether the patient takes antibiotics or not. However, a high percentage of false-positives has been detected, which may be caused by any type of contamination. In short, it is a technique that can be used as a complement to the previous ones and whose usefulness may increase in the future.

Radiographic evaluation in a suspected infected arthroplasty is rarely diagnostic and often normal. Radiographic evaluation, however, specifically focusing on sequential radiographic comparisons to discover progressive radiolucencies or the development of focal osteopenia or osteolysis around the prosthesis is advised. Periosteal new bone formation on radiographs is highly suggestive of infection.

Radioisotope scans may be helpful in the diagnosis of infected total joint arthroplasty. Indium[111] leukocyte scanning appears to be more accurate than technetium-99m diphosphonate scanning alone (78% versus 74%).[26] The accuracy of indium[111] leukocyte scanning combined with technetium-99m sulfur colloid marrow scintigraphy, however, provided a 95% accuracy. Rheumatoid arthritis and significant osteolysis are risk factors for false-positive results.[27] The sensitivity of indium scanning appears to be dependent on the activity of the infection with indolent and chronic infections having higher false-negative rates.

Aspiration of the painful joint arthroplasty is thought to be the gold standard and should be performed if infection is suspected. Fluid is typically sent for cell count with differential, gram stain, analysis for crystals, and aerobic and anaerobic cultures. Cultures should be obtained in the proper media for aerobic and anaerobic bacteria, fungal, and mycobacterial growth. If possible, multiple sets of cultures should be obtained to exclude the possibility of a false-positive contaminant. Multiple cut-off values with respect to synovial leukocyte count have been used to diagnose infection. Commonly accepted values range from a total leukocyte count of 1000 to 3500 with a neutrophil percentage of 60% and above.[28-30] Synovial fluid cell count and differential is a very useful diagnostic test. False-negatives are not uncommon in patients who received antibiotics prior to aspiration. For this reason antibiotics should be suspended, if possible, for 10 to 14 days before carrying out the aspiration. Ghanem et al have suggested a leukocyte threshold value of greater than 1100 cells/microliter and a neutrophil percentage of greater than 64% for the diagnosis of periprosthetic knee infection. Using these values in combination yields sensitivity of 85.0%, specificity of 99.2%, positive predictive value of 98.6%, and negative predictive value of 91.6%.[29]

A retrospective study presented at the Musculoskeletal Infection Society 19th Annual Open Scientific Meeting in August 2009 reported that the leukocyte cut-off value should be higher for patients with acute postoperative infections (defined as those less than 42 days in duration). Receiver operating characteristic curve analysis revealed a leukocyte count threshold of greater than 10,700 cells/microliter had a sensitivity of 96% and specificity of 90%. The neutrophil percent threshold of greater than 89% had a sensitivity of 82% and specificity of 68% for the diagnosis of acute postoperative total knee infections.[31]

At the time of surgery, an intraoperative frozen section of periprosthetic tissue obtained from multiple sites may be useful to help guide treatment. A value of 5 to 10 polymorphonuclear cells per high-powered field (400x) is commonly used to indicate infection.[32,33] The interpretation of this test is subject to pathologist and surgeon experience, and may be even more difficult in cases involving underlying inflammatory arthropathy or chronic antibiotic use.

While the gold standard for diagnosis is widely considered the culture and identification of an offending organism, so-called culture negative infections are not infrequently encountered.[34] This situation is commonly the result of concurrent antibiotic use leading to suppression of growth or organisms that are not easily cultured ex vivo.[35] As a result, most authors would recommend aspiration only following cessation of antibiotics for a period of at least 10 to 14 days. Gram stains can also frequently be misleading.[36] Various authors have recommended against routine aspiration of joint fluid for culture in the work-up of an asymptomatic total joint arthroplasty in the absence of other clinical indicators of infection (although cell count and differential may be of value). This is due to the poor predictive value of aspiration in the setting of low disease prevalence. Conversely, if infection is clinically suspected and other findings suggest the presence of infection, the predictive value of aspiration and culture is increased.[37]

The use of molecular techniques and sonication has been advocated as an alternative to more traditional tissue cultures to isolate organisms from the biofilm that coats the removed implant.[38-42]

Most surgeons now agree that the literature supports the use of cell count and differential as the most specific and sensitive test for the diagnosis of infection. It is often the combination of information from multiple studies, along with clinical judgment, that leads to the correct diagnosis.

CLASSIFICATION

Classification of periprosthetic infection is often related to the timing of onset from the initial index procedure and the use of the system is helpful in guiding appropriate management. Initially, Coventry described a 3-stage classification system based on timing of presentation and the presumed mode of infection, and this system has been recently updated and modified by Segawa et al.[43,44]

In this classification schema, an infection in the early postoperative period is acute (early postoperative). The patient with an acute infection typically presents during the first postoperative month, and a diagnosis is usually evident on history and physical examination. These patients may report wound complications and/or superficial cellulitis around the time of their index procedure. The etiology of acute infections may be wound colonization at the time of surgery, infected hematomas, or the spread of superficial infection. Many of these infections likely are potentially preventable with appropriate preoperative antibiotics and careful operative technique.

Chronic infections are also believed to originate during the index surgical procedure, but often due to a small inoculum or a low virulent organism, the onset of symptoms may be delayed. By definition, these patients present after the first month postoperatively. These patients typically present with a gradual deterioration in their function as well as an increase in their pain. They generally do not have clear systemic or local findings consistent with definitive infection. There may be a history of prolonged wound drainage at the time of the index procedure, a delay in discharge from the hospital, or previous prescriptions for ongoing courses of antibiotics that may have temporarily improved their symptoms. These infections may be the most difficult prosthetic infections to diagnose.

Acute hematogenous infections are typically presumed to be secondary to hematogenous spread to a previously asymptomatic and aseptic joint replacement. There may be a history of associated febrile illness or acute infection, such as a urinary tract infection or pneumonia, followed by deterioration in joint function. Invasive or semi-invasive procedures such as colonoscopy, dental procedures, or local treatment of cutaneous infections may be reported. These infections are more common in patients who are immunocompromised, have recurrent episodes of bacteremia such as would be seen in intravenous drug abusers or those requiring repeat chronic urinary catheterization, or those who have had single episodes of bacteremia such as was previously mentioned. Single episodes of bacteremia from dental manipulations, respiratory infection, remote prosthetic infection, open skin lesions, endoscopy, or contaminated operations are often associated with these prosthetic joint infections.[45-49]

Classification systems have expanded to include patients with positive intraoperative cultures. This group includes patients with positive intraoperative cultures found at the time of revision for presumed aseptic failure. In a report of 106 infections, 31 patients initially thought to have aseptic failures were diagnosed with deep infection on the basis of positive intraoperative cultures.[50] A minimum of 2 of 5 cultures was considered positive for infection. In this setting, culture results must be interpreted in conjunction with preoperative examination and laboratory studies, intraoperative culture results and frozen section, histology findings, and the overall clinical scenario. If positive culture results are deemed to be true positives, appropriate antibiotic therapy should be initiated.[51]

TREATMENT

Once the diagnosis of deep infection has been established, the treating physician must consider a number of factors when determining appropriate treatment. These factors include the duration of time between the index arthroplasty and the diagnosis of infection, consideration of the pathogen(s) and their subsequent antibiotic sensitivities responsible for the infection, clarification of host factors that may adversely affect successful treatment of the infection, status of the soft tissue envelope and the extensor mechanism, determination as to whether the arthroplasty is well fixed or loose, and assessment of the patient's expectations and functional demands. It is important that both the surgeon and treating institution are well equipped to handle this difficult problem.

Treatment goals for an infected TKA include the following:

- Eradication of infection
- Pain relief
- Maintenance of a functional lower extremity

As secondary attempts at infection eradication after a treatment failure are often hindered and adversely affected by progressive arthrofibrosis, devitalization of the soft tissue envelope, additional bone loss, and the possible development of antibiotic resistant organisms, it is important that the probability for a successful outcome after the first attempt is maximized.

The 6 basic treatment options for an infected TKA include the following:

- Antibiotic suppression without débridement
- Débridement with prosthesis retention
- Resection arthroplasty
- Arthrodesis
- Amputation
- Single- or two-stage resection and reimplantation of another prosthesis

Antibiotic Suppression Without Débridement

Antibiotic treatment alone will never eradicate deep periprosthetic infection. However, in very limited situations, suppressive antibiotic treatment alone may be reasonable and indicated when *all* of the following criteria are met:

- Prosthesis removal is not feasible, most commonly due to medical comorbidities that preclude an operative procedure
- Virulence of the microorganism is low and the micro-organism is susceptible to an oral antibiotic agent
- The antibiotics that are appropriate for suppression are without serious toxicity
- The prosthesis is not loose[52]

Relative contraindications to chronic antibiotic suppression would include the presence of other joint arthroplasties or the presence of other indwelling synthetic devices such as artificial heart valves or vascular grafts. In a multicenter study of 225 knees, antibiotic suppression was successful in only 18% of patients.[53] Combining several series indicates that antibiotic suppression is successful in 24% of patients (62 of 261 knees).[9,13,52-54] The use of a combined oral regimen of rifampicin in conjunction with a quinolone has been reported to be more successful than treatment with a single antibiotic agent for deep periprosthetic infection from *Staphylococcus*.[55]

It cannot be overemphasized that unless the long-term goal is antibiotic suppression without eradication of infection in a patient with a known organism, the practice of prescribing antibiotics empirically for patients with a potentially infected arthroplasty is strongly discouraged and typically only complicates future definitive treatment.

Débridement With Prosthesis Retention

Open débridement may be indicated for the acute infection in the early postoperative period or for acute hematogenous infection of a well-fixed and well-functioning prosthetic component that is diagnosed less than 2 to 4 weeks from the onset of symptoms. Suggested criteria for this treatment include a short duration of symptoms (preferably less than 2 weeks), susceptible organisms, the absence of prolonged postoperative drainage or a draining sinus tract, and a well-fixed, well-functioning implant.[56] As previously mentioned, a relative contraindication for component retention may be the presence of other joint replacements, indwelling prosthetic or synthetic devices, or the presence of a resistant organism. Overall results in series not following the suggested criteria are not encouraging, with control of infection achieved in only 18% to 24% of patients.[53,52,57] However, the single most important variable when considering the potential cure of infection is most likely the duration of infection prior to surgical débridement.[56,58] In a group of 35 patients who initially underwent débridement and prosthetic retention, infection was successfully controlled in 13 patients with a mean time to débridement of less than 5 days from the onset of symptoms compared to the 21 patients requiring additional surgical intervention whose mean time to surgery was 54 days.[58] In a more recent study from 2007, Chiu and Chen[59] sought to determine the prevalence of reinfection in 40 consecutive patients with deep infection after revision TKA. These patients had no prosthesis loosening or malalignment. Ten patients had acute postoperative infections, 20 patients had late chronic infections, and 10 patients had acute hematogenous infections. All had surgical débridement and parenteral antibiotics with retention of their existing prostheses. The patients were followed for a minimum of 3 years (range: 36 to 143 months). Overall successful implant salvage was achieved in 12 of the 40 patients (30%). However, likelihood of success depended on the type of infection: 70% success in patients with acute postoperative infections, 50% in patients with acute hematogenous infections, and 0% in patients with late chronic infections. The authors therefore recommend implant removal for all late chronic infections.

It cannot be overemphasized that the literature does not support the use of débridement with prosthetic component retention in cases of late chronic infections. Furthermore, multiple attempts at débridement and component retention to salvage the joint are typically counterproductive and lead to extensive peri-articular fibrosis, making subsequent revision surgery more difficult in addition to subjecting the patient to an undue number of procedures.

Resection Arthroplasty

Definitive resection arthroplasty is defined here as implant removal with no intention of subsequent knee reconstruction. The ideal candidate for this procedure is a patient with polyarticular rheumatoid arthritis with limited functional demands who is likely to have difficulty eradicating infection and/or tolerating more than one surgical procedure. Resection arthroplasty will allow the patient to sit more readily than with a knee arthrodesis. The primary disadvantage of resection arthroplasty is the frequent occurrence of knee instability and pain if the lower extremity is used for transfers or ambulation. This technique requires adequate initial débridement, removal of all infected and necrotic tissue and foreign debris, temporary fixation with pins to help maintain alignment and apposition of the tibia and femur to assist with reasonable stability to allow fibrosis to occur, and cast immobilization for a minimum of 6 months to allow fibrous stability to develop. Although eradication of infection has been well-documented with this technique, the suboptimal functional results cause this procedure to be rarely utilized except in very select patients with limited ambulatory demands.

Arthrodesis

Arthrodesis has been historically considered the gold standard treatment option for the infected TKA because of the excellent potential for resolving infection, alleviating pain, and providing a stable, painless joint. However, an arthrodesis precludes knee motion, thereby making sitting and other associated activities more difficult. Relative contraindications to arthrodesis include significant ipsilateral hip or ankle arthritis, contralateral knee arthritis, contralateral upper extremity amputation, and severe segmental bone loss. Indications for arthrodesis include individuals with a high functional demand, single joint disease, young physiologic age, extensor mechanism disruption, a poor soft tissue envelope requiring extensive soft tissue reconstruction, systemic immunocompromise, making successful aseptic reimplantation less likely, the presence of infection with microorganisms that require highly toxic antibiotic therapy or are resistant to conventional antibiotics, and patients who refuse amputation and are willing to accept a stiff, shortened, lower extremity. A variety of techniques have been used to obtain knee arthrodesis including the use of external fixators, plate fixation, and intramedullary nail fixation. The most important factor in obtaining union is the opposition of the ends of the bone.

Intramedullary nail fixation appears to provide a more reliable method of achieving union compared with external fixation. In a multicenter study by Waldman and associates, union was obtained with the initial surgical procedure in 20 of 21 (95%) patients using a modular titanium nail.[60] Most authors, however, would recommend a two-stage procedure, with the first stage consisting of thorough débridement and consideration of placement of an antibiotic spacer. The second stage would then involve insertion of the nail to avoid the intramedullary spread of infection and to minimize colonization of the hardware. In the presence of known active infection, the use of a biplanar external fixator is recommended.

Jacofsky et al reviewed knee arthrodesis for the infected total knee replacement using 2 different fixation techniques.[61] Eighty-five consecutive patients who underwent knee arthrodesis were followed until union, nonunion, amputation, or death. External fixation achieved successful fusion in 41 of 61 patients and was associated with a 4.9% rate of deep infection. Fusion was successful in 23 of 24 patients with intramedullary nailing and was associated with an 8.3% rate of deep infection. We observed similar fusion and infection rates with the 2 techniques. Complication rates are high irrespective of the technique, and one must consider the risks of both nonunion and infection when choosing the fixation method in this setting. Intramedullary nailing appears to have a higher rate of successful union but a higher risk of recurrent infection when compared with external fixation knee arthrodesis.

The optimum position for knee arthrodesis is 10 to 20 degrees of flexion to assist with foot clearance and prevent the need for hip circumduction during the swing phase of gait. However, the amount of knee flexion in this patient population should be decreased proportionally to the amount of shortening of the leg. In the presence of substantial bone loss, knee position near full extension will help maintain maximal extremity length and still allow foot clearance. The use of soft tissue flaps in the face of a poor soft tissue envelope should be liberally considered in order to help minimize wound healing complications, the rate of reinfection, and to provide healthy, well-vascularized tissue to the arthrodesis area.

Amputation

Amputation may be occasionally required for the management of an infected total knee replacement. It is typically indicated for life-threatening systemic sepsis, failed attempts at arthrodesis, situations in which the soft tissue envelope cannot be predictably restored, or in cases where the patient elects for amputation over arthrodesis or the prospect of multiple surgical procedures. Amputation should be performed at a level that maximizes function yet predictably eradicates infection. Following amputation, however, elderly patients may remain minimal or nonambulators due to the increased energy expenditure required for ambulation after amputation. Of 23 patients treated with above knee amputation for failed TKA, only 7 patients reported being able to ambulate regularly, whereas 20 used a wheelchair part of the day and 55% were confined to the wheelchair throughout the entire day.[62] However, many of these patients with multiple comorbidities may have been minimal ambulators even with reconstructive procedures.

Prosthesis Removal and Immediate Reimplantation (Single-Stage Exchange)

Removal of an infected TKA followed by débridement and immediate reimplantation of a new prosthesis has limited popularity in North America. The results are less successful for eradication of infection when compared with two-stage exchange protocols. In a series from the Endo-Klinic in Germany, 76 of 104 and 22 of 31 infected total knees were infection-free after a minimum of 2 years follow-up after 1-stage exchange. Cure rates in these 2 series were 73% and 71%, respectively.[63,64] The obvious advantage of this technique is the need for a single surgical procedure and the subsequent decreased costs and rehabilitation time associated with one operation. However, the financial and emotional costs for the 25% to 30% who fail this treatment modality must be considered, making this technique no more cost-effective than a two-stage exchange. Due to inferior results, the indications for single-stage exchange should be limited to patients who have a symptomatically loose prosthesis, would not tolerate staged surgical procedures, or in whom long-term antibiotic suppression is possible in the event they fail 1-stage exchange and require long-term suppression. This cohort of patients is typically the elderly patient with limited life expectancy and a bacterial infection that is sensitive to an oral nontoxic agent. Most experts in the area of infected arthroplasty do not believe that single-stage exchange has a role in the management of infected knee arthroplasty.

Prosthetic Removal and Delayed Reimplantation (Two-Stage Exchange)

Two-stage reimplantation protocols have become the gold standard for the treatment of late, chronic, periprosthetic knee infection. This technique gives the most predictable result for eradication of infection and the advantage of improved functional outcome compared with arthrodesis, definitive resection arthroplasty, or amputation. Contraindications for a two-stage reimplantation include persistent infection following the initial débridement procedure, medical contraindications precluding an additional surgical procedure, and a poor soft tissue envelope not amenable to reconstruction about the knee. Although a relative contraindication is the absence of a functional extensor mechanism, TKA with a drop lock knee brace may be preferable for some patients to an arthrodesis or an amputation.

Perhaps the most important treatment variable is the thoroughness of débridement with removal of all foreign material including all cement, and the presence of an immunocompetent host. Other important treatment factors include a sufficient delay from the time of resection arthroplasty to the time of reimplantation; the appropriate type, duration, and route of antimicrobial therapy; the use of local high-dose antibiotic impregnated polymethylmethacrylate spacers; the use of antibiotic containing polymethylmethacrylate at the time of reimplantation; and perhaps the use of an articulating antibiotic spacer that may improve function between stages and could possibly improve long-term functional outcomes. The ideal duration of time between the resection arthroplasty and the reimplantation remains poorly defined. However, a poor success rate of only 57% was reported in a small series of 14 patients in whom reimplantation was performed within several weeks of removal of the index implant.[14] In a more recent study of 89 infected total knee replacements, the use of antibiotic-impregnated polymethylmethacrylate at the time of reimplantation was the only variable that correlated with success of treatment in deep infection.[65] The two-stage treatment protocol described by Insall has been effective in the treatment of deep periprosthetic knee infections.[66,67] Our protocol consists of removal of the prosthesis and all nonviable tissue including all cement, débridement of soft tissues and bone followed by 6 weeks of parenteral antibiotics maintaining a minimum serum bactericidal titre of 1:8, and delayed reimplantation of a new prosthesis. A normal ESR and CRP after the patient has been off of his or her intravenous antibiotics for 7 to 14 days is certainly encouraging to support the diagnosis of eradication of deep infection. In many cases, these laboratory values do not normalize, but an improving trend off antibiotics is convincing evidence that the infection has been eradicated. Using a similar protocol, results were reported on 64 infected TKAs. At a minimum 2-year follow-up, 6 knees had become reinfected, but only 2 with the same organism. Including all reinfections, these results indicate an infection cure rate of 91%.[66]

The use of an antibiotic cement spacer placed in the knee joint after thorough débridement helps preserve length by maintaining the prosthetic space and helps reduce soft tissue contractures. Additionally, if an "anterior flange" is fashioned in the region of the anterior distal femur, excessive scarring of the extensor mechanism may be mitigated. Most importantly, the antibiotic spacer provides the delivery of high-dose local antibiotic therapy.[68,69]

A study of antibiotic elution concentrations from cement spacers in vivo reported highest elution concentrations when at least 3.6 g of tobramycin and 1 g of vancomycin were used per 40-g batch of cement.[66] Our recommendation is 3.6 to 4.8 g of tobramycin and 3 to 4 g of vancomycin per 40-g batch of cement. Some recommend the addition of 2 to 3 g of cefazolin per 40 g batch of cement to act as a porogen, thus increasing the elution of the other antibiotics. Cefepime can be used if a concern for *Pseudomonas* exists. It should be noted that there are no premixed antibiotic spacers currently available on the market that we consider to have adequate levels of antibiotics for treatment of periprosthetic infection.

The use of a block spacer, even if macrointerdigitated to prevent migration and erosion of the bone, still can allow excessive scarring to occur. In an attempt to help minimize stiffness and scar formation, some authors advocate articulating spacers. The PROSThesis of Antibiotic Loading Acrylic Cement (PROSTALAC) concept was first described by Duncan, but similar concepts were simultaneously developed by other authors.[70-72] The results of the PROSTALAC spacer for infected total knee replacement have been reported.[73] Forty-one of 45 patients (91%) were infection-free after a minimum follow-up of 20 months and a mean follow-up of 48 months. Only one patient remained infected with the original organism, thereby resulting in a "cure rate" for the original organism in 98% of patients. Additionally, the authors felt that the knee motion that was maintained between stages helped facilitate the reimplantation procedure.

Haleem et al reported on a series of 94 patients (96 knees) who underwent a two-stage reimplantation for treatment of an infected TKA.[74] All patients were treated with resection and placement of an interval antibiotic-loaded static cement spacer. At the time of reimplantation, antibiotic cement was utilized for cemented fixation. Patients were followed for a median of 7.2 years (range: 2.5 to 13.2 years). At final follow-up, 15 knees (16%) had required reoperation. Nine knees (9%) had component removal for reinfection and 6 knees (6%) were revised for aseptic loosening. The risk of recurrent infection was not correlated with the type of organism or patient demographics. The survivorship free of implant removal for any reason was 90% (confidence intervals: 83.9% to 96.4%) at 5 years and 77.3% (confidence intervals: 65.5% to 89.6%) at 10 years. The survivorship free of implant removal for reinfection was 93.5% (confidence intervals: 88.5% to 98.7%) at 5 years and 85% (confidence intervals: 73.8% to 96.3%) at 10 years. Survival free of revision for mechanical failure (aseptic loosening or radiographic loosening) was 96.2% (confidence intervals: 92% to 100%) at 5 years and 91% (confidence intervals: 80.8% to 98.3%) at 10 years. This series demonstrates that good results can be achieved with a two-stage resection protocol.

More recently, Anderson and associates analyzed 25 consecutive patients with chronic TKA deep infection who underwent two-stage articulating spacer surgery consisting of removal of the prosthesis and cement, thorough débridement, placement of an antibiotic-loaded articulating spacer, a course of intravenous antibiotics, and a delayed second-stage revision arthroplasty.[75] The second-stage procedure occurred at a mean of 11 weeks (range: 4 to 39 weeks) after insertion of

CLASSIFICATION OF INFECTION IN **TKA**

TYPE	CHARACTERISTICS	CRITERIA
I	Early postoperative	Wound infection (superficial or deep) that developed less than 4 weeks after the index operation.
II	Chronic	Developed 4 weeks or more after the index operation and had an insidious clinical presentation.
III	Acute hematogenous	Associated with a documented or suspected antecedent bacteremia and was characterized by an acute onset of symptoms in the affected joint with the prosthesis.
IV	Positive intraoperative cultures	Considered to have positive intraoperative cultures when the same organism grew on culture of at least 2 specimens that had been obtained at the time of a revision surgery.

the spacer, and mobilization was encouraged between stages. All patients were assessed at a minimum of 2 years after reimplantation. Only one patient (4%) was reinfected. The average range of motion prior to reimplantation was 5 to 112 degrees and 3 to 115 degrees at latest follow-up. The authors concluded that the knee motion that was maintained between stages helped facilitate the reimplantation procedure.

Fehring et al evaluated 25 patients treated with static nonarticulating spacers and 30 treated with tobramycin-laden articulating spacers.[76] The knee arthroplasties in 3 patients treated with a static spacer became reinfected (12%). The knee arthroplasty in one patient with an articulating spacer became reinfected (7%). Fifteen of the 25 patients with static spacers had unexpected bone loss between stages. No appreciable bone loss could be measured in the patients who received articulating spacers. The average Hospital for Special Surgery score was 83 points in the patients with static spacers and 84 points in the patients with articulating spacers. Range of motion at final follow-up averaged 98 degrees in the patients who received static spacers and 105 degrees in the patients who received articulating spacers. The authors felt the articulating spacers seemed to facilitate reimplantation of infected TKA without additional risk of infection. Unexpected bone loss was not a concern with this two-stage technique.

More recently, Freeman et al reported on the use of static and articulating spacers for two-stage reimplantation of infected TKA.[77] Seventy-six two-stage reimplantation included 28 static spacers and 48 articulating spacers. The eradication rate was 94.7% in the articulating group compared with 92.1% in the static group ($P = 0.7$). There were no significant differences in postoperative Knee Society pain scores. There were 28 (58%) good to excellent function scores in the articulating group and 10 (36%) in the static group ($P = .05$). This study demonstrates that the use of articulating spacers do not have an adverse effect on eradication of infection and may portend better functional outcomes.

SUMMARY

Infection is an uncommon but devastating complication following total joint arthroplasty. It carries significant consequences to the patient, surgeon, and society. Improvements in surgical technique have resulted in decreased infection rates. Nonetheless, periprosthetic infection remains a diagnostic and therapeutic challenge and the prevalence of this complication will likely increase as the number of joint arthroplasty procedures continue to rise.

Staged exchange arthroplasty is the gold standard for treatment of late and chronic infection after TKA. For early acute or hematogenous infections, meticulous débridement with exchange of modular components and implant retention may result in eradication of the offending organism. Future effort should focus on improvement of accurate diagnosis and success of treatment.

REFERENCES

1. Ong KL, Kurtz SM, Lau E, et al. Prosthetic joint infection risk after total hip arthroplasty in the Medicare population. *J Arthroplasty*. 2009;24(6 suppl 1):105-109.
2. Kurtz SM, Ong KL, Lau E, et al. Prosthetic joint infection risk after TKA in the Medicare population. *Clin Orthop Relat Res*. 2010;468(1):52-56.
3. Fitzgerald RH. Total hip arthroplasty sepsis. Prevention and diagnosis. *Orthop Clin North Am*. 1992;23(2):259-264.
4. Hanssen AD, Osmon DR, Nelson CL. Prevention of deep periprosthetic joint infection. *Instr Course Lect*. 1997;46:555-567.
5. Hanssen AD, Osmon DR. Prevention of deep wound infection after total hip arthroplasty: the role of prophylactic antibiotics and clean air technology. *Semin Arthroplasty*. 1994;5(3):114-121.
6. Bengtson S, Blomgren G, Knutson K, et al. Hematogenous infection after total knee arthroplasty. *Acta Orthop Scand*. 1987;58:529.
7. Bengtson S, Knutson K, Lidgren L. Revision of infected knee arthroplasty. *Acta Orthop Scand*. 1987;57:489.
8. Bengtson S, Knutson K, Lidgren L. Treatment of infected knee arthroplasty. *Clin Orthop Relat Res*. 1989;245:173-178.
9. Grogan TJ, Dorey F, Rollins J, et al. Deep sepsis following total knee arthroplasty: 10 year experience at the University of California at Los Angeles Medical Center. *J Bone Joint Surg*. 1986;68A:226-234.
10. Petty W, Bryan RS, Coventry MB, et al. Infection after total knee arthroplasty. *Orthop Clin North Am*. 1975;6:1005-1014.
11. Rand JA, Bryan RS. Reimplantation for the salvage of an infected total knee arthroplasty. *J Bone Joint Surg*. 1983;65A:1081-1086.
12. Schoifet SD, Morrey BF. Treatment of infection after total knee arthroplasty by debridement with retention of components. *J Bone Joint Surg*. 1990;72A:1383-1390.
13. Wilson MG, Kelley K, Thornhill TS. Infection as a complication of total knee replacement arthroplasty: risk factors in treatment in 67 cases. *J Bone Joint Surg*. 1990;72A:878-883.
14. Rand JA, Bryan RS, Morrey BF, et al. Management of the infected total knee arthroplasty. *Clin Orthop Relat Res*. 1986;205:75-85.
15. Blom AW, Brown J, Taylor AH, Pattison G, Whitehouse S, Bannister GC. Infection after total knee arthroplasty. *J Bone Joint Surg Br*. 2004;86:688-691.
16. Kurtz SM, Lau E, Schmier J, et al. Infection burden for hip and knee arthroplasty in the united states. *J Arthroplasty*. 2008;23(7):984-991.
17. Peersman G, Laskin R, Davis J, Peterson MG, Richart T. ASA physical status classification is not a good predictor of infection for total knee replacement and is influenced by the presence of comorbidities. *Acta Orthop Belg*. 2008;74:360-364.
18. Hanssen AD, Osmon DR, Nelson CL. Prevention of deep periprosthetic joint infection. *J Bone Joint Surg Am*. 1996;78:458-471.
19. Agarwal S, Kadhi SKM, Rooney RJ. Brucellosis complicating bilateral total knee arthroplasty. *Clin Orthop Relat Res*. 1991;267:179-181.
20. Windsor RE, Insall JN, Urs WK, et al. Two-stage reimplantation for the salvage of total knee arthroplasty complicated by infection: further follow-up and refinement of indications. *J Bone Joint Surg*. 1990;72A:272.
21. Parvizi J, Ghanem E, Sharkey P, Aggarwal A, Burnett RS, Barrack RL. Diagnosis of infected total knee: findings of a multicenter database. *Clin Orthop Relat Res*. 2008;466:2628-2633.
22. Sanzen L, Sundberg M. Periprosthetic low-grade hip infections. Erythrocyte sedimentation rate and C-reactive protein in 23 cases. *Acta Orthop Scand*. 1997;68:461-465.
23. Greidanus NV, Masri BA, Garbuz DS, et al. Use of erythrocyte sedimentation rate and C-reactive protein level to diagnose infection before revision total knee arthroplasty. A prospective evaluation. *J Bone Joint Surg Am*. 2007;89(7):409-416.

24. Di Cesare PE, Chang E, Preston CF, Liu CJ. Serum interleukin-6 as a marker of periprosthetic infection following total hip and knee arthroplasty. *J Bone Joint Surg Am.* 2005;87(9):1921-1927.

25. Mariani B, Tuan R. Advances in the diagnosis of infection in prosthetic joint implants. *Molecular Med Today.* 1998;4(5):207-213.

26. Palestro CJ, Swyer AJ, Kim CK, et al. Infected knee prosthesis: diagnosis with In-111 leukocyte, Pc-99m sulfur colloid and Tc-99m MDP imaging. *Radiology.* 1991;179:645.

27. Rand JA, Brown ML. The value of indium-111 leukocyte scanning in the evaluation of painful or infected knee arthroplasties. *Clin Orthop Relat Res.* 1990;259:179-182.

28. Spangehl MJ, Masri BA, O'Connell JX, Duncan CP. Prospective analysis of preoperative and intraoperative investigations for the diagnosis of infection at the sites of two hundred and two revision total hip arthroplasties. *J Bone Joint Surg Am.* 1999;81(5):672-683.

29. Ghanem E, Parvizi J, Burnett RS, et al. Cell count and differential of aspirated fluid in the diagnosis of infection at the site of total knee arthroplasty. *J Bone Joint Surg Am.* 2008;90(8):1637-1643.

30. Trampuz A, Hanssen AD, Osmon DR, et al. Synovial fluid leukocyte count and differential for the diagnosis of prosthetic knee infection. *Am J Med.* 2004;117(8):556-562.

31. Saxena A, Jacovides C, Siad J, et al. Cell count and differential of aspirated fluid in acute postoperative period total knee arthroplasty. Presented at the Musculoskeletal Infection Society 19th Annual Open Scientific Meeting; San Diego, CA; August 2009.

32. Athanasou NA, Pandey R, de Steiger R, Crook D, Smith PM. Diagnosis of infection by frozen section during revision arthroplasty. *J Bone Joint Surg Br.* 1995;77(1):28-33.

33. Lonner JH, Desai P, Dicesare PE, Steiner G, Zuckerman JD. The reliability of analysis of intraoperative frozen sections for identifying active infection during revision hip or knee arthroplasty. *J Bone Joint Surg Am.* 1996;78(10):1553-1558.

34. Berbari EF, Marculescu C, Sia I, et al. Culture-negative prosthetic joint infection. *Clin Infect Dis.* 2007;45(9):1113-1119.

35. Malekzadeh D, Osmon DR, Lahr BD, Hanssen AD, Berbari EF. Prior use of antimicrobial therapy is a risk factor for culture-negative prosthetic joint infection. *Clin Orthop Relat Res.* 2010;468(8):2039-2045.

36. Chimento GF, Finger S, Barrack RL. Gram stain detection of infection during revision arthroplasty. *J Bone Joint Surg Br.* 1996;78(5):838-839.

37. Bauer TW, Parvizi J, Kobayashi N, Krebs V. Diagnosis of periprosthetic infection. *J Bone Joint Surg Am.* 2006;88(4):869-882.

38. Tunney MM, Patrick S, Gorman SP, et al. Improved detection of infection in hip replacements. A currently underestimated problem. *J Bone Joint Surg Br.* 1998;80(4):568-572.

39. Tunney MM, Patrick S, Curran MD, et al. Detection of prosthetic joint biofilm infection using immunological and molecular techniques. *Meth Enzymol.* 1999;310:566-576.

40. Tunney MM, Patrick S, Curran MD, et al. Detection of prosthetic hip infection at revision arthroplasty by immunofluorescence microscopy and PCR amplification of the bacterial 16S rRNA gene. *J Clin Microbiol.* 1999;37(10):3281-3290.

41. Trampuz A, Piper KE, Jacobson MJ, et al. Sonication of removed hip and knee prostheses for diagnosis of infection. *N Engl J Med.* 2007;357(7):654-663.

42. Neut D, van Horn JR, van Kooten TG, van der Mei HC, Busscher HJ. Detection of biomaterial-associated infections in orthopaedic joint implants. *Clin Orthop Relat Res.* 2003;(413):261-268.

43. Coventry MB. Treatment of infections occurring in total hip surgery. *Orthop Clin North Am.* 1975;6:991-1003.

44. Segawa H, Tsukayama DT, Kyle RF, et al. Infection after total hip arthroplasty: a retrospective study of the treatment of eighty-one infections. *J Bone Joint Surg Am.* 1999;81:1434-1445.

45. Hughes PW, Salvati EA, Wilson PD, et al. Treatment of subacute sepsis of the hip by antibiotics and joint replacement: criteria for diagnosis and evaluation of 26 cases. *Clin Orthop Relat Res.* 1979;141:143-157.

46. Hunter D, Dandy D. The natural history of the patient with infected total hip replacement. *J Bone Joint Surg.* 1977;59B:293-297.

47. Rubin R, Salvati A, Lewis R. Infected total hip replacement after dental procedures. *Oral Surg.* 1976;41:18-23.

48. Stinchfield F, Bigliani L, Neu H, et al. Late haematogenous infection of total joint replacement. *J Bone Joint Surg.* 1980;62A:1345-1350.

49. Vandrhooft JE, Robinson RP. Late infection of a bipolar prosthesis following endoscopy. A case report. *J Bone Joint Surg.* 1994;76A:744-746.

50. Tsukayama DT, Estrada R, Gustilo RB. Infection after total hip arthroplasty: a study of the treatment of 106 infections. *J Bone Joint Surg.* 1996;78A:512-523.

51. Estrada R, Tsukayama DT, Gustilo RB. Management of total hip arthroplasty infections. A prospective study of 108 cases. *Orthop Trans.* 1994;17:1114-1115.
52. Tsukayama DT, Wicklund B, Gustillo RB. Suppressive antibiotic therapy in chronic prosthetic joint infections. *Orthopedics.* 1991;14:841-844.
53. Bengtson S, Knutson K. The infected knee arthroplasty. A six year follow-up of 357 cases. *Acta Orthop Scand.* 1991;62:301-311.
54. Johnson DP, Bannister GC. The outcome of infected arthroplasty of the knee. *J Bone Joint Surg Am.* 1986;68B:289-291.
55. Drancourt M, Stein A, Argenson JN, et al. Oral treatment of *Staphylococcus* SPP infected orthopedic implants with fusidic acid or ofloxacin in combination with rifampicin. *J Antimicrob Chemother.* 1997;39:235-240.
56. Brandt CM, Sistrunk WW, Duffy MC, et al. *Staphylococcus aureus* prosthetic joint infection treated with debridement and prosthesis retention. *Clin Infect Dis.* 1997;24:914-919.
57. Burger RR, Basch T, Hopson CN. Implant salvage in infected total knee arthroplasty. *Clin Orthop Relat Res.* 1991;273:105-112.
58. Tattevin P, Cremieux AC, Pottier P, et al. Prosthetic joint infection: when can prosthesis salvage be considered? *Clin Infect Dis.* 1999;29:292-295.
59. Chiu FY, Chen CM. Surgical débridement and parenteral antibiotics in infected revision total knee arthroplasty. *Clin Orthop Relat Res.* 2007;461:130-135.
60. Waldman BJ, Mont MA, Payman KR, et al. Infected total knee arthroplasty treated with arthrodesis using a modular nail. *Clin Orthop Relat Res.* 1999;367:230-237.
61. Mabry TM, Jacofsky DJ, Haidukewych GJ, et al. Comparison of intramedullary nailing and external fixation knee arthrodesis for the infected knee replacement. *Clin Orthop Relat Res.* 2007;464:11-15.
62. Pring DJ, Marks L, Angel JC. Mobility after amputation for failed knee replacement. *J Bone Joint Surg.* 1988;70B:770-771.
63. Siegel A, Frommelt L, Runde W. Therapy of bacterial joint infection by radical synovectomy in implantation of a cemented stabilized knee joint endoprosthesis. *Chirurg.* 2000;71:1385-1389.
64. von Foerster G, Kluber D, Kabler U. Mid- to long-term results after treatment of 118 cases of periprosthetic infections after knee joint replacement using one-stage exchange surgery. *Orthopade.* 1991;20:244-252.
65. Hanssen AD, Rand JA, Osmon DR. Treatment of the infected total knee arthroplasty with insertion of another prosthesis: the effect of antibiotic-impregnated bone cement. *Clin Orthop Relat Res.* 1994;309:116.
66. Goldman RT, Scuderi GR, Insall JN. Two-stage reimplantation for infected total knee replacement. *Clin Orthop Relat Res.* 1996;331:118-124.
67. Insall JN, Thompson FM, Brause BD. Two-stage reimplantation for salvage of infected total knee arthroplasty. *J Bone Joint Surg.* 1983;65A:1087-1098.
68. Masri BA, Duncan CP, Beauchamp CP. Long-term elution of antibiotics from bone cement: an in vivo study using the prosthesis of antibiotic-loaded acrylic cement (PROSTALAC) system. *J Arthroplasty.* 1998;13:331-338.
69. Penner MJ, Masri BA, Duncan CP. Elution characteristics of vancomycin and tobramycin combined in acrylic bone cement. *J Arthroplasty.* 1996;11:929-934.
70. Cadambi A, Jones RE, Maale GE. A protocol for staged revision of infected total hip and knee arthroplasties: the use of antibiotic-cement-implant composites. *Orthop Int.* 1995;3:133-145.
71. Duncan CP, Beauchamp CP, Masri B, et al. The antibiotic loaded joint replacement system: a novel approach to the management of the infected knee replacement. *J Bone Joint Surg.* 1992;74B(suppl III):296.
72. Hofmann AA, Kane KR, Tkach TK, et al. Treatment of infected total knee arthroplasty using an articulating spacer. *Clin Orthop Relat Res.* 1995;321:45-54.
73. Haddad FS, Masri BA, Campbell D, et al. The PROSTALAC functional spacer in two-stage revision for infected total knee replacements: prosthesis of antibiotic-loaded acrylic cement. *J Bone Joint Surg.* 2000;82B:807-812.
74. Haleem AA, Berry DJ, Hanssen AD. Mid-term to long-term followup of two-stage reimplantation for infected total knee arthroplasty. *Clin Orthop Relat Res.* 2004;(428):35-39.
75. Anderson JA, Sculco PK, Heitkemper S, Mayman DJ, Bostrom MP, Sculco TP. An articulating spacer to treat and mobilize patients with infected total knee arthroplasty. *J Arthroplasty.* 2009;24(4):631-635.
76. Fehring TK, Odum S, Calton TF, Mason JB. Articulating versus static spacers in revision total knee arthroplasty for sepsis. The Ranawat Award. *Clin Orthop Relat Res.* 2000;(380):9-16.
77. Freeman MG, Fehring TK, Odum SM, et al. Functional advantage of articulating versus static spacers in 2-stage revision for total knee arthroplasty infection. *J Arthroplasty.* 2007;22(8):1116-1121.

11

Stems
The "Religion" of Fixation Options?

Qais Naziri, MD; Harpal S. Khanuja, MD;
Michael A. Mont, MD; and Aaron J. Johnson, MD

The number of total knee arthroplasty (TKA) procedures is expected to increase to nearly 500,000 annually by the year 2030, with an estimated total number of revision procedures to be approximately 42,000 annually.[1] These revisions have the potential to translate into many complicated, time-consuming, and risky revision knee arthroplasty procedures. The most common reasons for revision include aseptic loosening, infection, and component malalignment.[2] Regardless of the cause of component failure, the surgeon may be forced to work with suboptimal bone stock including large bone deficits, weak metaphyseal bone, or areas of perforated cortex from previous hardware which all have the potential to compromise the structural integrity of the new component. One option for treating these complicated revision procedures is the implementation of components with intramedullary stems.

Intramedullary stems have many potential benefits. Biomechanically, they can provide diaphyseal fixation and relieve stress on deficient metaphyseal bone or allograft. The main mechanism by which this is achieved is through load transfer from the joint, through the intramedullary stem, and to the cortical bone surrounding the intramedullary canal. When patients have had prior knee hardware, perforations may exist in the cortical or metaphyseal bone. In these instances, stems have the advantage of load distribution beyond the cortical defect and consequently reduce the risk of stress risers leading to subsidence, or possibly a catastrophic fracture of the weakened metaphyseal bone.

However, despite these benefits, controversy remains over the appropriate fixation technique when implanting components with intramedullary stems. Some authors advocate the use of complete cementation of the condylar components and stem, while others are proponents of the use of press-fit stems in conjunction with cemented condylar components, and still others espouse completely noncemented components. Each has benefits and advantages unique to that particular technique, and all have enjoyed variable results published in the literature. The purpose of this chapter will be to review the biomechanics and advantages (both theoretical and practical) of using intramedullary stems, to discuss the 2 major cementing techniques, and to provide an overview of the published clinical results using each of these cementing methods.

Jacofsky DJ, Hedley AK, eds.
Fundamentals of Revision Knee Arthroplasty:
Diagnosis, Evaluation, and Treatment (pp 171-176).
© 2013 SLACK Incorporated.

Theoretical Advantages and Disadvantages of Stemmed Components

There are many biomechanical advantages that stems provide. The major concept of stem use is to provide diaphyseal fixation when there is insufficient metaphyseal bone stock or the remaining metaphyseal bone is structurally compromised. Diaphyseal fixation provides stress relief and transfers the load away from the weakened or absent metaphysis and additionally allows for the bypass of perforations from prior surgical fixation to prevent the formation of stress risers. These advantages are not without their risks. Load transfer can lead to stress shielding, bone resorption, and the potential for late implant failure. Additionally, some patients have reported pain that is localized to the stem tip.

The major theoretical advantage of stemmed components in TKA is load transfer away from metaphyseal bone,[3-6] which, in revision cases, can often be compromised. In a study by Reilly et al, cadaver knees were used to measure strains in the native knee, strains in the tibia after components were placed with diaphyseal stems, and strains seen in the stem itself.[6] The purpose of this study was to determine the amount of stress that was placed on the component and to determine the resultant stress that is absorbed by the cortical bone in an effort to calculate the percentage of load sharing that the stem provides. Both metal and plastic stems with a diameter of 16 mm and a length of 60 mm were used during testing and were implanted using both metaphyseal and diaphyseal cementing. The findings indicated that the strains near the component were lower with the metal stem, indicating that more load was transferred with a stiffer construct. Additionally, there was a directly proportional increase in the strains measured at the distal cortex due to load transfer from the stem. The amount of load sharing was also determined to be proportional to the length of the stem used. A study by Jazrawi et al[5] supported this conclusion, as their biomechanical testing of 6 cadaveric tibiae led to a decrease in the proximal strains seen as the stem length and diameter increased.

Because of the directly proportional effect of increasing load transfer as a function of stem length, stress shielding may be a concern, as its presence over time has been suggested to lead to progressive proximal bony resorption and ultimate component failure.[4-7] In a study by Innocenti et al, 500 patients who had undergone TKA had their radiographs reviewed for signs of tibial component subsidence.[7] Sixteen asymptomatic patients were identified who had radiographic subsidence, and their radiographs were then used to create finite element models in order to determine if their unique anatomy, combined with tibial component stem, could have created a stress shielding effect that could then ultimately have led to component subsidence and clinical failure. For both cemented and cementless fixation, the results of this study indicate that stress shielding—as had been previously theorized as a consequence of load transfer—can lead to bony resorption. However, of note is that despite the fact that stress shielding had led to slight subsidence of the tibial component, all patients were clinically asymptomatic and had excellent Knee Society pain and functional scores. While stress shielding remains a concern when using stemmed components, the clinical importance of this remains controversial. In a revision scenario, stress shielding may be preferred in an effort to decrease the amount of load that has to be supported by the weakened or absent metaphyseal bone.

Another purported advantage of the use of stemmed components is the ability to bypass cortical defects, and thereby theoretically reduce the risk of stress risers that can lead to periprosthetic fracture. Numerous studies have cited the occurrence of femoral fractures in the presence of cortical defects from biopsy sites, screw holes, cortical windows, or metastatic lesions.[8-12] However, despite the knowledge that these defects can lead to catastrophic failure, there is little scientific evidence to suggest what appropriate bypass distance is necessary in order to minimize stress fracture risk. In a study by Panjabi et al, 8 cadaver femora were used to determine the strain around a cortical defect when variable length stems were used to bypass the defect.[13] They determined that the use of a stem that bypasses the cortical defect by a minimum of 1.4 cortical diameters was sufficient to minimize the stress seen near the defect and was similar stress to that of an intact femur under the same loading conditions. Their recommendations were to bypass the defect by a minimum of 1.5 diameters; therefore, a femur with a diameter of 3 cm would require a stem to bypass the cortical defect by a minimum of 4.5 cm in order to minimize the risk of a stress fracture at the site of the defect.

With all stemmed components, regardless of how they are cemented into place, pain localized to the tip of the stem can be a problem unique to patients who have undergone revision with stemmed components and is something that patients should be warned about prior to the revision being performed.[14,15] In a study by Barrack et al of 143 revision knee arthroplasty procedures performed with stemmed components followed for a minimum of 2 years,[14] patients completed a drawing to indicate the specific location, on either the leg or thigh, where their pain was and were asked to describe the pain as occurring with (1) extreme activity, (2) moderate activity, (3) normal daily activity, or (4) at rest. Pain localized to the stem tip in solid stems was reported in 42 of 244 stems (18.8%), whereas only 5 of 62 slotted, fluted stems (8.1%) reported stem tip pain ($P < 0.05$). Of note, 36 of 112 patients (32%) with a solid stem reported pain related to the stem at either the femoral or tibial stem tip. Although the slotted stems appeared to cause less stem-related pain, there were still a large number of patients who reported stem pain, and patients should be warned of this possibility.

The major advantages of using stemmed revision TKA components are the structural benefits they provide when there is a lack of sufficient metaphyseal bone stock in revision scenarios. They provide load transfer away from this weakened area of bone and into the more structurally sound cortical bone as well as give the opportunity to bypass any cortical defects that may exist. These advantages are not without disadvantages, however, which include stress shielding, proximal bone resorption, and component subsidence, as well as leg or thigh pain directly related to stem use.

To Cement or Not to Cement?

Despite the advantages and disadvantages discussed above, controversy exists regarding the most appropriate fixation technique when using stemmed components in revision TKA. The first method is the use of cemented components, whereby all the condylar components and the diaphyseal stems are cemented into place. The alternative method is a hybrid technique in which the condylar components are cemented and the diaphyseal stems are press-fit or left freely in the canal. A third option is that the entire component may be press-fit without the use of any cement. Each of these methods has their own advantages and disadvantages, which will be discussed in depth in the following paragraphs. Additionally, clinical results of each of these fixation methods (summarized in Table 11-1) will be discussed.

Proponents of complete diaphyseal stem cementing argue that its use may be advantageous in patients who are extremely osteoporotic, who have extremely large femoral canals, or in whom malalignment cannot be avoided with modular offsets and press-fit stems.[16,17] An additional advantage of cemented diaphyseal stems is the ability to deliver antibiotic cement into the diaphyseal canal in infected TKA revisions. However, the major disadvantage associated with complete cementation that can be avoided with press-fit stems is difficult removal of the component and debris, should subsequent revision be required.[18,19]

Press-fit stems, when used with cemented condylar components, have purported advantages and disadvantages as well. The major advantage, as stated earlier, is their ease of removal should further revision be required. The biomechanical advantages discussed in the previous section all appear to hold true for either cemented or uncemented stems. The major disadvantage of press-fit stems is in the event of a large deformity of the femur or tibia secondary to a prior healed fracture, prior fracture or osteotomy, or excessive anatomic bowing of either the tibia or femur.[3,18-21] Modular stems allow the surgeon the ability to address mismatches with the distal femoral axis,

TABLE 11-1. SELECTED REPORTED SURVIVAL RATES OF THE 3 MAJOR REVISION FIXATION TECHNIQUES IN TOTAL KNEE ARTHROPLASTY

	AUTHOR (YEAR)	NUMBER OF KNEES (PATIENTS)	MEAN FOLLOW-UP (RANGE)	SURVIVAL
CEMENTED STEMS	Whaley (2003)[17]	38	121.2 months	96.7%
	Fehring (2003)	107	57 months (range: 24 to 142)	93%
CEMENTLESS STEMS	Haas (1995)[19]	76 (74)	42 months (range: 24 to 108)	92%
	Whiteside (1993)[20]	56 (56)	24 months (not reported)	98%
	Wood (2009)[21]	135 (not reported)	60 months (range: 24 to 144)	98% KMS* 12 years
	Fehring (2003)	95 (not reported)	57 months (range: 24 to 142)	71% (stable)
HYBRID FIXATION	Peters (2005)[15]	50 (47)	36 months (not reported)	91%
	Gofton (2002)	89 (84)	70.8 months (range: 4.1 to 8.6)	93.5% KMS 8.6 years

* Kaplan–Meier 36-month survivorship

as well as to correct the mediolateral and anteroposterior placement of the component in relation to the stem. Their use can also aid in balancing the flexion gap and can be used to either increase or decrease it with either more or less anterior placement of the component in relation to the intramedullary canal.

Chon et al[4] reviewed radiolucencies in revision components placed with and without diaphyseal cement. One hundred fifteen revision TKA procedures were reviewed with an average follow-up of 44 months (range: 24 to 126 months). Of the 75 revisions that were performed using press-fit stems, 67 (89%) had radiolucent lines less than 2 cm. By comparison, there were only 14 out of 24 (58%) that had radiolucencies in the group that had cemented stems. There was no difference in failure rates between the 2 groups.

Press-fit stemmed components have had excellent reported results. Peters et al reported on a series of 50 consecutive revision TKAs performed in 47 patients who had cemented condylar components and press-fit stems.[15] At a mean follow-up of 36 months (range: 24 to 96 months), there were no revisions for aseptic reasons. Eight patients died, and of the remaining 42 knees, 37 (88%) had good or excellent modified Hospital for Special Surgery knee scores. With revision for any reason as an endpoint, the Kaplan–Meier 36-month survivorship (KMS) was calculated to be 92%. Another study by Wood et al reviewed 135 knees in 127 patients who had undergone revision TKA with cemented condylar components and press-fit stems.[21] At a minimum 2-year follow-up (range: 2 to 12 years), the calculated KMS, with revision for any reason or radiographic loosening as the endpoint, was found to be 98% at 12 years, with 6 knees in 6 patients requiring further revision at a mean of 42 months (range: 12 to 96 months).

One study directly compared the outcomes of revision TKA with the use of cemented and uncemented stemmed components. Fehring et al reported on 113 revision procedures that were performed using stemmed components and had a minimum 2-year follow-up (range: 24 to 142 months).[22] Of those 113 revisions, there were 202 stemmed components placed. One hundred and seven of the stemmed components were cemented in place, whereas the remaining 95 were press-fit. At final follow-up, 100 of the 107 cemented stems (93%) were considered stable, in comparison to only 67 of the 95 press-fit stems (71%) that were considered stable. Although the authors concluded that cementless stems should be used with caution, these results are in contrast to the excellent results reported previously with the use of press-fit stems. Of note is that only 4 stemmed components in 3 patients required revision for aseptic loosening, despite the large number of components that were considered possibly loose, compared to none in the cemented cohort.

SUMMARY

The use of cemented stems is widely accepted as an adequate method of fixation in revision TKA procedures. Despite controversy that exists regarding the most appropriate cementing method, there are studies that support the use of both cemented and cementless diaphyseal stems. Despite the potential clinical success of both, there are risks to each method, which need to be weighed by the operative surgeon before a choice is made. Although cemented stems may prove to be a more difficult revision should subsequent surgery be necessary, they also provide the added benefit of being able to address cases of extreme osteoporotic bone or large femoral canals where press-fit stems may not be appropriate. Ultimately, the decision lies with the comfort level of the surgeon. There is no scientific evidence that strongly supports the use of one technique over another. However, surgeons are urged to carefully assess the risks of each method before making a decision. Additionally, longer-term studies that directly compare the performance of cemented versus press-fit stems are needed to assess whether there are definitive advantages of each method. A contraindication in cemented stems is the use of "off-setting" devices. These place the stem "off axis" to the implant and make simple linear disimpaction from the cement mantle impossible. If the stem diameter is appropriate they should never be indicated when cemented stems are used, as the cemented stem need not be centered in the intramedullary canal.

REFERENCES

1. Kurtz SM, Ong KL, Schmier J, et al. Future clinical and economic impact of revision total hip and knee arthroplasty. *J Bone Joint Surg Am.* 2007;89(suppl 3):144-151.
2. Bozic KJ, Kurtz SM, Lau E, et al. The epidemiology of revision total knee arthroplasty in the United States. *Clin Orthop Relat Res.* 2010;468(1):45-51.
3. Albrektsson BE, Ryd L, Carlsson LV, et al. The effect of a stem on the tibial component of knee arthroplasty. A roentgen stereophotogrammetric study of uncemented tibial components in the Freeman-Samuelson knee arthroplasty. *J Bone Joint Surg Br.* 1990;72(2):252-258.
4. Chon JG, Lombardi AV Jr, Berend KR. Hybrid stem fixation in revision total knee arthroplasty (TKA). *Surg Technol Int.* 2004;12:214-220.
5. Jazrawi LM, Bai B, Kummer FJ, Hiebert R, Stuchin SA. The effect of stem modularity and mode of fixation on tibial component stability in revision total knee arthroplasty. *J Arthroplasty.* 2001;16(6):759-767.
6. Reilly D, Walker P, Ben-Dov M, Ewald FC. Effects of tibial components on load transfer in the upper tibia. *Clin Orthop Relat Res.* 1982;165:273-282.

7. Innocenti B, Truyens E, Labey L, Wong P, Victor J, Bellemans J. Can medio-lateral baseplate position and load sharing induce asymptomatic local bone resorption of the proximal tibia? A finite element study. *J Orthop Surg Res.* 2009;4:26.

8. Burstein AH, Currey J, Frankel VH, Heiple KG, Lunseth P, Vessely JC. Bone strength. The effect of screw holes. *J Bone Joint Surg Am.* 1972;54(6):1143-1156.

9. Fidler M. Incidence of fracture through metastases in long bones. *Acta Orthop Scand.* 1981;52(6):623-627.

10. Johansson JE, McBroom R, Barrington TW, Hunter GA. Fracture of the ipsilateral femur in patients with total hip replacement. *J Bone Joint Surg Am.* 1981;63(9):1435-1442.

11. Kavanagh BF, Ilstrup DM, Fitzgerald RH Jr. Revision total hip arthroplasty. *J Bone Joint Surg Am.* 1985;67(4):517-526.

12. Taylor MM, Meyers MH, Harvey JP Jr. Intraoperative femur fractures during total hip replacement. *Clin Orthop Relat Res.* 1978;(137):96-103.

13. Panjabi MM, Trumble T, Hult JE, Southwick WO. Effect of femoral stem length on stress raisers associated with revision hip arthroplasty. *J Orthop Res.* 1985;3(4):447-455.

14. Barrack RL, Stanley T, Burt M, Hopkins S. The effect of stem design on end-of-stem pain in revision total knee arthroplasty. *J Arthroplasty.* 2004;19(7 suppl 2):119-124.

15. Peters CL, Erickson J, Kloepper RG, Mohr RA. Revision total knee arthroplasty with modular components inserted with metaphyseal cement and stems without cement. *J Arthroplasty.* 2005;20(3):302-308.

16. Hanssen AD. Cemented stems are requisite in revision knee replacement. *Orthopedics.* 2004;27(9):990,1003.

17. Whaley AL, Trousdale RT, Rand JA, Hanssen AD. Cemented long-stem revision total knee arthroplasty. *J Arthroplasty.* 2003;18(5):592-599.

18. Bertin KC, Freeman MA, Samuelson KM, Ratcliffe SS, Todd RC. Stemmed revision arthroplasty for aseptic loosening of total knee replacement. *J Bone Joint Surg Br.* 1985;67(2):242-248.

19. Haas SB, Insall JN, Montgomery W 3rd, Windsor RE. Revision total knee arthroplasty with use of modular components with stems inserted without cement. *J Bone Joint Surg Am.* 1995;77(11):1700-1707.

20. Whiteside LA. Cementless revision total knee arthroplasty. *Clin Orthop Relat Res.* 1993;(286):160-167.

21. Wood GC, Naudie DD, MacDonald SJ, McCalden RW, Bourne RB. Results of press-fit stems in revision knee arthroplasties. *Clin Orthop Relat Res.* 2009;467(3):810-817.

22. Fehring TK, Odum S, Olekson C, Griffin WL, Mason JB, McCoy TH. Stem fixation in revision total knee arthroplasty: a comparative analysis. *Clin Orthop Relat Res.* 2003;11(416):217-224.

Salvage of the Irretrievably Failed Total Knee Arthroplasty

David A. McQueen, MD and Christopher L. Anderson, MD

Rates of primary total knee arthroplasty (TKA), particularly in young active patients, and revision TKA are increasing at a rapid rate.[1] The need for salvage procedures to treat the inevitable associated failures will increase accordingly. The most common cause of the irretrievably failed TKA is recalcitrant infection persisting despite multiple previous attempts at treatment. Other common causes of failure include massive metaphyseal bone loss with associated ligamentous incompetence, deficient soft tissue coverage, and irreparable disruption of the extensor mechanism. The treatment of the irretrievably failed total knee has evolved over time. Amputation and resection arthroplasty have been replaced by arthrodesis and modular, mobile-bearing hinge arthroplasty with or without distal femoral replacement as the salvage procedures of choice. A thorough understanding of technical factors associated with each is a prerequisite to proceeding with these often complex reconstructive procedures.

The decision to proceed with a reconstructive procedure is a difficult one for both the patient and the surgeon. Modern two-stage reimplantation protocols, nonlinked constrained revision components with available augmentation, allograft and autograft techniques to address bony deficiency, and extensor mechanism reconstruction have considerably narrowed the definition of irretrievable failure. In general, patients can be divided into 2 categories. Younger, physically active patients in whom other reconstructive procedures have failed are candidates for knee arthrodesis. Older, more sedentary and physically infirm patients are candidates for modular, mobile-bearing hinge reconstruction. The expected outcome in both groups is eradication of infection and a pain-free, stable, sensate lower extremity that allows for independent function and ambulation.

ALTERNATIVE PROCEDURES

Although uncommonly performed, both above knee amputation (AKA) and resection arthroplasty remain viable treatment options in select patients. Medical infirmity that precludes a two-stage surgical procedure, life-threatening infection, and low-demand nonambulatory patients would be best served with these alternative forms of treatment. Functional results of these procedures tend to be uniformly poor.

Jacofsky DJ, Hedley AK, eds.
Fundamentals of Revision Knee Arthroplasty:
Diagnosis, Evaluation, and Treatment (pp 177-188).
© 2013 SLACK Incorporated.

Resection arthroplasty may be considered in severely disabled patients with polyarticular joint disease and low functional demands. With this technique, implants are removed and bone ends are contoured to allow maximal contact in full knee extension. Although this procedure was initially described as the first stage of a two-stage arthrodesis, no attempt at arthrodesis is made. Temporary fixation via suture or pinning is performed to maintain limb alignment, and a cast is worn for 6 months postoperatively. Weightbearing is allowed as tolerated. Benefits of this procedure include functional flexion of the knee; average range of motion is 40 to 53 degrees, which allows for easier sitting. Drawbacks include persistent knee instability and pain with associated difficulty in ambulation.[2] Falahee et al reported on a series of 28 knees undergoing resection arthroplasty for the treatment of failed septic TKA. Following the procedure, 15 patients were able to walk independently. Six patients with monoarticular disease were dissatisfied with the results of resection arthroplasty and underwent subsequent arthrodesis. Those patients with greater disability prior to the resection arthroplasty were more likely to be satisfied with the results of the procedure.[3]

AKA is an uncommonly performed salvage procedure following TKA. In one series of 18,443 primary arthroplasties, 0.14% went on to AKA for causes attributable to the arthroplasty. Amputation is typically a result of uncontrollable infection, pain, bone loss, and vascular complications.[4] Patients treated with amputation tend to be of overall poor health and functional capacity. In a retrospective review of 35 patients treated with AKA following septic failure of TKA, 15 patients (43%) had died during the mean 39-month follow-up.[5] Potential for independent ambulation following amputation is also quite poor, despite prosthetic fitting, and patients should expect to be dependent upon a wheelchair postoperatively. In one series of 23 amputations performed for failed TKA, only 7 of 23 were daily walkers, 20 of 23 used a wheelchair for part of the day, and 12 were confined to wheelchairs.[6]

Knee Arthrodesis

Knee arthrodesis has historically been performed as a primary treatment for pain and instability associated with a wide variety of pathologic knee conditions. Building upon the early work of Key, in 1958 Charnley and Lowe published a series of 171 cases of knee arthrodesis performed primarily for, in order of frequency, tuberculosis, osteoarthritis, and rheumatoid arthritis. These cases were treated with external fixation and Charnley compression clamps. The reported fusion rate in their series was 98.8%.[7] The introduction of modern TKA has significantly narrowed the common historical indications for arthrodesis while greatly expanding another. Currently, the most common indication for knee arthrodesis is the failed septic TKA.[8]

Arthrodesis in the face of failed TKA has historically been considerably less successful. In 1978, Hagemann et al published the first report on arthrodesis in patients with failed TKA. Using similar techniques as those of Charnley they obtained fusion in only 9 of 14 (74%).[9] The multiply operated knee with its associated difficulties serves to complicate knee arthrodesis following TKA. In order to address these issues and improve fusion rates, a variety of new arthrodesis techniques have been developed. These techniques may be broadly classified as intramedullary or extramedullary methods of fixation.

The ideal method of obtaining an arthrodesis in each clinical situation remains a matter of debate. The most commonly performed procedures are external fixation and intramedullary nailing. With failed TKA and associated bone loss as an indication, intramedullary devices have consistently shown better rates of union (80% to 100%) when compared to traditional external fixators (43% to 71%).[8] Newer forms of external fixation, Ilizarov devices, have been shown to be equally efficacious or better than intramedullary methods (93% to 100%).[10,11] The benefits and drawbacks of each method as well as patient-specific factors should be fully addressed prior to proceeding with arthrodesis.

Indications

Knee arthrodesis provides a stable, pain-free extremity at the expense of knee motion. Ideal candidates for this procedure are young, physically active patients with high functional demands following a failed TKA. Harris et al reviewed the functional results of amputation, arthrodesis, or arthroplasty in 22 patients following malignant skeletal tumor resection. Those patients undergoing arthrodesis were found to have a more stable limb that allowed for demanding physical work and recreational activities, compared to the TKA group that tended toward more sedentary lifestyles.[12] Salvage of the septic failed TKA remains the most commonly reported indication to perform arthrodesis. Other less common indications include aseptic loosening, poor soft tissues, deficient extensor mechanism, instability, and pain.[8]

Contraindications

Contraindications to knee arthrodesis are few and for the most part relative. Ipsilateral hip or ankle disease is frequently mentioned, as the joints adjacent to the fusion will experience increased stress related to compensatory alterations in gait mechanics. Bilateral knee involvement, contralateral amputation, and severe congenital anomalies are also relative contraindications.[13]

SURGICAL CONSIDERATIONS

Regardless of the method of fixation, adherence to basic surgical principles improves the chance of obtaining successful fusion. Preoperatively, a complete physical exam and medical history is obtained to assess for any comorbid conditions that might negatively affect wound healing and cardiopulmonary function. Oxygen consumption walking with an arthrodesis should be expected to be 25% to 30% higher than without.[14] Particular attention should be paid to the quality of soft tissue overlying the anterior knee. When the quality of overlying tissue is questionable, preoperative consultation with a plastic surgeon is recommended. Long leg standing radiographs are obtained to demonstrate overall limb alignment, quality of remaining bone stock, expected postoperative limb shortening, and the presence of other implants that would preclude the use of certain forms of fixation. A preoperative trial of knee immobilization may highlight potential difficulties that the patient may encounter postoperatively.[15] Patients with an arthrodesis tend to have difficulty climbing stairs, riding in automobiles, and with seating in arenas and theaters.[12]

The most critical surgical principle influencing successful fusion is rigid apposition of viable cancellous bone.[2] In cases with bone loss, obtaining rigidly opposed cancellous bone surfaces with sufficient surface area becomes progressively more difficult. This is highlighted in reports that include removal of more highly constrained TKA prostheses. In Hagemann's series, arthrodesis rates were 57% following removal of a hinged prosthesis versus 71% in those without.[9] In another early study of arthrodesis for failed TKA, Knutson reported a failure rate of 36% when salvaging hinge prostheses.[16]

Every attempt to eradicate infection should be made prior to the definitive arthrodesis procedure. Large retrospective reviews have shown that the successful treatment of infection results in higher fusion rates.[8] Multiple authors have advocated a two-stage procedure with removal of components and nonviable tissue followed by antibiotic-impregnated spacers and a course of intravenous antibiotics prior to definitive fusion. In a meta-analysis of 5 studies, Damron identified gram negative and polymicrobial infections as more likely to produce failure of arthrodesis.[13] Single-stage procedures, particularly those involving no gross purulence and gram positive organisms, have been successful and may be considered in patients who would not tolerate a second procedure.

Sagittal and coronal plane alignment are both important intraoperative considerations. Optimal sagittal alignment has been cited at 0 to 15 degrees of flexion. Limb shortening is inevitable with most methods of arthrodesis and averages 2.5 to 6.4 cm.[14] A moderate amount of shortening is beneficial as it allows for foot clearance in the swing phase of gait. Additional flexion of the fused knee contributes to further limb shortening; therefore, in cases with significant bone loss fusion in full extension is recommended. Coronal alignment should be in the physiologic range of 5 to 7 degrees of valgus.[14] The use of TKA cutting guides aids in obtaining optimal alignment and maximizing surface area available for fusion.

TECHNIQUES

Various techniques of knee arthrodesis for failed TKA have been developed with reported union rates of 43% to 100%.[8] Procedures may be broadly grouped into extramedullary and intramedullary type devices. Extramedullary devices include various forms of external fixators, compression plating, and compression screws. Intramedullary techniques include long intramedullary nails and short modular nails.

As arthrodesis is an uncommonly performed procedure, most evidence supporting the use of one type of fixation over another is anecdotal and provided by case series. The summation of these series does provide valuable information as to when a treating surgeon should proceed with a specific type of fixation. Information that should be obtained prior to the selection of a specific technique includes the presence of ongoing infection, degree of bone loss, soft tissue integrity, and functional demands of the patient following surgery.

EXTRAMEDULLARY DEVICES

External Fixation

External fixation for knee arthrodesis has a history that dates to 1932 when Key introduced the concept for treatment of knee tuberculosis. Traditional methods of external fixation include both uniplanar and biplanar. These traditional forms of external fixation have performed relatively poorly in the treatment of failed TKA with fusion rates ranging from 43% to 71%. More modern types of external fixators, Ilizarov devices, have improved fusion rates to 93% to 100% but have been associated with multiple complications.[8] In cases of TKA salvage, external fixation has been used primarily in the setting of uncontrollable infection. In this situation external fixation allows for fixation without the associated longstanding foreign body that is present with other types of fixation. Other proposed benefits include limited soft tissue dissection, better control of sagittal and coronal plane alignment, and the possibility of concomitant lengthening through distraction osteogenesis. Complications associated with external fixation are numerous and include pin tract infections, stress fracture, patient intolerance, and prolonged course of treatment.[15]

Uniplanar constructs have historically been the gold standard in knee arthrodesis. With the introduction of failed TKA as an indication, fusion rates fell significantly.[9] In an attempt to improve stability with regard to anteroposterior bending, biplanar techniques were developed. Despite the increased rigidity of biplane fixation when compared to uniplanar, fusion rates are not significantly different between the two. Hak et al published a series of 36 cases of arthrodesis performed with either a uniplanar or biplanar external fixator. In their series, the initial arthrodesis rate was only 61%. Comparable rates were obtained with both types of fixation. Complications were frequent and included 14 nonunions, 6 pin tract infections, 5 delayed unions, 1 stress fracture, and 1 persistent infection requiring amputation.[17]

The relative failure of traditional forms of external fixation led to the adaptation of modern Ilizarov techniques to attempt knee arthrodesis. The results of these devices have been largely successful despite their application in a single-stage procedure. Oostenbroek et al reported on the use of an Ilizarov device to obtain knee arthrodesis following failed septic TKA. In their series, the fixator was applied as a single-stage procedure following implant removal. All but one went on to successful fusion (93%) despite 8 patients (53%) having failed previous arthrodesis attempts. Mean duration of treatment was 28 weeks in the frame and 23 weeks of cast immobilization. Their complication rate was reported at 80% and was attributed to the advanced age of their patients. All had pin tract infections.[11]

Compression Plating

Compression plating, although used commonly in other orthopedic applications, remains relatively uncommonly reported in knee arthrodesis. Although reports are limited, fusion rates with this technique have been 100% in small series.[18,19] The purported benefits of this technique include rigid apposition of bone surfaces, familiarity of surgical technique, and early partial weightbearing. Potential drawbacks include more extensive soft tissue dissection, symptomatic hardware, and peri-implant stress fracture.

Lucas and Murray reported on the use of double plating for knee arthrodesis in 1961.[20] In a modification of their original technique, Nichols et al reported on the use of dual compression plating in a series of 11 patients following failed TKA. This technique involved the placement of 2 contoured dynamic compression plates to the anteromedial and anterolateral aspect of the knee. Their series included 7 septic TKA failures, 1 with an openly draining wound. Only the patient with the draining wound was managed with a two-stage procedure. Weightbearing as tolerated in an above-knee cast was allowed following discharge from the hospital. Union was achieved in all patients at an average of 5.6 months. Complications included persistent infection in one and femoral stress fracture in another. In order to reduce the rate of stress fracture, the authors recommended that the plates be placed in a staggered fashion.[18]

Pritchett et al proposed an alternative plating technique. Their series consisted of 26 patients, 6 with failed TKA, treated with a single anterior tension band plate construct. A 4.5-mm contoured plate was placed anteriorly and tensioned to allow compression along the concave joint surface and tension along the convex surface of the plate. Postoperatively partial weightbearing without supplemental immobilization was encouraged. Solid union occurred in all patients radiographically at an average of 16 weeks. Complications included persistent infection and deep aching that necessitated plate removal in 4 patients.[19]

INTRAMEDULLARY DEVICES

Long Intramedullary Nails

Intramedullary devices have a long history of use to achieve knee arthrodesis. In 1948, Chapchal reported on the use of intramedullary pinning for arthrodesis of the knee.[21] With the advent of failed TKA as an indication for arthrodesis, it was observed that intramedullary devices offered several distinct advantages when compared to external fixation methods. Intramedullary fixation typically allows for immediate weightbearing with axial compression across the arthrodesis site, improved mechanical stability, and superior rates (80% to 100%) of fusion.[8] Drawbacks include a more technically demanding procedure, less control of coronal and sagittal balance, and potential for intramedullary spread of infection.

Intramedullary devices are available in 2 forms. Long intramedullary nails and modular short nails are both currently available. Long nails have the theoretic benefit of greater stability over the long lever arm of the lower extremity. Modular nails offer the ability to perform fusion through a single incision, rigid compression through the locking mechanism of the nail, modularity in the ability to select different sizes of the femoral and tibial arms of the nail, and the ability to use the nail in patients with ipsilateral hip prostheses.

Early series highlight the technical difficulty and associated complications with placing long intramedullary nails. In a series of 20 patients, 8 with failed septic TKA, treated with long Kuntscher intramedullary nails, Donley reported an 85% fusion rate. The average estimated blood loss was 1574 mL, and the average operative time was 4.1 hours. Multiple complications were also described including intraoperative fracture, nail migration, and persistent gluteal pain.[22] With the advent of proximal locking screws, the migration issue has been addressed. Later series have documented similar fusion rates with significantly shorter operative times and EBL as surgeons have become more familiar with the technique.[23]

The use of intramedullary devices in the presence of infection is a subject of ongoing debate, despite the fact that there have been no documented cases of femoral or tibial osteomyelitis secondary to the use of intramedullary devices for knee arthrodesis.[14] The theoretic spread of infection throughout the medullary canal has prompted most to perform intramedullary nail arthrodesis as a staged procedure with treatment protocols similar to those of explanted TKA. Intramedullary nail arthrodesis can, however, be performed in the presence of infection as a single-stage procedure. In Puranen et al's series of 33 knees treated with long intramedullary nails, 7 of 8 infected TKA were treated in a single stage. All eventually went on to union despite the presence of a preoperative fistula and soft tissue defect in three.[24] More recent series of predominately long intramedullary nails used for the treatment of failed septic TKA describe two-stage protocols with successful fusion rates of 83% in 41 patients.[25,26]

Modular Intramedullary Nails

Modular devices include both the Neff nail (Zimmer, Warsaw, Indiana) and the Wichita Fusion Nail (WFN; Stryker Orthopaedics, Mahwah, NJ). These devices incorporate a coupling mechanism between the femoral and tibial arms of the nail allowing for retrograde insertion of the femoral component and antegrade insertion of the tibial component through a single knee incision. The WFN also allows for compression across the arthrodesis site with a compression screw. Modularity of these devices allows for better canal fit in cases of femoral and tibial canal width discrepancy. Reported union rates with these devices have ranged from 90% to 100%, and in the case of the WFN more rapid rates of union have been reported[27,28] (Figure 12-1).

Arroyo et al reported on a series of 21 patients, 5 with failed TKA, treated with the Neff nail. Their reported fusion rate was 90% at an average of 8.4 months. Complications included stress fracture, peroneal nerve palsy, superficial wound infection, and reflex sympathetic dystrophy.[27] In another series of 44 patients, 26 with septic TKA, the WFN was successful in obtaining arthrodesis in 100% at an average of 15.5 weeks. Major complication rate was 20% with delayed union, deep infection, and peri-implant fracture reported.[28] Should modular short nail removal be required, the nail may need to be sectioned and removed through anterior cortical windows.

The WFN has also had favorable results when used in series utilizing other types of fixation. In one series of 32 fusions performed following failed TKA, successful fusion was obtained in 10 of 11 cases utilizing the WFN at an average of 4.5 months. External fixation was utilized in 15, plating in 3, and long intramedullary nail in three. Of these remaining 21 patients, fusion was obtained in only 11 after a mean duration of 6.5 months.[29]

HINGE RECONSTRUCTION

Walldius first described hinged knee reconstruction in 1951 for the primary treatment of arthritis. Regarding patient selection, he stated that risk reduction had been maximized by

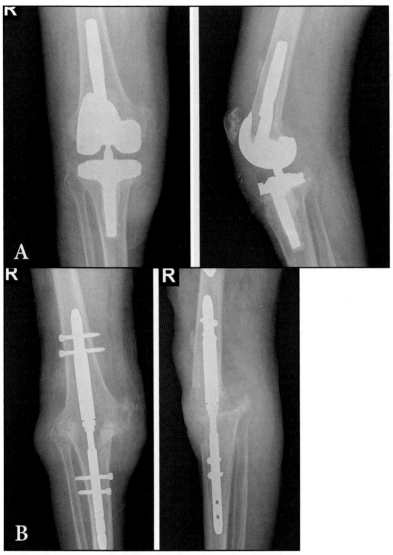

Figure 12-1. (A) Ninety year old with recurrent septic total knee, absent patellar tendon, and failed medial gastrocnemius flap. (B) Sound arthrodesis after explantation, antibiotic spacer placement, and subsequent arthrodesis.

"choosing those patients who are already so disabled that an unsuccessful operation could hardly cause a change for the worse." In an 8-year follow-up of his original series, he reported very good results in 41 (64%), good results in 6 (10%), and poor results in 17 (26%). Very good results were defined as a stable, pain-free joint with a range of motion from 50 to 90 degrees. Failures were primarily the result of infection.[30] Despite these promising early results, hinge arthroplasty was largely abandoned in nontumor applications due to less than optimal clinical outcomes associated with first- and second-generation devices. Early designs were true fixed hinges that allowed for motion only in the sagittal plane. This led to transmission of force to the bone-cement interface and unacceptably high rates of aseptic loosening. Other common problems included deep infection and common patellofemoral complications.[31] Modern third-generation designs have attempted to address these issues and have led to a resurgence in the use of hinged devices for a variety of indications.

Third-generation designs have incorporated numerous design changes in an attempt to address previous causes of failure. The most important of these changes includes the ability to rotate.[32,33] Theoretically, this decrease in constraint should allow for more natural kinematics of the knee,

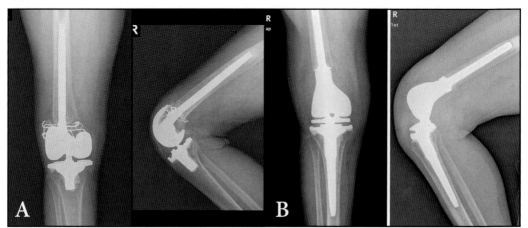

Figure 12-2. (A) Sixty-two year old with nonunion of distal femur, broken intramedullary stem distal femoral stress shielding. (B) Reconstruction with hinged modular replacement system.

thus leading to decreased wear and stress that has been associated with aseptic loosening. Other changes include deeper, more anatomic trochlea to address patellofemoral issues as well as modular fluted stems to allow for press-fit fixation. Despite these changes, rotating hinge reconstruction is still plagued by high complication rates and should be reserved for salvage-type situations.[33]

Indications

Rotating hinge reconstruction remains an uncommonly performed procedure. In one series covering 18 years at one institution, a rotating hinge device with distal femoral replacement was used for nonneoplastic limb salvage in only 0.14% of cases.[34] In most primary and revision TKA cases the stability imparted by nonlinked constrained implants provides sufficient stability for good functional outcomes while continuing to allow peri-articular soft tissues to absorb force.[35] In revision cases with massive metaphyseal bone loss and ligamentous insufficiency, a linked device may be required (Figure 12-2).

Common indications for rotating hinge arthroplasty have varied considerably between authors and institutions. In the salvage of the irretrievably failed TKA, rotating hinge reconstruction is indicated in the revision of previous hinged implant, severe bone loss including the epicondylar attachment of collateral ligaments, gross ligamentous insufficiency, and distal femoral periprosthetic fracture and nonunion.[36]

The addition of distal femoral replacement to rotating hinge arthroplasty may be considered in select patients, particularly those elderly low-demand patients in which adequacy of distal femoral bone stock precludes other forms of treatment. Demographics from multiple series have shown that the elderly female with associated osteopenia has represented the majority of patients selected for distal femoral replacement.[34,36] Periprosthetic fracture of the femoral component continues to pose a significant treatment dilemma. Prolonged periods of immobilization and limited physical activity may have a considerable negative effect on an otherwise frail elderly individual. In one recent series of periprosthetic femoral fractures after TKA, only 28 of 41 patients returned to their prefracture level of activity, 10 had significant limitations in gait and ability to perform activities of daily living, and 3 died as a result of surgery.[37] The immediate stability and return to independent ambulation provided by distal femoral replacement justifies its use in these types of situations (Figure 12-3).

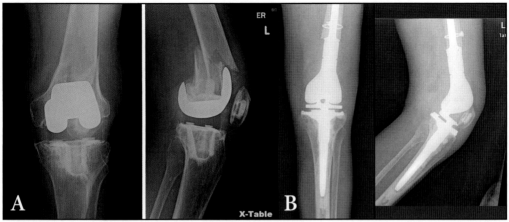

Figure 12-3. (A) Eighty-three year old with fall from standing. Observe widening of interepicondylar distance indicating level of comminution behind the implant. (B) Reconstruction with hinged modular replacement system.

Contraindications

Contraindications to hinge reconstruction with or without distal femoral replacement are similar to those of standard revision cases. Physical infirmity that precludes a surgical procedure, uncontrollable ongoing infection, and those with very low functional demands may be better treated with alternative procedures such as amputation or resection arthroplasty.

Outcomes

Outcomes following hinged reconstruction with or without distal femoral replacement have generally been satisfactory in short- to midterm follow-up, though complication rates, including deep infection, tend to be higher than those of primary TKA and revision TKA.[33] Berend and Lombardi recently reported a series of 39 rotating hinge TKAs, most of which also had distal femoral replacement. At a mean follow-up of 46 months they noted no failures from aseptic loosening. There were 5 reoperations; 2 recurrent infections, 1 periprosthetic fracture, 1 late infection, and 1 bearing exchange. Knee scores improved from 39 to 87, and pain scores improved from 18 to 43. The authors attributed their improved results to improvements in design, fixation, and modularity.[36]

Quality of life and clinical outcomes are also similar between hinge revisions and total condylar designs. Fuchs et al reported on 26 salvage revision TKAs, 10 of which were hinge designs. Outcomes were evaluated using Hospital for Special Surgery score, Knee Society score, and the Visual Analogue Scale for pain among others. Total condylar replacement had a significantly different greater range of motion, but there were no other significant differences among the previously listed scores.[38]

SUMMARY

The salvage of the irretrievably failed TKA poses a significant treatment dilemma for both surgeon and patient. Young, physically active patients may be treated successfully with arthrodesis using a variety of techniques. In more sedentary, frail, elderly patients, reconstruction with a hinge arthroplasty with or without distal femoral replacement is a viable treatment option. The goals of both are a stable, pain-free, sensate lower limb that allows for continued independent function and ambulation.

REFERENCES

1. Kurtz S, Ong K, Lau E, Mowat F, Halpern M. Projections of primary and revision hip and knee arthroplasty in the United States from 2005 to 2030. *J Bone Joint Surg Am.* 2007;89:780-785.

2. Rand JA. Alternatives to reimplantation for salvage of the total knee arthroplasty complicated by infection. *Instr Course Lect.* 1993;42:341-347.

3. Falahee MH, Matthews LS, Kaufer H. Resection arthroplasty as a salvage procedure for a knee with infection after a total arthroplasty. *J Bone Joint Surg Am.* 1987;69:1013-1021.

4. Sierra RJ, Trousdale RT, Pagnano MW. Above-the-knee amputation after a total knee replacement: prevalence, etiology, and functional outcome. *J Bone Joint Surg Am.* 2003;85-A:1000-1004.

5. Fedorka CJ, Chen AF, McGarry WM, Parvizi J, Klatt BA. Functional ability after above-the-knee amputation for infected total knee arthroplasty. *Clin Orthop Relat Res.* 2011;469:1024-1032.

6. Pring DJ, Marks L, Angel JC. Mobility after amputation for failed knee replacement. *J Bone Joint Surg Br.* 1988;70:770-771.

7. Charnley J, Lowe HG. A study of the end-results of compression arthrodesis of the knee. *J Bone Joint Surg Br.* 1958;40-B:633-635.

8. Wiedel JD. Salvage of infected total knee fusion: the last option. *Clin Orthop Relat Res.* 2002;404:139-142.

9. Hagemann WF, Woods GW, Tullos HS. Arthrodesis in failed total knee replacement. *J Bone Joint Surg Am.* 1978;60:790-794.

10. David R, Shtarker H, Horesh Z, Tsur A, Soudry M. Arthrodesis with the Ilizarov device after failed knee arthroplasty. *Orthopedics.* 2001;24:33-36.

11. Oostenbroek HJ, van Roermund PM. Arthrodesis of the knee after an infected arthroplasty using the Ilizarov method. *J Bone Joint Surg Br.* 2001;83:50-54.

12. Harris IE, Leff AR, Gitelis S, Simon MA. Function after amputation, arthrodesis, or arthroplasty for tumors about the knee. *J Bone Joint Surg Am.* 1990;72:1477-1485.

13. Damron TA, McBeath AA. Arthrodesis following failed total knee arthroplasty: comprehensive review and meta-analysis of recent literature. *Orthopedics.* 1995;18:361-368.

14. Conway JD, Mont MA, Bezwada HP. Arthrodesis of the knee. *J Bone Joint Surg Am.* 2004;86-A:835-848.

15. MacDonald JH, Agarwal S, Lorei MP, Johanson NA, Freiberg AA. Knee arthrodesis. *J Am Acad Orthop Surg.* 2006;14:154-163.

16. Knutson K, Lindstrand A, Lidgren L. Arthrodesis for failed knee arthroplasty. A report of 20 cases. *J Bone Joint Surg Br.* 1985;67:47-52.

17. Hak DJ, Lieberman JR, Finerman GA. Single plane and biplane external fixators for knee arthrodesis. *Clin Orthop Relat Res.* 1995;316:134-144.

18. Nichols SJ, Landon GC, Tullos HS. Arthrodesis with dual plates after failed total knee arthroplasty. *J Bone Joint Surg Am.* 1991;73:1020-1024.

19. Pritchett JW, Mallin BA, Matthews AC. Knee arthrodesis with a tension-band plate. *J Bone Joint Surg Am.* 1988;70:285-288.

20. Lucas DB, Murray W. Arthrodesis of the knee by double-plating. J Bone Joint Surg Am. 1961;43A:795-808.

21. Chapchal G. Intramedullary pinning for arthrodesis of the knee joint. J Bone Joint Surg Am. 1948;30A:728-734.

22. Donley BG, Matthews LS, Kaufer H. Arthrodesis of the knee with an intramedullary nail. *J Bone Joint Surg Am.* 1991;73:907-913.

23. Incavo SJ, Lilly JW, Bartlett CS, Churchill DL. Arthrodesis of the knee: experience with intramedullary nailing. *J Arthroplasty.* 2000;15:871-876.

24. Puranen J, Kortelainen P, Jalovaara P. Arthrodesis of the knee with intramedullary nail fixation. *J Bone Joint Surg Am.* 1990;72:433-442.

25. Talmo CT, Bono JV, Figgie MP, Sculco TP, Laskin RS, Windsor RE. Intramedullary arthrodesis of the knee in the treatment of sepsis after TKR. *HSS J.* 2007;3:83-88.

26. Bargiotas K, Wohlrab D, Sewecke JJ, Lavinge G, Demeo PJ, Sotereanos NG. Arthrodesis of the knee with a long intramedullary nail following the failure of a total knee arthroplasty as the result of infection. *J Bone Joint Surg Am.* 2006;88:553-558.

27. Arroyo JS, Garvin KL, Neff JR. Arthrodesis of the knee with a modular titanium intramedullary nail. *J Bone Joint Surg Am.* 1997;79:26-35.

28. McQueen DA, Cooke FW, Hahn DL. Knee arthrodesis with the Wichita Fusion Nail: an outcome comparison. *Clin Orthop Relat Res.* 2006;446:132-139.

29. Domingo LJ, Caballero MJ, Cuenca J, Herrera A, Sola A, Herrero L. Knee arthrodesis with the Wichita Fusion Nail. *Int Orthop.* 2004;28:25-27.

30. Walldius B. Arthroplasty of the knee using an endoprosthesis. 8 years' experience. *Acta Orthop Scand.* 1960;30:137-148.

31. Hui FC, Fitzgerald RH. Hinged total knee arthroplasty. *J Bone Joint Surg Am.* 1980;62:513-519.

32. Barrack RL. Evolution of the rotating hinge for complex total knee arthroplasty. *Clin Orthop Relat Res.* 2001;392:292-299.

33. Pour AE, Parvizi J, Slenker N, Purtill JJ, Sharkey PF. Rotating hinged total knee replacement: use with caution. *J Bone Joint Surg Am.* 2007;89:1735-1741.

34. Springer BD, Sim FH, Hanssen AD, Lewallen DG. The modular segmental kinematic rotating hinge for nonneoplastic limb salvage. *Clin Orthop Relat Res.* 2004;421:181-187.

35. Lombardi AV, Berend KR. Posterior cruciate ligament-retaining, posterior stabilized, and varus/valgus posterior stabilized constrained articulations in total knee arthroplasty. *Instr Course Lect.* 2006;55:419-427.

36. Berend KR, Lombardi AV. Distal femoral replacement in nontumor cases with severe bone loss and instability. *Clin Orthop Relat Res.* 2009;467:485-492.

37. Platzer P, Schuster R, Aldrian S, et al. Management and outcome of periprosthetic fractures after total knee arthroplasty. *J Trauma.* 2010;68:1464-1470.

38. Fuchs S, Sandmann C, Gerdemann G, Skwara A, Tibesku CO, Bottner F. Quality of life and clinical outcome in salvage revision total knee replacement: hinged vs total condylar design. *Knee Surg Sports Traumatol Arthrosc.* 2004;12:140-143.

13

Special Topic
Stress Shielding and Osteolysis

Michael T. Manley, FRSA, PhD; Steven M. Kurtz, PhD; and Kevin L. Ong, PhD

Approximately 580,000 primary total knee replacements (TKRs) are performed annually in the United States.[1] The number of revision knee procedures, now about 53,000 each year, is steadily increasing. The survivorship of revision knee joint replacement is generally worse than for primary knee replacement and becomes steadily worse if rerevision is necessary.[2] Recent analysis of survivorship data show that if revision is required, patients undergoing a second or later revision are approximately 6 times more likely to require rerevision than patients undergoing a first revision.[2] In addition, the costs and risks associated with revision surgery means that there is both financial and emotional incentives to increase the longevity of primary TKR.[3]

The most common indications for revision knee surgery are infection (25.2%) and mechanical loosening (16.1%). Periprosthetic osteolysis and wear accounts for 3.2% and 4.9% of the reasons for revision, respectively.[4] All of these factors can be interrelated. For example, a diagnosis of mechanical loosening may be due to a loss of fixation caused by one or more factors such as adverse periprosthetic bone remodeling, osteolysis, and stress shielding. In total hip arthroplasty, increased interest in bearing wear and the recognition of wear-related osteolysis as a causative factor for failure over the past decade means that osteolytic bone loss is commonly reported as the reason for hip revision. Clinical data available for osteolysis in total knee arthroplasty (TKA) suggest the incidence is less common than in the hip, probably due to the difference in joint conformity and wear patterns between hip and knee. It is known that wear particles released from knee replacements are larger in size and less granular than those released from replaced hips.[5] Nonetheless, osteolysis can occur can occur in the knee,[6,7] producing lesions that can compromise the mechanical support for the implant components. Bone remodeling and stress shielding are often more apparent in the hip than in the knee, but loss of bone behind the anterior portion of the knee femoral component is now recognized as an increasing problem if revision is necessary.

The difficulties of revision surgery in hip and knee are often complicated by bone defects, regardless of how they are caused. Bone defects may lead to the need for extensive reconstruction with morselized allograft or autograft or by defect filling with allograft, xenograft, synthetic bone graft substitutes, or metal wedges and block augments. All of these reconstruction methods

Jacofsky DJ, Hedley AK, eds.
*Fundamentals of Revision Knee Arthroplasty:
Diagnosis, Evaluation, and Treatment* (pp 189-204).
© 2013 SLACK Incorporated.

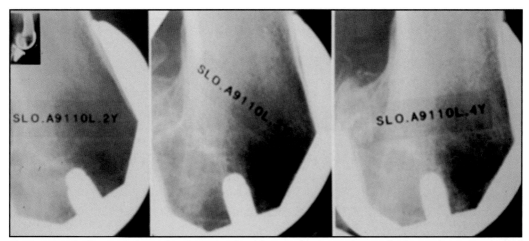

Figure 13-1. Reduction in bone density in the distal femur adjacent to the patella-femoral joint. (Reprinted with permission of Jean-Alain Epinette, MD.)

can lead to a successful revision. However, augments may fail due to lack of incorporation at the interface with bone or may collapse due to excessive stress. With allograft and xenograft, the augment may fail due to adverse biologic response. Mechanical augments may fail due to inadequate support from the host bone, the presence of the augment may lead to further stress shielding of surrounding bone, or interfaces between the augment and bone may be compromised by ingress of wear particles.

The purpose of this chapter is to provide a review of the scientific evidence regarding the prevalence, etiology, prevention, and treatment of stress shielding, osteolysis, and bone remodeling following knee arthroplasty.

STRESS SHIELDING

In contrast to total hip femoral components, stress shielding around total knee femoral components is not well studied. Adverse bone remodeling associated with the femoral component of TKR is particularly difficult to evaluate due to the anterior flange of the femoral component obscuring the radiographic field of view. Lateral views of the resurfaced distal femur may show a reduction in bone density in the distal femur adjacent to the patella-femoral joint (Figure 13-1). Additionally, a region of compromised bone behind the anterior femoral flange is seen often when the femoral component is removed during revision surgery. At moderate survivorship, this pocket of compromised bone may not unduly affect the revision procedure. An attempt to quantify distal femoral bone loss was made by Soininvaara et al who utilized dual x-ray absorptiometry to assess the periprosthetic bone mineral density for 16 patients up to 2 years after cemented TKA with 1 of 3 different knee designs.[8] Rapid bone loss around the femoral component of up to 25.5% (central metaphyseal region) was detected during the first 6 postoperative months. This bone loss was still present 24 months post surgery. It is unclear whether distal femoral stress shielding in the knee is to due to protection of the underlying bone from patella-femoral stresses or to the bypassing of the distal femur as weightbearing loads are transmitted from the mid-femur through the stiff femoral component to the tibia or to both mechanisms. It seems probable that for very long survivorship, stress shielding of the distal femur may affect component fixation or lead to collapse of femoral structures (see Figure 13-1).

Measurements of bone density changes in the proximal tibia following TKR also have been relatively limited. Lonner et al[9] measured the effect of tibial stem design on bone densities in the proximal tibia at an average of 94 months post-surgery. The bone quality around the Miller-Galante I prosthesis (Zimmer, Warsaw, IN), which has 4 0.5-cm pegs, was compared with the bone quality under a Press-Fit Condylar prosthesis (DePuy Orthopaedics, Warsaw, IN) with a single 4-cm stem. The authors found that there was a greater degree of metaphyseal bone density loss (up to 70%) associated with the use of a cemented stem compared with an unstemmed design. The effects of stemmed components in TKA have also been demonstrated in laboratory experiments. Completo et al[10] performed strain gauging tests of synthetic tibiae before and after implantations with cemented and press-fit stem augments for the PFC Sigma Modular Knee System (DePuy Orthopaedics). With the cemented stem augment, a pronounced strain-shielding effect in the proximal "bone" level close to tibial tray was found. The press-fit stem presented a minor effect of strain shielding as stress was transmitted more extensively throughout the stem.

The potential for bone resorption has also been demonstrated in computational models of the implanted knee. Most contemporary TKR designs use a metal tray to provide more even distribution of weightbearing stresses across the tibial plateau. However, the presence of a metal tray may elevate the risk of stress shielding. Au et al[11] used a finite element model to show that the inclusion of medial and lateral pegs in addition to a central fixation post cause localized stress shielding in the periphery of the tibia. In general, tibial implant models show a reduction of cancellous bone stress together with abnormal compressive stresses beneath central fixation posts. The computational model by van Lenthe et al[12] showed that revision prostheses tend to cause more bone resorption than primary ones, especially in the most distal regions due to stress transmission through a stem. While the use of a stemmed component may provide resistance to lift-off and shear, the stem may contribute to proximal bone resorption and subsequent tibial component loosening in the long term.

All-polyethylene tibial components have been proposed as "less stiff" implants that could reduce stress shielding. Dalury et al[13] conducted a prospective study involving the use of an all-polyethylene tibial component in elderly patients aged 70 years and older. After a minimum follow-up of 7 years, stress shielding was seen in 8 of the 120 knees (6.6%). There were no incidents of osteolysis. Harrison et al[14] prospectively followed 41 patients aged 60 years or younger who underwent TKA with cementless trabecular metal tibial components that are less stiff than solid metal tray designs. Dual-energy x-ray absorptiometry scans of the operated and nonoperated proximal tibiae were performed preoperatively and at 2 months, 1 year, and 2 years postoperatively. In the region between the pegs immediately beneath the baseplate and in the region immediately beneath the pegs, there were no changes in bone mineral density between the operated and nonoperated knees at all time points. In contrast, the bone mineral density in the region directly below the tibial baseplate decreased by an average of 6.7% at 2 months in the operated knees, ($P = 0.0001$), although there was no difference in bone mineral density at 1 and 2 years in this region between the operated and nonoperated knees. However, the operated knees exhibited reduced densities relative to their preoperative states at 1- and 2-year follow-up. It is unclear as yet whether less stiff tibial implants of conventional design will reduce stress shielding enough to have long-term clinical benefit.

Clinical experience and the results of these few studies suggest that stress shielding and bone density loss following TKR is real. The presence of stiff femoral and tibial components redistribute stresses in the periprosthetic bone, leading to stress shielding of the bone as it responds to the reduced mechanical loads. Maintenance of the quality and integrity of the host bone is important in providing structural support to the prostheses over the long term. In addition, stress shielded bone loses density and structural integrity and thus is less able to prevent the intrusion of joint fluids and particles. Stress shielded bone may be the precursor to the cascade that leads to osteolysis and device failure.

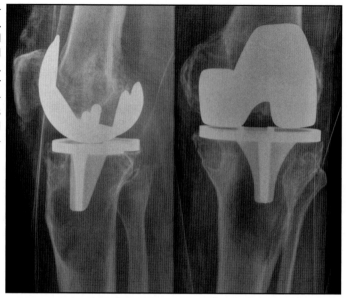

Figure 13-2. Severe osteolysis around a cementless TKA. (Reprinted with permission and copyright of the British Editorial Society of Bone and Joint Surgery. Baker PN, Khaw FM, Kirk LMG, Esler CNA, Gregg PJ. A randomised controlled trial of cemented versus cementless press-fit condylar total knee replacement: 15-year survival analysis. *J Bone Joint Surg [Br].* 2007;89-B:1608-1614.)

Osteolysis

Incidence

In TKR, the quality and the processing of the polyethylene used to manufacture the tibial and patella bearings have a large role to play in osteolysis. In the 1990s it was recognized that the sterilization methods used in knee polyethylene could affect the mechanical properties of the material and lead to its degradation in vivo. Collier et al[7] conducted a radiographic review of 365 posterior cruciate ligament-retaining Anatomic Modular Knee primary TKAs (DePuy Orthopaedics). Osteolysis was identified in 34% of 242 knees treated with a tibial-bearing insert that had been gamma-irradiated in air and affixed to a rough tibial tray surface. In contrast, osteolysis was found in 9% of 98 knees that were treated with an insert that had been gamma-irradiated in an inert gas, or had not been irradiated, and affixed to a polished surface. Osteolysis was found to be associated with factors such as surface finish within the tibial tray, the specific polyethylene of the tibial insert (the material from which it was machined, the sterilization method, and the shelf age), and surgical placement (hyperextension of the femoral component relative to the tibial component).

Cemented fixation of knee components can provide an effective barrier to the migration of wear debris into the periprosthetic joint space if the cement mantle is in proper contact with the bone cuts and with the implant. For cementless knees, inadequate component design or inadequate bone cuts may prevent proper contact between implant and bone and prohibit full development of ingrowth or ongrowth fixation. Gaps at cemented or cementless fixation interfaces that communicate with the joint space allow fluid and particles to penetrate between the implants and bone. An excessive particle accumulation in the fixation interface can lead to a cellular response, osteolysis, and adverse bone remodeling (Figure 13-2).[15]

A wide range in the incidence of osteolysis following TKR has been reported in the literature with a variety of knee designs and with different polyethylene bearing formulations. Osteolysis rates as high as 90% are reported,[16] but most commonly when authors have studied osteolysis in the knee, the incidence is generally between 10% to 20%. The determination of the presence of osteolysis in a given patient does not necessarily mean that the knee will go on to revision, at least in the time frame of the study design. Often the presence of an osteolytic lesion is determined radiographically and rarely confirmed as such by histologic analysis.

Arora and Ogden[17] identified the presence of osteolytic lesions in 13 of the 82 knees (16%) that were implanted with a cemented modular Freeman-Samuelson Knee (Zulzer Orthopaedics AG, Baar, Switzerland) after an average of 7.25 years. The lesions were found primarily around the tibial component in 12 knees and were only found around the femoral component in 2 knees. The most common site was anterior to the tibial stem (*n* = 9) followed by the medial tibial condyle (*n* = 7). O'Rourke et al[18] evaluated the prevalence of radiographic osteolysis around 105 posterior cruciate-substituting TKAs (Insall-Burstein II system, Zimmer) in which a cemented modular tibial component had been used. While no knees were revised because of loosening or osteolysis in this series, osteolysis was present in 17 knees (16%). Cadambi et al[19] reported an 11.1% incidence of femoral osteolysis (30 cases in 28 patients) in a series of 271 primary TKAs that were implanted with minimally constrained total knee designs (Synatomic [DePuy Orthopaedics] or Porous-Coated Anatomic [PCA, Howmedica, Rutherford, NJ]). Femoral osteolysis was observed in 26 Synatomic and 4 PCA knees after an average follow-up period of 52 months. The average time to the diagnosis of femoral osteolysis was 31 months (range: 7 to 96 months).

Following the theme of minimal femoral/tibial bearing constraint, Huang et al[20] compared the prevalence of osteolysis after failed TKA with a mobile-bearing prosthesis and with a fixed-bearing prosthesis. The prevalence of osteolysis was significantly higher in the mobile-bearing group (47%; 16 of 34 knees) than in the fixed-bearing group (13%; 6 of 46 knees) (*P* = 0.003). The distal part of the femur was involved in 13 knees in the mobile-bearing group and in 4 knees in the fixed-bearing group. Osteolysis was predominantly on the femoral side; 17 knees had osteolysis in the posterior aspect of the femoral condyle. Of these, 12 knees had no evidence of osteolysis on prerevision radiographs. In contrast, Kim and Kim[6] found that the prevalence of osteolysis associated with mobile-bearing knees (Low Contact Stress, DePuy Orthopaedics) was no higher than for fixed-bearing knees (Anatomic Modular Knee, DePuy Orthopaedics) in 61 patients younger than 55 years who had bilateral simultaneous primary knee replacements. Osteolysis was identified in both radiographs and computed tomography scans in 6 knees (10%) in the Anatomic Modular Knee group and 4 knees (7%) in the Low Contact Stress group. Hooper et al[21] examined the outcome of 400 consecutive patients who underwent TKR with the Low Contact Stress mobile-bearing system after a minimum follow-up of 10 years. Clinical and radiological assessment of 238 patients (244 knees) indicated that polyethylene wear was more common in the meniscal-bearing component, with 5 knees requiring revision and a further 8 demonstrating early wear. Osteolysis was not seen in the rotating platform component, but was present in 3 of the meniscal-bearing knees.

For different polyethylene formulations, Weber et al[22] performed a retrospective review of more than 1000 TKAs performed with the AGC prosthesis (Biomet, Warsaw, IN) using a uniform surgical technique with a 5- to 11-year follow-up. Of tibial components, 698 were of compression-molded monoblock design and 353 were of ram-extruded modular assembly design. Higher rates of osteolysis (1.7% versus 0.1%), radiolucent lines (19% versus 5.6%), and revision (3.1% versus 1.4%) were found with the ram-extruded modular design, although it is unclear whether the difference is due to modularity, polyethylene type, or both factors.

For cementless knees, no occurrences of osteolysis were observed in a series of cementless trays without screw holes[23] or in a series of cemented knees without the use of screws.[24] The authors suggest that the absence of screws or screw holes may limit the pathways for wear debris to penetrate the fixation space, while the absence of screws caused no deleterious effect on implant stability or bone ingrowth. In a prospective study of 118 hydroxyapatite-coated, cementless TKRs at a mean follow-up of 7.9 years in patients who were 55 years old and younger,[25] there were 2 revisions of the tibial component because of aseptic loosening and 1 case of polyethylene wear requiring further surgery. No osteolysis or progressive radiological loosening of any other component was identified, suggesting that uncemented interfaces are capable of resisting intrusion of wear particles.

Patient factors such as obesity[26] show a significant influence on the incidence of osteolysis. Spicer et al[26] conducted a matched study of 326 TKRs in 285 osteoarthritic patients with body mass index (BMI) greater than 30 kg/m^2 and 425 TKRs in 371 patients with BMI less than 30 kg/m^2. Revision rates showed 4.9% of the obese patient group underwent revision surgery, compared with 3.1% of the nonobese group. Although linear osteolysis (radiolucency) rates were comparable, focal osteolysis rates (6.8%) were 5 times those of the nonobese patients (1.2%) when the BMI exceeded 40 kg/m^2.

With contemporary knee designs and contemporary bearings, recent studies report no radiographic evidence of osteolysis at early follow-up.[27,28] Rossi et al[28] observed no signs of component loosening or osteolysis in a prospective consecutive series of 50 rotating platform, cemented TKRs (NexGen LPS, Zimmer) in 43 patients after a mean follow-up of 46 months. In a review of 279 primary TKAs with a modular, cemented, third-generation, posterior stabilized prosthesis (average 4-year follow-up),[27] no radiographic evidence of loosening or osteolysis was found and no revisions were performed or recommended for loosening, osteolysis, instability, or polyethylene wear.

Etiology

Although osteolysis was initially termed as cement disease, it is now well accepted that osteolysis occurs as the result of a foreign body response to particulate wear and corrosion debris. These particles may consist of polyethylene, bone cement, and metal, all of which have been shown to elicit an inflammatory response. The particles become phagocytosed by macrophages and giant cells in the synovial or periprosthetic tissue. These cells, in turn, become activated and can cause osteolysis. The macrophages can directly induce the immobility of osteoclasts, resulting in the formation of resorption pits. Osteolysis is more commonly initiated by the activation of cytokine production following the stimulation of synovial or periprosthetic macrophages. Cytokines such as interleukin-1b, which is proinflammatory and causes osteoclastic stimulation, are released by these activated macrophages. The cytokines also cause decreased osteoblastic bone formation.

Hydrodynamics factors may also play a role in the transport of wear particles and contribute to osteolysis. Local fluid pressure gradients around the prostheses are believed to provide a mechanism for the migration of particulate debris, forcing fluid and particles into the surrounding bone. Fluid pressure changes during joint motion can produce very high intra-articular pressures, which can induce osteocyte death and subsequent osteoclast-induced bone resorption.[29,30]

The size, shape, type, and concentration of wear particles also play an important role in determining whether an osteolytic response may be provoked. Large particles are engulfed or surrounded by giant cells and often invested in a fibrous sheath. In comparison, small particles, those sized smaller than 1 micron, are ingested by macrophages, provoking an inflammatory response.[31] In TKA, the predominant mode of bearing failure and "wear" is material fatigue. This mechanism produces polyethylene particles that are larger and more irregular in shape when compared with those after total hip arthroplasty, in which the predominant mode of failure is abrasive and adhesive wear. Wear particulate debris retrieved from failed TKA has shown that the mean particle size is an average of 3 times larger than those in total hip arthroplasty.[5] Schmalzried et al[32] analyzed the polyethylene wear debris and the cellular response in periprosthetic tissues from 19 failed TKRs and 24 failed total hip replacements. The foreign-body inflammatory reaction in the failed total hip replacements was characterized by plump macrophages in the presence of multiple submicron particles of pulmonary embolism (PE). The majority of particles were less than 1 micron in size. In contrast, the foreign-body inflammatory reaction in the TKR cases was characterized by giant cells with fewer macrophages and particles generally between 2 and 20 microns. Since particle size plays an important role in influencing the magnitude of the biological response, the larger-sized TKR debris results in a diminished mediator release, which in turn may account for the lower incidence of osteolysis and aseptic loosening in some designs of TKR.

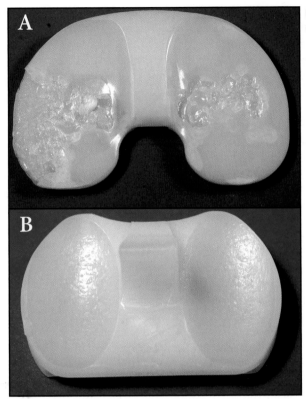

Figure 13-3. (A) Severe delamination and (B) pitting modes of damage.

Wear particles may be generated at the articulating surface between the femoral component and polyethylene tibial insert. Surface damage on polyethylene components may arise from 7 different modes of damage, which have been observed in retrieved total knee prostheses.[33] These include pitting, embedded debris, scratching, delamination, surface deformation, burnishing, and abrasion. Pitting is a mode of fatigue wear that is characterized by the formation of millimeter-sized craters and is considered to be a more benign wear mechanism that does not provoke an osteolytic response due to its large particle sizes (Figure 13-3). Embedded debris may arise from bone cement, bone chip, or metallic bead fragments becoming embedded in the polyethylene component, possibly leading to third body wear, as well as scratching of the surfaces of the metallic counterface. Scratching is a mode of abrasive wear that is characterized by linear features that are produced by plowing of microscopic asperities. Delamination is a severe form of fatigue wear, involving the removal of sheets of polyethylene and can result in catastrophic wear (see Figure 13-3). Surface deformation, which corresponds to permanent changes in the surface geometry or "creep" or "cold flow," does not result in material removal and therefore does not strictly correspond to wear. Burnishing is a mode of adhesive/abrasive wear that produces wear debris from a polishing effect, of particle sizes that can elicit an osteolytic response. Abrasion is characterized as a shredding of the polyethylene surface and is classified as a mode of abrasive wear. The surface damage to components seen with in vivo oxidation of the gamma-air sterilized polyethylene of the late 20th century should be a concern of the past with modern polymer processing methods.

While wear at the articulating surface between the femoral component and polyethylene tibial insert have been the primary focus of attention by researchers, backside wear between the inferior surface of the tibial insert and the metal tray is also a potential source of wear particles.[18,34,35] Backside wear is typically characterized by burnishing or scratching of the polyethylene component, sometimes removing the machining marks from the surface. Polyethylene may also extrude into screw holes of recesses of the tray. The rates of backside wear in some designs have been as high as 100 mg/year, which is 2 to 4 times higher than the rates associated with total hip replacements.[35] Backside wear may be a significant contributor to polyethylene wear and development of osteolysis; therefore, great emphasis has been placed on limiting the relative motion between the tibial insert and metal tray or baseplate with rigid locking mechanisms,[36,37] which minimize the generation of wear particles.

Post damage in posterior stabilized condylar components has also been identified as a potential source of polyethylene wear and debris generation in TKA.[18,38,39] Although the tibial post is designed to articulate with the cam in the femoral component during flexion, the post may impinge with the femoral component during hyperflexion, leading to anterior wear. In more severe cases, fatigue damage or post fracture may be encountered. Post fractures have been attributed to a number of factors such as joint instability/laxity or lack of ligamentous balancing,[40-43] posterior slope of the tibial component,[38,39,41] flexed position of the femoral component,[38,39,41] failure to use a thick enough insert to avoid hyperextension,[44] cement extrusion (overhang of cement overriding the femoral component),[45] and tissue ingrowth causing impingement.[45] Surgical positioning of the components can play a critical role in the generation of polyethylene wear and potential for osteolysis. For example, the risk of anterior impingement of the post against the intercondylar notch during hyperextension increases with each additional angle that the tibial component is placed with a posterior slope and/or that the femoral component is placed in a flexed position because the knee does not need to rotate as much before hyperextension occurs. It is unclear if post damage is also related to wear in other regions of the polyethylene component, as it has been suggested that post-cam impingement may be associated with the application of rotational torques to the tray-insert interface and subsequent backside wear.[39]

Prevention

Particulate debris from the articular and backside surfaces of the polyethylene inserts of modular tibial components remains an issue in the survivorship of TKR. The possibility that particles can be generated at the tibial bearing-tibial tray interface has led to contemporary knee designs where the polyethylene insert is securely locked to the tray. Since the underlying mechanism for osteolysis is the inflammatory response to wear debris, survivorship strategies now focus on minimizing wear production. Contemporary polyethylene components are mostly highly cross-linked polyethylene with or without a contained free radical scavenger (at the time of writing usually vitamin E[46-48]) while the femoral counterface is either cobalt chromium alloy or ceramic.[49-55]

Cross-linking polyethylene knee bearings have been studied extensively. Williams et al[51] tested mildly cross-linked (35 kGy radiated) and highly cross-linked (70 kGy radiated) polyethylenes against cobalt chromium and zirconia femoral counterfaces in a wear simulator. The average submicron volume fraction of the polyethylene wear particles were found to decrease from about 65% to 45% with increased cross-linking and also with changing the counterface material from cobalt chrome to zirconia. The averaged number of generated particles decreased by approximately 4-fold with increased cross-linking and 3-fold with changing the counterface material to zirconia. Through knee simulator wear testing and customized tibial post testing, Stoller et al[49] compared the use of conventional polyethylene and highly cross-linked polyethylene in a posterior stabilized total knee design. They found that the wear volume was reduced by 67% to 75% for aged highly cross-linked polyethylene compared with aged conventional polyethylene. The highly cross-linked polyethylene tibial posts, somewhat surprisingly, demonstrated improved durability. Popoola et al[50] compared the wear, delamination, and fatigue resistance of aged gamma irradiation sterilized conventional polyethylene and gas plasma sterilized melt-annealed highly cross-linked polyethylene tibial inserts, using a variety of wear tests and edge loading fatigue testing. The study showed that the highly cross-linked polyethylene inserts had higher wear and fatigue resistance, with an average wear rate reduction of about 80% compared with the conventional polyethylene components. Wear simulator testing by Wang et al[53] of highly cross-linked polyethylene cruciate retaining and posterior stabilized knee inserts manufactured by a sequential irradiation and annealing process also demonstrated about 60% to 70% less wear compared to conventional polyethylene inserts. Clearly modern highly cross-linked polyethylenes do reduce wear in the knee. However, the cross-linking reduces the toughness, ductility, and fracture resistance of the polymer. Retrieval analyses will show in the future whether these reduced mechanical properties lead to different modes of failure in the knee.

Ceramic bearings are widely used for hip replacements because they offer the advantage of low wear when compared to the standard metal polyethylene bearings. The manufacture of ceramic components for knee replacements is challenging due to the complex geometry of the components and risk of fracture. Alumina ceramic has been used extensively for TKR in Japan. Nakamura et al[56] described the use of a unique ball-and-socket knee joint with an alumina ceramic femoral component, which was designed to improve deep knee flexion and long-term bearing durability. Zirconia ceramic femoral components have also been developed and utilized, with Bal et al[57] reporting on the 2-year clinical results of 39 posterior stabilized TKAs performed with a zirconia ceramic femoral component. Only one revision for persistent knee instability after trauma was encountered in this series. Oxidized zirconia, manufactured by diffusing oxygen into a zirconium-niobium alloy, produces a hardened ceramic surface (Oxinium, Smith & Nephew, Memphis, TN). Revisions linked specifically to the use of oxidized zirconia in TKA have not been reported.[58,59] Survivorship of 98.7% at 7 years postoperatively has been observed in 98 primary TKAs with oxidized zirconia femoral components.[58] Heyse et al[59] also examined 16 retrieved TKAs with an oxidized zirconia femoral component for wear and surface damage after an average in situ use of 16.4 ± 11.9 months. No major wear of the polyethylene components was found, while there were no failures directly related to the oxidized zirconia.

Careful attention to surgical preparation and implant positioning can also improve the longevity of TKR by limiting abnormal wear. For example, the avoidance of femoral component flexion and posterior tibial slope will minimize anterior tibial post impingement in posterior stabilized designs.[39] An increase in the posterior slope of the tibial component can also significantly increase the instability of the tibial component.[60,61] The increased instability may manifest as an increase in the anterior micromotion of the polyethylene insert relative to the baseplate,[60] possibly increasing backside wear.

Pharmaceutical agents, such as bisphosphonates, have been used for preventing and managing postmenopausal osteoporosis and also have been explored in improving the durability of joint arthroplasty.[62,63] Because of their anabolic effect on osteoblasts, bisphosphonates have the potential to enhance periprosthetic bone ingrowth, prevent bone resorption under adverse conditions, and dramatically extend the long-term durability of joint arthroplasties. A meta-analysis of 6 randomized controlled trials suggest that bisphosphonates have a beneficial effect with regard to maintaining more periprosthetic bone mineral density than in controls following total hip replacement or TKR.[62] At 3, 6, and 12 months, bisphosphonate-treated patients had lower weighted mean reductions in periprosthetic bone loss by 3.3% ($P < 0.01$), 4.5% ($P < 0.001$), and 4.2% ($P = 0.03$), respectively. Bisphosphonates also appeared to have a greater effect on replaced knees than hips at some follow-up intervals; the difference in bone loss between controls and bisphosphonates was 14.0% at 6 months following TKR compared with 2.5% following THA ($P < 0.001$). However, the difference in the effect of bisphosphonates between total hip arthroplasty and TKA was not significant at 3 or 12 months. The long-term effects of bisphosphonate use are still unclear. Along with improvements in implant design and material properties, bisphosphonates and other pharmaceutical agents may be used in the future to help improve the longevity of joint arthroplasties.

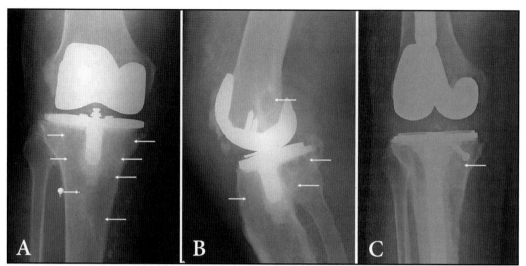

Figure 13-4. (A) Preoperative anteroposterior and (B) lateral radiographs of a patient with a large non-contained ostolytic defect (arrows). The defect was managed with a (C, arrowed) structural allograft in the proximal tibia and revision of the components. (Reprinted with permission of Burnett RS, Keeney JA, Maloney WJ, Clohisy JC. Revision total knee arthroplasty for major osteolysis. *Iowa Orthop J.* 2009;29:28-37.)

Treatment

Revision TKA presents complex challenges of bone loss and ligamentous insufficiency. Periprosthetic bone loss is frequently encountered at the time of revision TKA, and the outcome of the revision often depends on the management of this bone deficiency. Bone loss patterns can be anatomically categorized, and the surgical treatment can be algorithmically approached based on the bone loss pattern.[64] The patterns of bone loss can be classified as cystic, epiphyseal, cavitary, or segmental. Cystic bone loss is characterized by small defects in the trabecular bone that are in the area of the bone-implant interface and may be filled with bone grafting (particularly with larger cysts) or cement. Epiphyseal defects involve cortical bone loss in the tibial plateau or femoral condyles and are addressed with modular tibial or femoral augments. Augments offer the advantage of reconstructing the deficient bone, while still being stable enough to allow immediate weightbearing. However, additional bone removal is usually necessary to fit the augment within the existing bone stock. Cavitary bone loss is usually seen in severe cases of osteolysis and is characterized by large, intracortical bone loss in the metaphyseal region of the distal femur and/or proximal tibia. Trabecular metal cones or allograft reconstruction with bulk and/or morselized allograft can be used for reconstructing cavitary defects. Allograft reconstruction is generally less expensive than metaphyseal filling implants but requires protected weightbearing and may also produce implant instability if bony incorporation is not achieved. Segmental defects refer to combined patterns of epiphyseal and cavitary bone loss that are missing large portions of distal femoral and/or proximal tibia bone. Similar to cavitary bone loss, these are often treated with bulk allograft reconstruction or implantation of rotating platform, hinged prostheses. The hinged type implant is often used to provide additional constraints on the joint when ligamentous insufficiency is present.

The literature suggests that major osteolytic defects may be effectively addressed with a variety of bone grafting techniques. Burnett et al[65] reported on 28 knees in 26 patients that underwent revision surgery. The majority of the knees (*n* = 17) were treated with standard revision implants with the use of augments and/or morselized allograft, but not structural allograft. Eight of the remaining knees were treated with structural allograft reconstruction and a stemmed component (Figure 13-4), while the remaining 3 knees with well-fixed components were managed with insert exchange and impaction cancellous bone grafting. At a minimum radiographic follow-up of 2 years, 24 of the knees (86%) demonstrated component stability and incorporation of both cancellous and structural allografts. The use of bone grafting has been recommended for tibial defects involving 50% or more of the bony support of either tibial plateau.[66] In a 3- to 6-year follow-up of 24 knees with bone grafts for tibial defects at the time of either primary or revision TKA, 22 of the grafts demonstrated bony union and revascularization with no clinical collapse.[66] Lotke et al[67] prospectively evaluated the clinical outcomes of 48 consecutive revision TKAs with substantial bone loss treated with impaction allograft after an average follow-up of 3.8 years. There were no mechanical failures of the revisions, and all radiographs have shown incorporation and remodeling of the bone graft. Although impaction grafting may be expensive, time consuming, and is technically demanding, it avoids donor site morbidity and can address variable and irregular defects. Impaction grafting in revision TKA is reported to have excellent durability and versatility and can be used to effectively manage major osteolytic defects.[67]

Bone allografts that anatomically match the site of the defect may not be routinely available. Shaped femoral heads have been used as structural allografts following severe tibial bone loss.[68,69] In a case series of 15 patients (15 knees) who were treated with shaped femoral head allograft along with long-stemmed components,[68] 13 knees did not require further surgery after a mean follow-up of 5.4 years. These knees demonstrated allograft incorporation after an average of 1.9 years with no component migration. Engh and Ammeen[69] evaluated the outcomes following 49 revision knees in which a structural allograft had been used to reconstruct a severe tibial bone defect. Polyethylene wear and osteolysis was present in 24 of the 49 knees. In 45 knees, femoral head allografts were used to reconstruct the tibial bone deficiency, while proximal tibial allograft and distal femoral allograft were used in the remaining 3 knees and 1 knee, respectively. Radiographic review of 33 unrevised knees showed no evidence of graft collapse or aseptic loosening associated with the structural allograft after an average 7.9 years postoperatively. An osteolytic lesion greater than 2 cm was found in 2 knees, while an additional 4 knees had a small amount of osteolysis smaller than 2 cm. However, the osteolysis did not involve the tibial regions that were repaired with the structural allograft, and none of these patients required additional surgery because of osteolysis. The repair of tibial bone defects with structural allografts instead of a fully cemented stem during revision surgery, particularly a longer diaphyseal-engaging stem, may help avoid a more challenging repeat revision surgery, if it is subsequently encountered.

Modular polyethylene exchange during revision knee arthroplasty for the treatment of wear and osteolysis provides the benefit of avoiding full revision of well-fixed components. Griffin et al[70] evaluated the results of isolated polyethylene exchange for wear and/or osteolysis in 68 press-fit condylar (PFC) TKAs. At the time of component exchange, accessible osteolytic lesions were treated with bone grafting in 35 knees and cement augmentation in 32 knees. At a minimum of 24 months after polyethylene exchange surgery (average: 44 months), there were 11 failures (16.2%) involving aseptic loosening in 10 knees (8 femoral components, 3 tibial trays) and infection in 1. Radiographic review demonstrated no progression of osteolytic lesions in 66 of the 68 knees (97%), while the lesion size progressed in the remaining 2 knees. Despite the limited follow-up of the study, the lack of progression of osteolysis in the majority of the knees is encouraging. The outcomes of 67 revision TKA with and without the retention of a secure, cemented femoral component were assessed by Mackay and Siddique.[71] The original femoral component was secure and was retained in 25 knees, with no evidence of abrasion or osteolysis. Both components were revised in the remaining 42 knees. After a mean follow-up of 4 years, rerevision for loosening was required in 28% ($n = 7$) of the knees where the original femoral component was retained, compared with 7% ($n = 3$) in the other group where both components were originally revised ($P < 0.01$). The remaining knees functioned well with no radiological evidence of osteolysis. The high rate of failure after retaining a secure femoral component may be attributed to the accumulation of fatigue cracks in the supporting cement mantle, the presence of polyethylene wear debris, or less than ideal alignment of the components and ligamentous instability.[71] Further studies are needed to better understand the consequences of retaining a secure femoral component.

Options for the method of stem fixation in revision TKA include variable length stems that are designed to engage in the metaphysis or diaphysis. The use of extended stems can enhance stability by transferring stress from the bone-deficient tibial plateau to the shaft, but this can also compromise the existing bone stock through stress shielding. Fehring et al[72] compared the use of cemented and uncemented metaphyseal engaging stems in 113 revision TKAs with a minimum follow-up of 2 years. Of the 202 stems, 107 were cemented (54 femoral, 53 tibial), while the remaining 95 were press-fit (47 femoral, 48 tibial). After an average follow-up of 4.8 years, the implants with cemented stems were more radiographically stable than those with press-fit stems ($P = 0.0001$). In contrast, 71% of the implants with uncemented stems were considered stable, 19% were possibly loose requiring close follow-up, and 10% were loose, raising concerns about the use of cementless metaphyseal engaging stems. Whiteside et al[73] reported favorable outcomes following the use of cementless fixation of both the femoral and tibial components in 92 patients with severe bone loss. With follow-up ranging from 60 to 127 months postoperatively, increase in radiodensity and evidence of bone healing occurred in the bone defects that could be seen on radiographs for 31 tibiae and 28 femurs. With the exception of 1 tibial component loosening, none of the remaining components had radiographic appearances of migration, progressive radiolucencies, or pedestal formation around the stem.

For almost 2 decades, modular revision knee systems have been used to provide a wide array of surgical options to repair the bone loss and instability encountered at revision surgery. More contemporary designs allow the independent augmentation of the distal and posterior femoral condyles as well as the medial and lateral tibial plateaus. However, the outcomes following the use of modular revision systems have been mixed. At a minimum follow-up of 5 years following the use of the Coordinate (DePuy Orthopaedics) revision TKA,[74] 9 knees failed and required either revision or component removal, while 8 additional knees were considered clinical failures. The most common reason for failure in this series was infection, followed by aseptic loosening, pain, and stiffness. Despite the use of metallic augmentation in 85% of these cases, large structural allografts were required in 48% of the knees. Revisions with bone loss that required bulk allograft failed less often (19.2%) than revisions managed without bulk allografts (42.9%). While the authors of this study concluded that modular augments alone did not effectively address the bone loss and instability encountered in many instances at revision surgery, they suspected that the quality of bone and lack of sufficient cancellous bone structure may have led to an inadequate cement bond at the host bone-allograft interface.

Summary

The development of osteolytic lesions can pose challenges for surgical reconstruction during revision arthroplasty. Osteolysis around TKRs may arise from a variety of design, surgical, and patient factors. Backside wear remains a concern with some fixed bearing designs. Improper component placement may cause contact between components and unforeseen failure modes. Bearing materials such as ceramics and highly cross-linked polyethylene have promise for minimal wear and the reduction in particle-induced osteolysis. The issue of polyethylene oxidation in vivo is addressed by a reduction in free radicals in contemporary highly cross-linked polyethylene materials especially formulated for use in the knee. Free radical scavengers as a polyethylene additive are present in some polyethylenes to further reduce oxidation potential. However, their presence may also reduce the cross-linked density of the materials. All highly cross-linked polyethylenes suffer degradation of some mechanical properties when compared to the virgin material. Only time will tell if these properties are important to TKR survival in patients at long periods of follow-up.

References

1. Agency for Healthcare Research and Quality. HCUP Databases. Healthcare Cost and Utilization Project (HCUP). 2008 January 9, 2009; Available at: http://www.hcup-us.ahrq.gov/nisoverview.jsp.

2. Ong KL, Lau E, Suggs J, Kurtz SM, Manley MT. Risk of subsequent revision after primary and revision total joint arthroplasty. *Clin Orthop Relat Res.* 2010;468(11):3070-3076.

3. Bozic KJ, Durbhakula S, Berry DJ, et al. Differences in patient and procedure characteristics and hospital resource use in primary and revision total joint arthroplasty: a multicenter study. *J Arthroplasty.* 2005;20(7 suppl 3):17-25.

4. Bozic, KJ, Kurtz SM, Lau E, et al. The epidemiology of revision total knee arthroplasty in the United States. *Clin Orthop Relat Res.* 2010;468(1):45-51.

5. Shanbhag AS, Bailey HO, Hwang DS, Cha CW, Eror NG, Rubash HE. Quantitative analysis of ultrahigh molecular weight polyethylene (UHMWPE) wear debris associated with total knee replacements. *J Biomed Mater Res.* 2000;53(1):100-110.

6. Kim YH, Kim JS. Prevalence of osteolysis after simultaneous bilateral fixed- and mobile-bearing total knee arthroplasties in young patients. *J Arthroplasty.* 2009;24(6):932-940.

7. Collier MB, Engh CA Jr, McAuley JP, Ginn SD, Engh GA. Osteolysis after total knee arthroplasty: influence of tibial baseplate surface finish and sterilization of polyethylene insert. Findings at five to ten years postoperatively. *J Bone Joint Surg Am.* 2005;87(12):2702-2708.

8. Soininvaara T, Nikola T, Vanninen E, Miettinen H, Kröger H. Bone mineral density and single photon emission computed tomography changes after total knee arthroplasty: a 2-year follow-up study. *Clin Physiol Funct Imaging.* 2008;28(2):101-106.

9. Lonner JH, Klotz M, Levitz C, Lotke PA. Changes in bone density after cemented total knee arthroplasty: influence of stem design. *J Arthroplasty.* 2001;16(1):107-111.

10. Completo A, Fonseca F, Simoes JA. Strain shielding in proximal tibia of stemmed knee prosthesis: experimental study. *J Biomech.* 2008;41(3):560-566.

11. Au AG, Liggins AB, Raso VJ, Amirfazli A. A parametric analysis of fixation post shape in tibial knee prostheses. *Med Eng Phys.* 2005;27(2):123-134.

12. van Lenthe GH, Willems MM, Verdonschot N, de Waal Malefijt MC, Huiskes R. Stemmed femoral knee prostheses: effects of prosthetic design and fixation on bone loss. *Acta Orthop Scand.* 2002;73(6):630-637.

13. Dalury DF, Pomeroy DL, Gonzales RA, Gruen TA, Adams MJ, Empson JA. Midterm results of all-polyethylene tibial components in primary total knee arthroplasty. *J Arthroplasty.* 2009;24(4):620-624.

14. Harrison AK, Gioe TJ, Simonelli C, Tatman PJ, Schoeller MC. Do porous tantalum implants help preserve bone?: evaluation of tibial bone density surrounding tantalum tibial implants in TKA. *Clin Orthop Relat Res.* 2010;468(10):2739-2745.

15. Baker PN, Khaw FM, Kirk LM, Esler CN, Gregg PJ. A randomised controlled trial of cemented versus cementless press-fit condylar total knee replacement: 15-year survival analysis. *J Bone Joint Surg Br.* 2007;89(12):1608-1614.

16. Kim YH, Oh JH, Oh SH. Osteolysis around cementless porous-coated anatomic knee prostheses. *J Bone Joint Surg Br.* 1995;77(2):236-241.

17. Arora J, Ogden AC. Osteolysis in a surface-cemented, primary, modular Freeman-Samuelson total knee replacement. *J Bone Joint Surg Br.* 2005;87(11):1502-1506.

18. O'Rourke MR, Callaghan JJ, Goetz DD, Sullivan PM, Johnston RC. Osteolysis associated with a cemented modular posterior-cruciate-substituting total knee design: five to eight-year follow-up. *J Bone Joint Surg Am.* 2002;84-A(8):1362-1371.

19. Cadambi A, Engh GA, Dwyer KA, Vinh TN. Osteolysis of the distal femur after total knee arthroplasty. *J Arthroplasty.* 1994;9(6):579-594.

20. Huang CH, Ma HM, Liau JJ, Ho FY, Cheng CK. Osteolysis in failed total knee arthroplasty: a comparison of mobile-bearing and fixed-bearing knees. *J Bone Joint Surg Am.* 2002;84-A(12):2224-2229.

21. Hooper G, Rothwell A, Frampton C. The low contact stress mobile-bearing total knee replacement: a prospective study with a minimum follow-up of ten years. *J Bone Joint Surg Br.* 2009;91(1):58-63.

22. Weber AB, Worland RL, Keenan J, Van Bowen J. A study of polyethylene and modularity issues in >1000 posterior cruciate-retaining knees at 5 to 11 years. *J Arthroplasty.* 2002;17(8):987-991.

23. Cooke C, Walter WK, Zicat B. Tibial fixation without screws in cementless total knee arthroplasty. *J Arthroplasty.* 2006;21(2):237-241.

24. Ezzet KA, Garcia R, Barrack RL. Effect of component fixation method on osteolysis in total knee arthroplasty. *Clin Orthop Relat Res.* 1995;(321):86-91.

25. Tai CC, Cross MJ. Five- to 12-year follow-up of a hydroxyapatite-coated, cementless total knee replacement in young, active patients. *J Bone Joint Surg Br.* 2006;88(9):1158-1163.
26. Spicer DD, Pomeroy DL, Badenhausen WE, et al. Body mass index as a predictor of outcome in total knee replacement. *Int Orthop.* 2001;25(4):246-249.
27. Fuchs R, Mills EL, Clarke HD, Scuderi GR, Scott WN, Insall JN. A third-generation, posterior-stabilized knee prosthesis: early results after follow-up of 2 to 6 years. *J Arthroplasty.* 2006;21(6):821-825.
28. Rossi R, Ferro A, Bruzzone M, Bonasia DE, Garzaro G, Castoldi F. NexGen LPS rotating platform total knee arthroplasty: medium-term results of a prospective study. *Chir Organi Mov.* 2009;93(2):65-70.
29. Skripitz R, Aspenberg P. Pressure-induced periprosthetic osteolysis: a rat model. *J Orthop Res.* 2000;18(3):481-484.
30. Van der Vis HM, Aspenberg P, Marti RK, Tigchelaar W, Van Noorden CJ. Fluid pressure causes bone resorption in a rabbit model of prosthetic loosening. *Clin Orthop Relat Res.* 1998;(350):201-208.
31. Ingham E, Fisher J. The role of macrophages in osteolysis of total joint replacement. *Biomaterials.* 2005;26(11):1271-1286.
32. Schmalzried TP, Jasty M, Rosenberg A, Harris WH. Polyethylene wear debris and tissue reactions in knee as compared to hip replacement prostheses. *J Appl Biomater.* 1994;5(3):185-190.
33. Hood RW, Wright TM, Burstein AH. Retrieval analysis of total knee prostheses: a method and its application to 48 total condylar prostheses. *J Biomed Mater Res.* 1983;17(5):829-842.
34. Wasielewski RC, Parks N, Williams I, Surprenant H, Collier JP, Engh G. Tibial insert undersurface as a contributing source of polyethylene wear debris. *Clin Orthop Relat Res.* 1997;(345):53-59.
35. Li S, Scuderi G, Furman BD, Bhattacharyya S, Schmieg JJ, Insall JN. Assessment of backside wear from the analysis of 55 retrieved tibial inserts. *Clin Orthop Relat Res.* 2002;(404):75-82.
36. Galvin A, Jennings LM, McEwen HM, Fisher J. The influence of tibial tray design on the wear of fixed-bearing total knee replacements. *Proc Inst Mech Eng H.* 2008;222(8):1289-1293.
37. Engh GA, Lounici S, Rao AR, Collier MB. In vivo deterioration of tibial baseplate locking mechanisms in contemporary modular total knee components. *J Bone Joint Surg Am.* 2001;83-A(11):1660-1665.
38. Banks SA, Harman MK, Hodge WA. Mechanism of anterior impingement damage in total knee arthroplasty. *J Bone Joint Surg Am.* 2002;84-A(suppl 2):37-42.
39. Callaghan JJ, O'Rourke MR, Goetz DD, Schmalzried TP, Campbell PA, Johnston RC. Tibial post impingement in posterior-stabilized total knee arthroplasty. *Clin Orthop Relat Res.* 2002;(404):83-88.
40. Bal BS, Greenberg D. Failure of a metal-reinforced tibial post in total knee arthroplasty. *J Arthroplasty.* 2007;22(3):464-467.
41. Jung KA, Lee SC, Hwang SH, Kim SM. Fracture of a second-generation highly cross-linked UHMWPE tibial post in a posterior-stabilized scorpio knee system. *Orthopedics.* 2008;31(11):1137.
42. Mestha P, Shenava Y, D'Arcy JC. Fracture of the polyethylene tibial post in posterior stabilized (Insall Burstein II) total knee arthroplasty. *J Arthroplasty.* 2000;15(6):814-815.
43. Puloski SK, McCalden RW, MacDonald SJ, Rorabeck CH, Bourne RB. Tibial post wear in posterior stabilized total knee arthroplasty. An unrecognized source of polyethylene debris. *J Bone Joint Surg Am.* 2001;83-A(3):390-397.
44. Lim HC, Bae JH, Hwang JH, Kim SJ, Yoon JY. Fracture of a polyethylene tibial post in a scorpio posterior-stabilized knee prosthesis. *Clin Orthop Surg.* 2009;1(2):118-121.
45. Silva M, Kabbash CA, Tiberi JV 3rd, et al. Surface damage on open box posterior-stabilized polyethylene tibial inserts. *Clin Orthop Relat Res.* 2003;(416):135-144.
46. Oral E, Ghali BW, Rowell SL, Micheli BR, Lozynsky AJ, Muratoglu OK. A surface crosslinked UHMWPE stabilized by vitamin E with low wear and high fatigue strength. *Biomaterials.* 2010;31(27):7051-7060.
47. Lerf R, Zurbrugg D, Delfosse D. Use of vitamin E to protect cross-linked UHMWPE from oxidation. *Biomaterials.* 2010;31(13):3643-3648.
48. Kurtz SM, Dumbleton J, Siskey RS, Wang A, Manley M. Trace concentrations of vitamin E protect radiation crosslinked UHMWPE from oxidative degradation. *J Biomed Mater Res A.* 2009;90(2):549-563.
49. Stoller AP, Johnson TS, Popoola OO, Humphrey SM, Blanchard CR. Highly crosslinked polyethylene in posterior-stabilized total knee arthroplasty in vitro performance evaluation of wear, delamination, and tibial post durability. *J Arthroplasty.* 2011;26(3):483-491.
50. Popoola OO, Yao JQ, Johnson TS, Blanchard CR. Wear, delamination, and fatigue resistance of melt-annealed highly crosslinked UHMWPE cruciate-retaining knee inserts under activities of daily living. *J Orthop Res.* 2010;28(9):1120-1126.
51. Williams PA, Brown CM, Tsukamoto R, Clarke IC. Polyethylene wear debris produced in a knee simulator model: effect of crosslinking and counterface material. *J Biomed Mater Res B Appl Biomater.* 2010;92(1):78-85.

52. Utzschneider S, Harrasser N, Schroeder C, Mazoochian F, Jansson V. Wear of contemporary total knee replacements: a knee simulator study of six current designs. *Clin Biomech (Bristol, Avon)*. 2009;24(7):583-588.

53. Wang A, Yau SS, Essner A, Herrera L, Manley M, Dumbleton J. A highly crosslinked UHMWPE for CR and PS total knee arthroplasties. *J Arthroplasty*. 2008;23(4):559-566.

54. Bal BS, Garino J, Ries M, Oonishi H. Ceramic bearings in total knee arthroplasty. *J Knee Surg*. 2007;20(4):261-270.

55. Oonishi H, Ueno M, Kim SC, Oonishi H, Iwamoto M, Kyomoto M. Ceramic versus cobalt-chrome femoral components; wear of polyethylene insert in total knee prosthesis. *J Arthroplasty*. 2009;24(3):374-382.

56. Nakamura S, Kobayashi M, Ito H, Nakamura K, Ueo T, Nakamura T. The Bi-Surface total knee arthroplasty: minimum 10-year follow-up study. *Knee*. 2010;17(4):274-278.

57. Bal BS, Greenberg DD, Buhrmester L, Aleto TJ. Primary TKA with a zirconia ceramic femoral component. *J Knee Surg*. 2006;19(2):89-93.

58. Innocenti M, Civinini R, Carulli C, Matassi F, Villano M. The 5-year results of an oxidized zirconium femoral component for TKA. *Clin Orthop Relat Res*. 2010;468(5):1258-1263.

59. Heyse TJ, Davis J, Haas SB, Chen DX, Wright TM, Laskin RS. Retrieval analysis of femoral zirconium components in total knee arthroplasty preliminary results. *J Arthroplasty*. 2011;26(3):445-450.

60. Bai B, Baez J, Testa N, Kummer FJ. Effect of posterior cut angle on tibial component loading. *J Arthroplasty*. 2000;15(7):916-920.

61. Sah AP, Scott RD, Iorio R. Angled polyethylene insert exchange for sagittal tibial malalignment in total knee arthroplasty. *J Arthroplasty*. 2008;23(1):141-144.

62. Bhandari M, Bajammal S, Guyatt GH, et al. Effect of bisphosphonates on periprosthetic bone mineral density after total joint arthroplasty. A meta-analysis. *J Bone Joint Surg Am*. 2005;87(2):293-301.

63. Shanbhag AS. Use of bisphosphonates to improve the durability of total joint replacements. *J Am Acad Orthop Surg*. 2006;14(4):215-225.

64. Huff TW, Sculco TP. Management of bone loss in revision total knee arthroplasty. *J Arthroplasty*. 2007;22(7 suppl 3):32-36.

65. Burnett RS, Keeney JA, Maloney WJ, Clohisy JC. Revision total knee arthroplasty for major osteolysis. *Iowa Orthop J*. 2009;29:28-37.

66. Dorr LD, Ranawat CS, Sculco TA, McKaskill B, Orisek BS. Bone graft for tibial defects in total knee arthroplasty. *Clin Orthop Relat Res*. 2006;(446):4-9.

67. Lotke PA, Carolan GF, Puri N. Impaction grafting for bone defects in revision total knee arthroplasty. *Clin Orthop Relat Res*. 2006;(446):99-103.

68. Lyall HS, Sanghrajka A, Scott G. Severe tibial bone loss in revision total knee replacement managed with structural femoral head allograft: a prospective case series from the Royal London Hospital. *Knee*. 2009;16(5):326-331.

69. Engh GA, Ammeen DJ. Use of structural allograft in revision total knee arthroplasty in knees with severe tibial bone loss. *J Bone Joint Surg Am*. 2007;89(12):2640-2647.

70. Griffin WL, Scott RD, Dalury DF, Mahoney OM, Chiavetta JB, Odum SM. Modular insert exchange in knee arthroplasty for treatment of wear and osteolysis. *Clin Orthop Relat Res*. 2007;(464):132-137.

71. Mackay DC, Siddique MS. The results of revision knee arthroplasty with and without retention of secure cemented femoral components. *J Bone Joint Surg Br*. 2003;85(4):517-520.

72. Fehring TK, Odum S, Olekson C, Griffin WL, Mason JB, McCoy TH. Stem fixation in revision total knee arthroplasty: a comparative analysis. *Clin Orthop Relat Res*. 2003;(416):217-224.

73. Whiteside LA. Cementless fixation in revision total knee arthroplasty. *Clin Orthop Relat Res*. 2006;446:140-148.

74. Hockman DE, Ammeen D, Engh GA. Augments and allografts in revision total knee arthroplasty: usage and outcome using one modular revision prosthesis. *J Arthroplasty*. 2005;20(1):35-41.

Periprosthetic Fractures
Knee

Adam J. Schwartz, MD and Henry D. Clarke, MD

INCIDENCE AND ETIOLOGY

Periprosthetic fracture following total knee arthroplasty (TKA) is estimated to occur in 0.1% to 2% of primary cases.[1,2] As the demand for TKA procedures performed in the United States is estimated to increase by more than 600% by the year 2030, the diminishing number of specialized joint arthroplasty surgeons will undoubtedly encounter this complication more frequently in the future.[3]

Risk factors for periprosthetic fracture around a TKA include poor bone quality, history of a neurologic disorder, chronic steroid use, revision knee surgery, and other technical factors.[4] Bone quality can be compromised in cases of advanced age, osteoporosis, rheumatoid arthritis, or other inflammatory arthropathies. Bogoch et al reviewed 16 cases of periprosthetic supracondylar fracture and noted 12 had rheumatoid arthritis.[5] Similarly, Figgie et al reviewed the results of 24 supracondylar periprosthetic fractures in 22 patients.[6] Twelve of 22 patients (54.5%) occurred in patients with rheumatoid arthritis.

Neurologic conditions have also been identified as an independent risk factor for complications following TKA. Gait disturbance, muscle imbalance, and poor proprioception may lead to falls, abnormal joint forces, and poor knee kinematics. The result is an increased incidence of periprosthetic fracture. In a review of 61 supracondylar fractures above a total knee replacement, Culp et al found that 17 patients (27.9%) had a pre-existing neurologic disorder such as epilepsy, Parkinson's, or neuropathic joint, among others.[7]

In a review of more than 19,000 TKA procedures from the Mayo Clinic database, Berry found a higher incidence of periprosthetic fracture in the revision setting.[1] Intraoperatively, fractures were found to occur in 0.2% of primary cases compared to 1.9% of revision cases. Postoperatively, the risk of periprosthetic fracture was more than double for revision cases versus primary cases (4.4% versus 2.1%, respectively). Large wear-induced osteolytic defects and bone loss following component removal likely account for the higher incidence of periprosthetic fracture in the revision setting.

Jacofsky DJ, Hedley AK, eds.
Fundamentals of Revision Knee Arthroplasty:
Diagnosis, Evaluation, and Treatment (pp 205-214).
© 2013 SLACK Incorporated.

Although anterior notching of the femur has been reported as a risk factor for postoperative periprosthetic fracture,[7,8] more recent literature has failed to show a strong correlation.[9-11] Ritter et al reviewed a consecutive series of 1089 total knee replacements.[9] Despite the fact that femoral notching was identified on the lateral radiograph of 325 knees (29.8%), only 2 supracondylar femur fractures occurred, both in cases without evidence of notching. The authors concluded that no correlation exists between femoral notching and periprosthetic supracondylar femur fracture. In a recent biomechanical analysis, Shawen et al demonstrated that the combination of low bone density and anterior femoral notching was associated with the highest significant correlation with periprosthetic supracondylar fracture.[12] Other technical factors that may predispose patients to periprosthetic fracture include the presence of bone defects from instrumentation or previous hardware, the use of cementless press-fit stems, and the presence of a thin patellar remnant (12 mm or less) following patellar resurfacing. Transection of the lateral geniculate artery at the time of lateral release has been identified as a potential cause for patellar fracture.[13] Additionally, recent case reports have described both femoral and tibial periprosthetic fractures resulting from stress risers caused by pin sites used during computer navigation.[14-17]

CLASSIFICATION

Periprosthetic fractures can occur intraoperatively or postoperatively. Those that occur postoperatively are typically the result of low-energy falls.[18]

A variety of classification systems exist to describe periprosthetic femur fractures following TKA.[19-23] The system of Rorabeck and Taylor[23] incorporates the integrity of the prosthesis into the classification system and addresses the need for revision arthroplasty at the time of fracture fixation. Type I fractures are undisplaced with an intact prosthesis. Most classification systems would characterize fractures as nondisplaced if they are angulated less than 5 degrees or displaced less than 5 mm. These fractures are amenable to nonoperative management in select cases. Type II and III fractures are displaced (greater than 5 degrees of angulation or 5 mm displacement). Type II fractures demonstrate a well-fixed, well-functioning prosthesis, while type III fractures occur in conjunction with a loose prosthesis, or one that demonstrates evidence of impending failure.

Fractures of the tibia are less frequently encountered.[2] The classification system described by Felix et al is based upon component integrity and anatomic location.[24] The 4 types of fractures are based on anatomic location and include the following:

- Type I fractures involve the tibial plateau
- Type II fractures are adjacent to the tibial stem if present
- Type III fractures are distal to the prosthesis
- Type IV fractures occur involve the tibial tubercle

Type I fractures were the most commonly encountered pattern, thought to be the result of component malalignment or implant loosening. All fracture types are subcategorized as occurring around (A) a well-fixed implant, (B) a loose implant, or (C) intraoperatively.

The incidence of patellar fracture has decreased due to modifications in implant design, particularly patellar component thickness and geometry and improved femoral trochlear depth.[25] Patellar fractures are classified as displaced or nondisplaced with an intact or loose component.[26] These fractures can be further classified based upon the integrity of the extensor mechanism.

TREATMENT

A number of considerations should be addressed prior to selecting a treatment modality. A complete history and physical examination will reveal any predisposing risk factors, previous prosthetic issues or complications, and the presence of multiple scars or poor vascularity, which may lead to wound healing problems. If a question exists regarding the healing potential of the soft tissue envelope, a plastic surgeon may be enlisted to help with wound closure or for local flap coverage. The patient's medical comorbidities, prefracture functional status, and perioperative risk should be addressed and the goal of surgery clearly defined.

Treatment of periprosthetic fracture is based on fracture pattern, displacement, and implant stability. Nondisplaced fractures that occur in the setting of a well-fixed, well-functioning prosthesis may be considered for nonoperative management. A long leg cast is used for 6 to 8 weeks with frequent radiographic evaluation to ensure fracture stability and maintenance of alignment. After this period of immobilization, patients may be transitioned to a hinged knee brace and begin gentle range of motion exercises along with increased weightbearing.

The most frequently encountered type of periprosthetic fracture is a low-energy displaced supracondylar fracture with an intact prosthesis (Figure 14-1).[2] Nonsurgical management of a displaced supracondylar fracture is rarely indicated for elderly patients with very short life expectancy or poor prefracture function and limited baseline ambulatory capacity.[27] Surgical options include open reduction and plate fixation, closed reduction and percutaneous locking plate fixation, or retrograde intramedullary nailing. The choice of fixation technique is largely dependent upon fracture location, pattern, and bone quality. The surgical approach for open reduction utilizes the previous anterior knee incision, which may be extended proximally and laterally as necessary. If multiple incisions exist, the most laterally based incision is typically chosen to maximize blood flow to the medial soft tissues. A lateral parapatellar arthrotomy may be performed, with care taken to avoid ligation of the lateral geniculate artery. The fascia lata is incised, revealing the underlying vastus lateralis, which may be elevated off the intermuscular septum. Perforating vessels are ligated and the lateral femoral cortex exposed. Reduction may be obtained manually or with the use of a femoral distractor if assistance is limited. A simple configuration involves pin placement in the proximal lateral femur and another in the distal femur, taking into account the location of future plate fixation. Once adequate reduction has been achieved, fixation may be achieved with a 90-degree blade plate, a dynamic condylar screw, a conventional condylar buttress plate, or a peri-articular locking plate that allows for multiple fixed-angle screws to be placed in the distal fragment. Alternatively, reduction may be obtained prior to exposure and a laterally based plate placed percutaneously. This technique has the advantage of preserving the biological soft tissue envelope at the fracture site, thus improving healing potential.

Retrograde intramedullary nail fixation is useful for transverse fractures with a large enough distal fragment to accept adequate locking screw placement. A particular advantage of nail fixation is the avoidance of varus collapse in the setting of severe posteromedial cortical comminution.[27] Preoperative planning is of vital importance if intramedullary nail fixation is chosen. The procedure can be performed on a radiolucent table with a bump or radiolucent triangle to aid with fracture reduction. The approach utilizes the same skin and extensor mechanism approach that was performed at the time of the original arthroplasty procedure. The patella is retracted laterally, thus exposing the intercondylar notch. It is also of vital importance to preoperatively determine the intercondylar distance of the femoral implant. The authors would direct the reader to the review article published by Su et al,[4] which includes a detailed table that documents the most commonly encountered femoral components and intercondylar distances. Reduction is achieved either with manual traction or a femoral distractor that uses a slightly different pin configuration. To avoid interference with nail placement, the distal pin is placed in the proximal tibia, while the proximal pin may be placed in the dense bone of the proximal femoral calcar, away from the intramedullary canal. Alternatively, the proximal pin may be placed unicortically either anteriorly or posteriorly to the path of the nail. Once adequate reduction has been achieved, the distal femur is opened, and the femoral canal reamed to a size slightly larger than the final nail to be placed (typically 1.5 to 2 mm larger than the nail diameter chosen). The length of the nail is measured by recording the distance of the guidewire from the intercondylar notch to a location just proximal to the

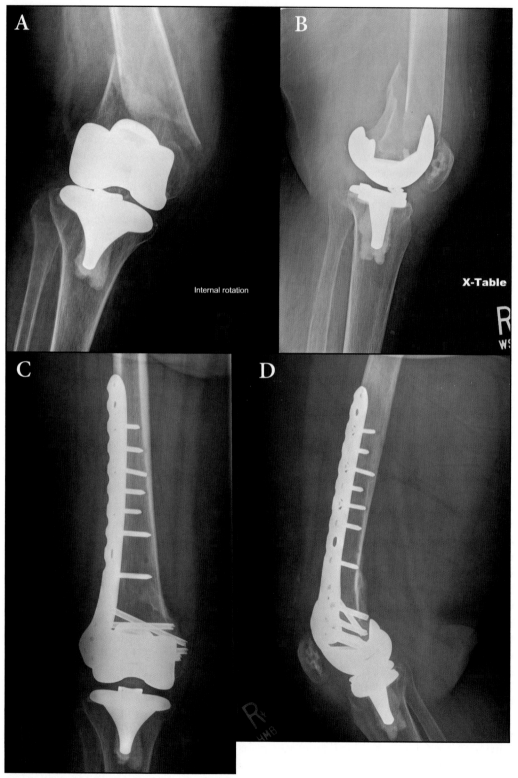

Figure 14-1. (A, B) AP and lateral radiographs of a type II periprosthetic femur fracture. Note the well-fixed posterior-stabilized implant. (C, D) AP and lateral images taken 3 months after fixation using a laterally placed peri-articular locking plate.

lesser trochanter. The proximal tip of the retrograde nail should end at a location well proximal to the lesser trochanter to avoid causing a stress riser in the subtrochanteric region. The nail is placed, and the distal locking screws are placed using the attached drill guide. Compression may be applied through the fracture manually prior to locking the nail proximally. The proximal screws are placed freehand from anterior to posterior using a "perfect-circle" technique. Radiolucent drills and outrigger guides are available to facilitate proximal locking. One company recently developed a magnetic device to help localize freehand screw placement without the need for fluoroscopy. Various distal locking configurations are available for retrograde nails. It is advantageous to utilize an implant that allows for several screws to be placed in multiple planes.

Periprosthetic femoral fractures that involve a loose knee arthroplasty implant are frequently associated with large osteolytic defects that require revision of the prosthesis and simultaneous fracture fixation.[29,30] Both goals may typically be achieved by revision to a long-stemmed implant with supplemental plate or cerclage wire fixation and defect augmentation with metal or allograft. A stepwise approach to knee revision should be followed.[31] A full complement of instruments designed to remove well-fixed total knee components should be available, if necessary.[32] Removal of the patellar component is typically not required unless patellar fracture is the main indication for surgery or there is suspicion of component loosening or malfunction. After removal of all knee arthroplasty components, the fracture is assessed for axial and rotational stability. Transverse fracture patterns are typically stable in the axial plane, but are rotationally unstable. Such fractures may be amenable to intramedullary fixation with a long stem that engages the diaphyseal bone. This fixation may be supplemented with a conventional condylar plate or a laterally based peri-articular locking plate. Low profile cerclage wires may provisionally provide fixation as the canal is reamed, particularly in oblique fracture patterns.

In cases of severe fracture comminution, fixation is difficult to achieve with intramedullary stems alone. An alternative to fracture fixation is revision to a modular hinged endoprosthesis. The approach for distal femoral replacement is either direct anterior, through a medial parapatellar arthrotomy, or anteromedial, exploring the interval between the vastus medialis muscle and the medial intermuscular septum. The latter approach provides direct access to identify and protect the neurovascular bundle and maintains the integrity of the entire extensor mechanism, but may result in significant undermining of the medial soft tissue sleeve, particularly in the multiply-operated knee. The tibial component will almost always need to be revised if the periprosthetic fracture involves a primary knee implant and revision to a hinged endoprosthesis is planned. While an all-polyethylene tibial component may provide durable fixation in the primary setting, a metal-backed tibial implant that allows for the placement of stem extensions should be used when converting from a primary implant to a hinged endoprosthesis. After establishing a stable tibial platform, the remainder of the fracture fragments are removed proximally, and the femoral canal exposed. Knowledge of the cranial-caudal dimensions of the smallest body segment helps to determine the exact amount of bone necessary to resect in order to prevent overlengthening of the affected limb. Templating the opposite normal extremity may be useful to determine the level of resection in cases of severe bone loss and comminution. Additionally, the position of the patella in relation to the joint line is noted with the knee held in full extension. As a final confirmatory test, the assembled modular femoral implant may be compared to the length of the resected bone on the back table. Femoral component rotation is difficult to determine after resection of the metaphyseal portion of the distal femur. If possible, a mark should be placed on the anterior femur prior to resection of the metaphysis to provide a guide for femoral rotation. In cases of severe comminution, or if the metaphysis has already been removed, the linea aspera proximally should provide a rough estimate of the posterior aspect of the femur, although this is not an exact reference point. Trial implants are placed, and rotation of the femoral component may also be determined based on patellar tracking.

OUTCOMES

The majority of literature regarding periprosthetic knee fractures is retrospective in design and addresses supracondylar fractures as these are the most commonly encountered. Bezwada et al reviewed the results of 30 supracondylar fractures fixed with either retrograde intramedullary nailing (18 fractures) or open reduction and internal fixation (12 patients).[33] Both operative time and blood loss were greater for the open reduction and internal fixation group compared to intramedullary nailing. One patient underwent above-knee amputation due to deep infection, and another experienced nonunion, successfully treated with autogenous bone graft and revision open reduction and internal fixation. All patients returned to ambulatory capacity except for the one patient who underwent amputation. Han et al reported uniformly excellent results in 9 patients with supracondylar femur fracture above a well-fixed knee implant treated with retrograde nailing.[34]

More recent literature has focused on the efficacy of locking plates, particularly for elderly patients with poor bone. Large et al compared the results of 50 periprosthetic supracondylar femur fractures fixed with either a locking (29 fractures) or conventional plate or intramedullary nailing (21 fractures).[35] The patients treated with locked plating demonstrated lower intraoperative blood loss, better maintenance of alignment, and an overall decreased complication rate. Both malunions and nonunions were more frequent in the conventional fixation group (47% and 16%, respectively) compared to the locked plating group (20% and 0%, respectively). Anakwe et al reviewed the results of 28 periprosthetic fractures fixed with the less invasive stabilization system (LISS).[36] Fifteen fractures occurred around a well-fixed hip implant, 11 occurred above a well-fixed knee prosthesis, and another 2 interprosthetic fractures between hip and knee implants were included. Five patients died within the follow-up period. Among the patients who survived longer than 16 weeks, however, all achieved radiographic and clinical union. Similarly, Sah et al reported the results of 22 consecutive patients with interprosthetic femur fracture treated with single-locked plating.[37] None of the cases required supplemental allograft struts. At a mean 13.8 weeks postoperatively, all fractures achieved bony union, and at the time of most recent clinical follow-up all patients had regained their prefracture ambulatory capacity.

Modular distal femoral endoprosthetic devices have been increasingly utilized for highly comminuted, unstable fracture patterns particularly in low-demand patients. In the oncologic setting, long-term survival rates of up to 86% have been reported.[38] An excellent review of the available literature regarding nononcologic indications is provided by Harrison et al.[39] The 20-year survivorship for nononcologic applications also approaches 90%. Springer et al reviewed the results of 26 modular segmental endoprostheses implanted for nononcologic indications.[40] The cohort included 11 patients with chronic periprosthetic nonunion and 1 acute periprosthetic fracture. At a mean follow-up of 58.5 months, no patient required revision, although 4 knees demonstrated evidence of loosening. While long-term survival rates are significantly lower than for conventional knee implants, modular endoprosthetic devices may be the only salvage option in cases of chronic malunion or nonunion, where severe bone and/or soft tissue defects preclude the use of more conventional implants.

PEARLS FOR PREVENTION

Prevention of periprosthetic fracture begins with preoperatively identifying any risk factors that may predispose the patient to this complication. Patients with poor bone quality, neurologic conditions, rheumatoid arthritis, or those on chronic steroid therapy should be identified. Stemmed implants that allow for additional fixation into the diaphysis should be available if the surgeon expects problems with metaphyseal fixation alone due to poor bone quality. A minimum of 10 to 12 mm of bone should remain following patellar resection for resurfacing.[41] If this is not possible, leaving the patella unresurfaced should be considered.

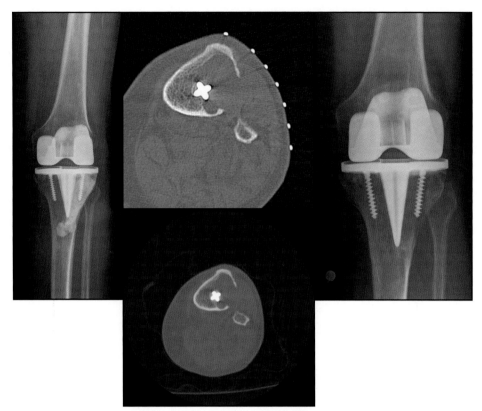

Figure 14-2. This 91-year-old low-demand patient presented with a well-functioning but painful left total knee arthroplasty 20 years following his original surgery. Plain radiographs and computed tomography scan revealed a well-fixed femoral and tibial component with advanced polyethylene wear and severe osteolysis of the proximal tibia. Laboratory evaluation and aspiration was negative for infection. The patient was taken for exchange of the polyethylene liner and extended intralesional curettage and cementation of the large area of osteolysis.

The use of "less invasive" or "minimally invasive" techniques has been associated with an increased risk of early knee failure.[42] Exposure should be adequate to avoid excessive retraction on bony structures and to allow for even, complete bony cuts. Poor visualization and forceful retraction may lead to bony avulsions, cortical perforations, and metaphyseal fracture. This is particularly problematic in patients with patella baja, limited preoperative flexion, or severe deformity. To facilitate the use of smaller incisions, many implant manufacturers have developed low-profile instrumentation and cutting jigs. These devices often require completion of bony cuts to be performed freehand following jig removal. Attempt to remove uncompleted bone cuts may result in fracture of large portions of adherent metaphyseal bone. To avoid such a scenario, the surgeon should ensure that the cut has been completed prior to removal of a bone fragment. Side-cutting or reciprocating saws can be particularly useful in achieving a true complete cut.

Late periprosthetic fracture is best prevented with routine radiographic follow-up and treatment of large symptomatic osteolytic lesions prior to fracture (Figure 14-2). Osteolytic lesions around well-fixed implants may be treated with bone grafting, cementation, or with exchange of the worn polyethylene liner. Impending fractures in the setting of a nonmodular implant, or one that demonstrates evidence of femoral and/or tibial component damage, should be revised to a long-stemmed or metaphyseal engaging stem.

REFERENCES

1. Berry DJ. Epidemiology: hip and knee. *Orthop Clin North Am.* 1999;30(2):183-190.
2. Kim K, Egol KA, Hozack WJ, Parvizi J. Periprosthetic fractures after total knee arthroplasties. *Clin Orthop Relat Res.* 2006;446:167-175.
3. Kurtz S, Ong K, Lau E, Mowat F, Halpern M. Projections of primary and revision hip and knee arthroplasty in the United States from 2005 to 2030. *J Bone Joint Surg Am.* 2007;89(4):780-785.
4. Su ET, DeWal H, Di Cesare PE. Periprosthetic femoral fractures above total knee replacements. *J Am Acad Orthop Surg.* 2004;12(1):12-20.
5. Bogoch E, Hastings D, Gross A, Gschwend N. Supracondylar fractures of the femur adjacent to resurfacing and MacIntosh arthroplasties of the knee in patients with rheumatoid arthritis. *Clin Orthop Relat Res.* 1988;(229):213-220.
6. Figgie MP, Goldberg VM, Figgie HE, Sobel M. The results of treatment of supracondylar fracture above total knee arthroplasty. *J Arthroplasty.* 1990;5(3):267-276.
7. Culp RW, Schmidt RG, Hanks G, et al. Supracondylar fracture of the femur following prosthetic knee arthroplasty. *Clin Orthop Relat Res.* 1987;(222):212-222.
8. Lesh ML, Schneider DJ, Deol G, et al. The consequences of anterior femoral notching in total knee arthroplasty. A biomechanical study. *J Bone Joint Surg Am.* 2000;82-A(8):1096-1101.
9. Ritter MA, Thong AE, Keating EM, et al. The effect of femoral notching during total knee arthroplasty on the prevalence of postoperative femoral fractures and on clinical outcome. *J Bone Joint Surg Am.* 2005;87(11):2411-2414.
10. Ritter MA, Faris PM, Keating EM. Anterior femoral notching and ipsilateral supracondylar femur fracture in total knee arthroplasty. *J Arthroplasty.* 1988;3(2):185-187.
11. Gujarathi N, Putti AB, Abboud RJ, et al. Risk of periprosthetic fracture after anterior femoral notching. *Acta Orthop.* 2009;80(5):553-556.
12. Shawen SB, Belmont PJ Jr, Klemme WR, Topoleski LD, Xenos JS, Orchowski JR. Osteoporosis and anterior femoral notching in periprosthetic supracondylar femoral fractures: a biomechanical analysis. *J Bone Joint Surg Am.* 2003 Jan;85-A(1):115-21.
13. Tria AJ, Harwood DA, Alicea JA, Cody RP. Patellar fractures in posterior stabilized knee arthroplasties. *Clin Orthop Relat Res.* 1994;(299):131-138.
14. Massai F, Conteduca F, Vadalà A, et al. Tibial stress fracture after computer-navigated total knee arthroplasty. *J Orthop Traumatol.* 2010;11(2):123-127.
15. Ossendorf C, Fuchs B, Koch P. Femoral stress fracture after computer navigated total knee arthroplasty. *Knee.* 2006;13(5):397-399.
16. Jung H, Jung Y, Song K, Park S, Lee J. Fractures associated with computer-navigated total knee arthroplasty. A report of two cases. *J Bone Joint Surg Am.* 2007;89(10):2280-2284.
17. Wysocki RW, Sheinkop MB, Virkus WW, Della Valle CJ. Femoral fracture through a previous pin site after computer-assisted total knee arthroplasty. *J Arthroplasty.* 2008;23(3):462-465.
18. Healy WL, Siliski JM, Incavo SJ. Operative treatment of distal femoral fractures proximal to total knee replacements. *J Bone Joint Surg Am.* 1993;75(1):27-34.
19. Chen F, Mont MA, Bachner RS. Management of ipsilateral supracondylar femur fractures following total knee arthroplasty. *J Arthroplasty.* 1994;9(5):521-526.
20. Neer CS, Grantham SA, Shelton ML. Supracondylar fracture of the adult femur. A study of one hundred and ten cases. *J Bone Joint Surg Am.* 1967;49(4):591-613.
21. DiGioia AM, Rubash HE. Periprosthetic fractures of the femur after total knee arthroplasty. A literature review and treatment algorithm. *Clin Orthop Relat Res.* 1991;(271):135-142.
22. Rorabeck CH, Taylor JW. Classification of periprosthetic fractures complicating total knee arthroplasty. *Orthop Clin North Am.* 1999;30(2):209-214.
23. Rorabeck CH, Taylor JW. Periprosthetic fractures of the femur complicating total knee arthroplasty. *Orthop Clin North Am.* 1999;30(2):265-277.
24. Felix NA, Stuart MJ, Hanssen AD. Periprosthetic fractures of the tibia associated with total knee arthroplasty. *Clin Orthop Relat Res.* 1997;(345):113-124.
25. Sheth NP, Pedowitz DI, Lonner JH. Periprosthetic patellar fractures. *J Bone Joint Surg Am.* 2007;89(10):2285-2296.
26. Hozack WJ, Goll SR, Lotke PA, Rothman RH, Booth RE. The treatment of patellar fractures after total knee arthroplasty. *Clin Orthop Relat Res.* 1988;(236):123-127.

27. Engh GA, Ammeen DJ. Periprosthetic fractures adjacent to total knee implants: treatment and clinical results. *Instr Course Lect.* 1998;47:437-448.

28. Davison BL. Varus collapse of comminuted distal femur fractures after open reduction and internal fixation with a lateral condylar buttress plate. *Am J. Orthop.* 2003;32(1):27-30.

29. Berry DJ. Periprosthetic fractures associated with osteolysis: A problem on the rise. *J Arthroplasty.* 2003;18(3 Pt 2):107-111.

30. Beals RK, Tower SS. Periprosthetic fractures of the femur. An analysis of 93 fractures. *Clin Orthop Relat Res.* 1996;(327):238-246.

31. Dennis DA. A stepwise approach to revision total knee arthroplasty. *J Arthroplasty.* 2007;22(4 suppl 1):32-38.

32. Mason JB, Fehring TK. Removing well-fixed total knee arthroplasty implants. *Clin Orthop Relat Res.* 2006;446:76-82.

33. Bezwada HP, Neubauer P, Baker J, Israelite CL, Johanson NA. Periprosthetic supracondylar femur fractures following total knee arthroplasty. *J Arthroplasty.* 2004;19(4):453-458.

34. Han HS, Oh KW, Kang SB. Retrograde intramedullary nailing for periprosthetic supracondylar fractures of the femur after total knee arthroplasty. *Clin Orthop Surg.* 2009 Dec;1(4):201-6. Epub 2009 Nov 25.

35. Large TM, Kellam JF, Bosse MJ, et al. Locked plating of supracondylar periprosthetic femur fractures. *J Arthroplasty.* 2008;23(6 suppl 1):115-120.

36. Anakwe RE, Aitken SA, Khan LAK. Osteoporotic periprosthetic fractures of the femur in elderly patients: outcome after fixation with the LISS plate. *Injury.* 2008;39(10):1191-1197.

37. Sah AP, Marshall A, Virkus WV, Estok DM, Della Valle CJ. Interprosthetic fractures of the femur: treatment with a single-locked plate. *J Arthroplasty.* 2010;25(2):280-286.

38. Schwartz AJ, Kabo JM, Eilber FC, Eilber FR, Eckardt JJ. Cemented distal femoral endoprostheses for musculoskeletal tumor: improved survival of modular versus custom implants. *Clin Orthop Relat Res.* 2010;468(8):2198-2210.

39. Harrison RJ, Thacker MM, Pitcher JD, Temple HT, Scully SP. Distal femur replacement is useful in complex total knee arthroplasty revisions. *Clin Orthop Relat Res.* 2006;446:113-120.

40. Springer BD, Sim FH, Hanssen AD, Lewallen DG. The modular segmental kinematic rotating hinge for nonneoplastic limb salvage. *Clin Orthop Relat Res.* 2004;(421):181-187.

41. Reuben JD, McDonald CL, Woodard PL, Hennington LJ. Effect of patella thickness on patella strain following total knee arthroplasty. *J Arthroplasty.* 1991;6(3):251-258.

42. Barrack RL, Barnes CL, Burnett RSJ, et al. Minimal incision surgery as a risk factor for early failure of total knee arthroplasty. *J Arthroplasty.* 2009;24(4):489-498.

Financial Disclosures

Dr. Christopher L. Anderson has no financial or proprietary interest in the materials presented herein.

Dr. Wael K. Barsoum is a consultant to Stryker Orthopaedics and Shukla Medical and receives research support from Stryker Orthopaedics, Zimmer, Salient Surgical Technologies, CoolSystems, Orthovita, DJO, Active Implants, and Recothrom. Dr. Barsoum receives royalties from Stryker Orthopaedics, Zimmer, Exactech, Wright Medical Technology, and Shukla Medical and stock options in OtisMed Corporation, Custom Orthopaedic Solutions, and iVHR. Dr. Barsoum has 2 issued patents and 30 applications.

Dr. Michael R. Bloomfield has no financial or proprietary interest in the materials presented herein.

Dr. John J. Bottros has no financial or proprietary interest in the materials presented herein.

Dr. Mark D. Campbell is a consultant for Arthrex and Bacterin.

Dr. Robert M. Cercek has no financial or proprietary interest in the materials presented herein.

Dr. Henry D. Clarke has a consulting agreement with Biomet and receives institutional research support from Stryker Orthopaedics.

Dr. Dermot Collopy is a consultant to and receives research assistance from Stryker Orthopaedics.

Dr. Craig J. Della Valle is a consultant for Biomet and Smith & Nephew and receives research support from Smith & Nephew and Stryker Orthopaedics. Dr. Della Valle receives institutional research support from Zimmer and stock options for his work on the Scientific Advisory Board for CD Diagnostics.

Dr. Douglas A. Dennis receives royalties for transfer of intellectual property from Depuy Inc and Innomed. Dr. Dennis is a consultant to Depuy Inc and Porter Adventist Hospital.

Dr. Ian M. Gradisar has no financial or proprietary interest in the materials presented herein.

Dr. Curtis W. Hartman receives research support from Smith & Nephew.

Dr. Anthony K. Hedley has several patents with Synvasive Technology Inc and Stryker Orthopaedics and receives financial compensation for his work as a consultant with Stryker Orthopaedics.

Dr. Kirby D. Hitt consults for and receives royalties from Stryker Orthopedics.

Dr. David J. Jacofsky is a consultant for Bacterin, Comprehensive Care Solutions, Safe Independence, Stryker Orthopaedics, Smith & Nephew, and Technology Capital Investors. Dr. Jacofsky receives research support from Biomet, DePuy, Stryker Orthopaedics, Smith & Nephew, and VQ Ortho Care and receives royalties from Stryker Orthopaedics.

Dr. Aaron J. Johnson has no financial or proprietary interest in the materials presented herein.

Dr. Vamsi K. Kancherla has no financial or proprietary interest in the materials presented herein.

Dr. Harpal S. Khanuja has no financial or proprietary interest in the materials presented herein.

Dr. Raymond H. Kim is a consultant for Stryker Orthopaedics and receives royalties from Innomed Inc and institutional research support from DePuy.

Dr. Viktor E. Krebs has not disclosed any relevant financial relationships.

Dr. Steven M. Kurtz works for an institution that receives grants from Stryker Orthopaedics.

Dr. Michael T. Manley has not disclosed any relevant financial relationships.

Dr. David A. McQueen is a consultant for Stryker Orthopedics.

Dr. R. Michael Meneghini is a consultant for and receives fees and royalties from Stryker Orthopaedics.

Dr. Michael A. Mont has no financial or proprietary interest in the materials presented herein.

Dr. Trevor G. Murray has no financial or proprietary interest in the materials presented herein.

Dr. Qais Naziri has no financial or proprietary interest in the materials presented herein.

Dr. Kevin L. Ong works for an institution that receives grants from Stryker Orthopaedics.

Dr. Adam J. Schwartz has no financial or proprietary interest in the materials presented herein.

Dr. Scott M. Sporer is a consultant for Zimmer and Smith & Nephew and receives research support from Zimmer.

Dr. Bryan D. Springer is a consultant for Stryker Orthopaedics and Convatec Surgical.

Dr. Joseph F. Styron has no financial or proprietary interest in the materials presented herein.

Dr. Creighton C. Tubb has no financial or proprietary interest in the materials presented herein.

Index

ZERO
DEFECTS

A New Dimension

JAMES F. HALPIN
Director of Quality, Martin Company
Orlando, Florida

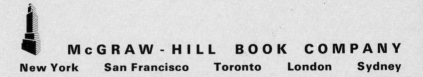

McGRAW-HILL BOOK COMPANY
New York   San Francisco   Toronto   London   Sydney

55,340

ZERO DEFECTS

DEFECTS

in Quality Assurance

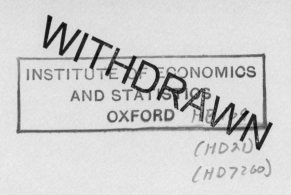
ZERO DEFECTS

Foreword

The reader of this book and I probably have two important things in common: We are both interested in learning more about Zero Defects, and we are both contemplating the possibility of having such a program within our own organizations. A number of executives in our company were fortunate enough to receive briefings from the author during a series of visits to his office at the Martin Company's Orlando, Florida Division. While the reader may not have this advantage, he can get the next best thing to it in one evening in the comfort of his easy chair.

Zero Defects is an organized, effective effort to reverse the tendency of modern specialization and production techniques to undermine the traditional American pride in craftsmanship. The experiences of Martin Company, and the many other organizations in industry, the military, and government, that have adopted this "do it right the first time" idea demonstrate its success.

Under the Zero Defects program accepted motivational techniques have been molded together ingeniously by the author to produce a simple, straightforward program to ensure quality products and services. Mr. Halpin's knowledge of his subject ranges from top-management insight all the way to intimate knowledge of each specific detail of the program.

There is no doubt in my mind that Mr. Halpin's techniques for implementation, measurement, recognition, and sustaining a ZD program can be of great value to anyone considering starting such an effort within his own organization. The fact that thousands of organizations with millions of employees have put such programs to very profitable use since Martin originated the program four years ago has long since answered the question: "Does it work?"

The key to the entire program, as the author points out, is the individual, his needs, his desires, and his achievements. Zero Defects uses these things for the benefit of the individual and his company. Posters and banners can help, but true success depends on the close, personal management-employee contact that is emphasized.

If, after reviewing Mr. Halpin's techniques for employee motivation, you decide to go forward with the program, it may be the most important quality step your organization has ever taken. Past results indicate that the savings achieved during the first few months more than offset the cost of the entire program.

My company, Montgomery Ward, is convinced that ZD can make a great contribution to improving the quality of our customer service and can add to our total performance. It provides something that is seriously lacking in American industry. Zero Defects is, in my opinion, the outstanding quality program of the decade, if not the century.

Robert E. Brooker
PRESIDENT, MONTGOMERY WARD

Preface

This book was written in response to the thousands of requests I have received for more information about the Zero Defects concept and its implementation. It is directed to the man who is considering a Zero Defects program, the man who has a Zero Defects program, and the man who is simply interested in hearing more about this common-sense method of quality assurance through prevention rather than detection.

For the person considering the implementation of such a program, it is my hope that this book will offer a step-by-step guide to the successful realization of his established quality goals. For the person who is involved in an established Zero Defects program, this book should offer a checklist for the elimination of possible program gaps and some new ideas about recognition, measurement, and sustaining factors. For our last potential reader—the man who is stimulated to read the book through intellectual curiosity about the program—this volume will chart a complete review of Zero Defects from its earliest days to its future application.

I would like to think that this is a book about people because people are the essence of the Zero Defects concept. Zero Defects is simply a method of assuring that each individual within an organization realizes his importance to that organization's product or service and, conversely, that each member of management realizes and recognizes the important contribution of each person reporting to him.

I define Zero Defects as a management tool aimed at the reduction of defects through prevention. It is directed at motivating people to prevent mistakes by developing a constant, conscious desire to do their job right the first time.

The key to this definition is the word "people." To be successful the program must center on the individual, for over the long haul, the quantity of errors *each* of us makes is directly proportional to the importance *each* of us places on the function of the moment.

Consider a letter typed by your secretary, for your signature, to the chief executive of the company which is your principal customer. Would you expect, or tolerate, two errors per page? One? Zero? This is the secret: She knows the standard—Zero Defects; she knows her work will receive your personal attention; she knows she'll be apprised of the results, and so (almost without exception) she types a perfect letter.

Good. Now why not apply this method across the board? Unless you believe secretaries are different from other people.

You see, competent secretaries have been schooled in Zero Defects (whether they know it or not) since their employment. This book is intended to re-school those multitudes who are not secretaries.

Incidentally, I am certain many readers will be tempted to search the pages of this book for an error in spelling, grammar, or punctuation. If you look at Zero Defects in this way, our cause is lost. We are perfectionists, but not perfect. Our goal is not to prove we have done our job perfectly—but that it is definitely worth while for everyone to try.

One final thought. Zero Defects is not the answer to all your quality ailments. It won't permanently solve your customer/product quality problems. It will help temporarily. But as your performance increases, your customer's tolerance level will decrease proportionately. In my opinion that's as it should be. It's an American road to progress.

James F. Halpin

Acknowledgments

It goes without saying that a program of this magnitude cannot be the work of a single individual. Hundreds of people have been directly involved in the birth, feeding, and care of *Zero Defects*. I wish to express specific thanks to the following: G. T. "Tom" Willey (Martin Company Vice President, Orlando Division General Manager, and my strongest supporter these many years), E. J. "Ed" Cottrell (Martin-Orlando's capable Director of Public Relations and my chief counselor), and P. B. "Phil" Crosby (who was there from the start, but now heads his own quality operation with the International Telephone and Telegraph Company), and to R. M. "Bob" Buck, who has supervised promotion for the ZD program, and whose editorial services were very valuable in the preparation of this book. By acknowledging the assistance of these four dedicated men, I hope to convey some of my appreciation to all my colleagues and fellow workers at Martin-Orlando. It is a simple fact: Without the help of all of them, *Zero Defects* would not exist.

I would also like to give special thanks to Dr. Paul Beall, President of Oglethorpe University, who suggested and in fact, insisted that the book be written in the first place, because of his strong convictions that the Zero Defects philosophy ought to be shared with all of American industry.

James F. Halpin

Definitions of Terms

The following definitions of key words used in this book are intended to eliminate misinterpretation due to varied usage throughout business and industry:

Organization   The industrial, business, or governmental unit actually initiating a Zero Defects program. An example is the author's own Orlando, Florida, Division of the Martin Company (not the Martin Company as a whole, which includes many divisions throughout the United States). All techniques in this book are based on this physical unit or organization type of implementation.

Senior Executive   The top member of management within the implementing organization. In a single-location company it may be the president—in a larger corporation it could be a plant or division general manager.

Top Management   Those members of the Senior Executive's staff who report directly to him and who, with him, direct the policy of the implementing organization.

Middle Management   Those areas of management that stand between top management and the first line supervisor.

Contents

xii   CONTENTS

PART 1

The Concept and Status of the Program

The History and Philosophy of Zero Defects

> *To err is human. . . .* ALEXANDER POPE, 1711
>
> *. . . your goal of defect-free performance is both imperative and attainable.* LYNDON JOHNSON, 1965

Zero Defects:
A Search for Perfection

To comprehend fully the basic philosophy of the Zero Defects program, one must first look into the nature of the defect itself. Defects, or worker errors, are caused primarily by three situations:

Lack of knowledge

Lack of proper facilities

Lack of attention

The first cause is easily detected and can be corrected by modern training techniques. The second can be eliminated through periodic facility and tool surveys and activities such as the Error Cause Removal phase covered in Chapters 7 and 9. The last is the subject of this book and the object of the Zero Defects program; it is the problem of improper employee attitudes: The problem is difficult to detect except in extreme cases. Management can show the individual how to do it and provide the best possible tools to accomplish the task properly, and if the employee doesn't care whether or not he makes a mistake, he will probably err. This raises the question: "Why shouldn't he care about mistakes?"

THE ZERO DEFECTS PHILOSOPHY

Throughout their lives, people are conditioned to accept the fact that they are not perfect and thus make mistakes. You might say people have accepted a standard requiring a few mistakes each day in order to be certified as human beings: "To err is human. . . ." We term this the "passing-grade complex."

From his earliest days, the individual has been required by society to achieve only a passing grade. At home the mere fact that he got his chores done was enough to spread a smile on his parents' faces. In school there was always the passing C. In the service, there was the "qualifying score," and in college he was back on the passing-grade routine again. You would think that once out in the competitive world, he would be expected to approach perfection in his chosen field. But here again he finds the "to err is human" alibi; he meets acceptable quality levels; and he sees permanent rework and repair operations, levels of reliability, and all the other performance goals that indicate that management, like mother and dad, doesn't expect perfection. Small wonder the individual never looks for perfection in anything he does—but doesn't he?

The originators of the Zero Defects concept asked themselves this same question. They concluded that in some things—those things that affect the individual personally—he does in fact seek perfection. For instance, will a man who has a 5 percent error rate on the job be short-changed 5 percent of the time in his monetary transactions? Will he wear one black and one brown shoe to work 5 percent of the time? Will he accidentally go home to the wrong house once or twice a month? In all cases the answer is a resounding no! If he wrecked his car 5 percent of the time he drove it, we would soon stop hearing about the population explosion.

Extending this line of inquiry, the early program organizers asked themselves if the individual ever expected perfection from other people. For instance, would he say, "To err is human," if his dentist pulled the wrong tooth? Would he shrug his shoulders if the auto mechanic failed to replace oil in his car during an oil change? How understanding would he be if his wife broke that one and only bowling trophy? Obviously, if the thing affected him personally, he would expect a high degree of perfection.

Here we have brought up the double standard. If our "everyworker" demands perfection from his mechanic, doctor, dentist, lawyer, and all the rest, why doesn't he demand the same of himself in his own job? The answer is obvious: perfection in his own job does not seem to affect him personally. If he makes one or two mistakes a month, no one will fire him for that. Besides, doesn't management hire quality checkers, proofreaders, and the like just to catch his errors? His supervisor has often said: "Just as long as we keep the errors down, the manager will stay out of our hair." Thus, an error or two here and there really doesn't matter. In fact, management seems to expect some mistakes.

How can this conditioning be reversed? The answer is simple: by reconditioning the employee to take a personal interest in *everything* he does; by convincing him that his job is just as important as the task of the doctor or the dentist. The technique for this reconditioning is called "Zero Defects."

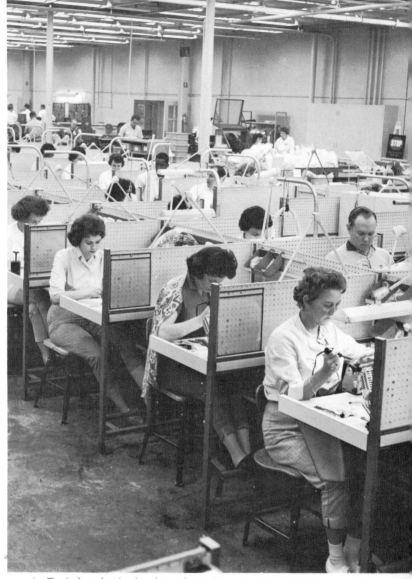

FIG. 1 Typical production in a large electronics operation. This type of worker is at times removed from final assembly by as many as 500 steps and in many cases has never seen the end product.

And in thousands of companies and government organizations around the country, it has progressed toward its goal.

THE ZERO DEFECTS CONCEPT

The Zero Defects concept promotes a *constant, conscious desire to do a job (any job) right the first time!* The attainability of this goal is directly proportional to the attitude or desire of the individual. What will give him this de-

5

ELEMENTARY SHCOOL GRADES

Reporting Period

	1	2	3	4	5	6
1st Semester						
Days Present	35	30	36	35	30	35
Days Absent	0	5	4	3	2	3
Times Tardy	1	0	1	0	0	1
Conduct	Good	Good	Good	Good	Fair	Good
Subjects						
Reading	A	B	C	A	A	B
English	A	B	B	A	A	A
Spelling	B	C	B	A	B	B
Writing	C	B	B	C	B	A
Social Studies	A	C	B	C	C	A
Arithmetic	B	C	B	C	B	B
Science	B	B	C	C	B	B
Following Subjects are Marked S or U						
Art	S	U	S	U	S	S
Music	S	U	U	S	S	S
Health	S	S	U	S	S	S
Phys. Ed.	U	S	U	U	S	S

Explanation of Grading Symbols:

A Excellent   D Poor
B Good   E Failing
C Satisfactory   S Satisfactory
R Incomplete   U Unsatisfactory

Parents Signature

Mrs Henry Jones
Harry Jones
Mrs Harry Jones

Harry Jones
Mrs Harry Jones
Harry Jones

FIG. 2 Many parents would accept a report card such as this with little question—after all, the grades are "above average." In many cases, this "passing-grade" complex extends into later life, causing the individual to look only for performance that "gets by."

sire? The answer is constant awareness: awareness that his task is important; awareness that the product he is working on is important; awareness that management thinks his efforts are important.

This awareness has been missing in American industry and business for some time. The lack of awareness is due, for the most part, to mass-production techniques and the virtual removal of the individual from proximity to the end product (see Figure 1). The enormous requirements for equipment during World War II introduced mass-production to almost all modern industries. High production rates could be obtained only by simplifying each task to permit the training of unskilled individuals to perform basic repetitive duties.

The term "specialist" was broadened to include workers without skills as well as highly trained technicians. To an appreciable degree, quantity replaced quality as a measure of productiveness. If four out of five units were acceptable, this was satisfactory. Fast delivery of goods in quantity took top priority.

Much of this operational doctrine still holds true. In many instances the customer has become the actual quality inspector. Many consumer items are purchased, taken home, and then returned to the store because of a flaw.

6

ZERO DEFECTS: A SEARCH FOR PERFECTION   7

These errors not only make customers dissatisfied with both manufacturer and merchandiser but cost both organizations money. A supplemental merchandising system for "seconds" (articles with minor flaws) has emerged, but obviously this is only an attempt to secure a partial return from manufacturing already completed.

Naturally, as workers became more specialized and much product inspection was delegated to customers, the outlook of industrial management changed. Management lost sight of the important fact that the workers themselves are a tremendous quality resource and are capable of much more than functioning as machines on assembly lines or in offices. People became little more than arms and legs performing certain motions at certain times.

Many members of industrial management served in the armed forces during World War II. Wartime requirements of military service called for subjugating individual skills for the common good. These wartime practices spread to industry during and following the conflict. In many areas standards of craftsmanship and individual judgment all but ceased to exist.

These changes in management viewpoint also affected the worker. He became accustomed to meeting only the standards he was asked to meet—and at times these were far from perfection. If a particular task was difficult, the worker usually wondered how badly the extra effort was needed. He failed to react to a potential challenge. At home, the same worker might praise his child for receiving passing marks in his school courses. If the child gained praise and rewards for C's, why seek A's? (See Figure 2.) The obvious result was a generation of people seeking security, but striving only to "get by."

Ultimately, industry began to react to this climate of mediocrity. The study of human behavior became more popular, and behavioral scientists advocated various methods and programs to increase human performance. Many of these programs helped employees feel happier about their work and lives and generally resulted in fewer resignations—but not in increased performance. Other programs, founded in industrial engineering doctrine, strove to convince employees to work harder, faster, safer, and more regularly. Since wages are a strong motivating force, various incentive programs were adopted widely.

Most company-sponsored programs retained three basic flaws, however. First, many motivational programs were intended to convince employees to do what management wanted without creating an honest, personal desire in the minds of the employees. Second, virtually all incentive-type programs encouraged employee dishonesty, since the eventual goal became "beating the system" rather than improving work quality. And third, many programs implied a threat to the employee: in the event a certain action is *not* attained, a reward will be withheld or punitive action will occur. Any parent is aware the most a threat can accomplish is simple conformity—and that only as long as the threat remains present and active.

DIRECTED MANAGEMENT ACTION

It seems that management was aware it had a problem; the big question seemed to be what to do with it. Zero Defects gives management the answer. The solution is found in the program's basic concept and is accomplished without threat or punishment. Through careful guidance and direction it is possible for management to get that intangible "something extra" out of each employee on a day-to-day basis. Zero Defects accomplishes its ends by working on the one attribute of an employee that always remains his own—*his* attitude, *his* desire.

With respect to personal performance on the job, the employee's attitude is usually confused. As far as his job is concerned, he doesn't know what to think of himself or his task. Once he has left work for the day, he tries to think as little about it as possible. The Zero Defects program is a management technique beamed at getting the employee to *think*—getting him to think positively about each and every task. The principles behind the concept are not new; they are the same basic ideas behind most successful management or leadership. But in Zero Defects, these principles are applied to the most significant roadblock to industrial excellence today: the relationship between management and the individual employee.

The experiences of thousands of successful ZD organizations have proved that if management follows a relatively simple series of positive steps, the individual employee will respond with an exhibition of craftsmanship that hasn't been seen since Stradivari closed his shop. The process is as follows:
1. Present a challenge.
2. Back the challenge with action of your own.
3. Establish standards.
4. Check results.
5. Act in accordance with the results to recognize accomplishment.

To put it in narrative form: Management explains just how important each task is and asks the employee to strive for perfection. Management makes it obvious that it does seek perfection in the product or service offered and sets an example by encouraging nothing less. Management establishes standards of performance and states them to the individual employee. Management checks the results of employee effort and lets the individual know where he stands. When these standards are met, management takes positive action to give the employee recognition and let him know it has confidence that more of the same will be forthcoming.

Stated in this manner, Zero Defects seems like a cold, dull routine. Quite the opposite—Zero Defects is in fact a warm, intimate, business relationship between management and employee. The individual knows what is expected of him and where he stands in the eyes of management. In turn, management knows its position and what the employee expects from it. The employee is no longer a little individual on a big production line. He is now as important a part of the entire organization as any member of management. Together they have become a single force, working toward an important goal—Zero Defects.

It makes no difference what type of employee you are dealing with. Zero Defects is an across-the-board program. The basic challenge is the same for the president of the organization as it is for the sweeper. The program techniques apply not only to production workers but to secretaries, scientists, bookkeepers, administrators, maintenance men, and every other group that makes up the implementing organization. There has never been a case where "partial" Zero Defects has been more than partially successful. Program discrimination can only reflect the message that either management does not believe enough in the program to present it company-wide or that the program is necessary in only one or two areas. Both images are negative and defeat all the basic elements of the Zero Defects–program concept.

The one factor that takes the Zero Defects program out of the "simple routine" classification is the key to the whole program—the individual. Throughout our discussion of the philosophy and concept, the plural terms "employees" and "individuals" are purposely avoided. Both words are used only in the singular. Management can never put Zero Defects across by beaming it at the work force as a whole. The program must be sold individually to every employee in the organization before it can fully succeed. That is the challenge of Zero Defects.

No one will ever tell you that Zero Defects implementation is an easy task. "Simple," "uncomplicated," "effective," "inexpensive," "rewarding" are all adjectives commonly used in connection with the program name—but "easy," never!

Before any organization adopts Zero Defects, it should seriously consider all the ramifications of the program. An unrealistic or cynical attitude toward it at the start will probably mean limited success. In this day and age of strong competition, no company can stay on top very long without almost absolute quality assurance achieved at a realistic cost. Zero Defects adds that assurance to any organization that will accept it.

2

Let me tell you how it got started. If I can reconstruct for you the birth of this idea, it may help you to understand it better. Like all great ideas, it is a simple one. And, it had a simple beginning. . . .

G. T. WILLEY, VICE PRESIDENT, MARTIN COMPANY

The Evolution of Zero Defects

Like most worthwhile ideas or discoveries, Zero Defects was born of necessity. To fully comprehend this necessity, we must first look into the industry that introduced the program—the American defense industry.

The defense of our nation depends on the quality of the goods and services produced for its purposes. It is conceivable that a single defect can cause damage to the entire defense posture of our nation. The thought of the loss of even a single life because of defective material is intolerable. As a result, the government has over 50,000 people involved in the inspection of purchased goods and services. The defense industry has another 250,000 people controlling processes and checking products before delivery. In fact, an excess of 1 billion dollars is spent on detection of defects and corrective action in the defense industry every year.

It is only natural, then, that a program such as Zero Defects was given birth and nurtured in the most complex area of defense contracting—the missile industry. The program did, in fact, originate with the United States Army Pershing missile system (see Figure 3), developed and produced by Martin Marietta Corporation's Martin Company at its Orlando, Florida, division.

Every other area of American business and industry was facing the same problems. Every consumer has at one time experienced some sort of defect in the items he has purchased. While service guarantees do afford protection for

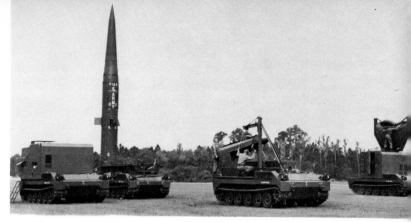

FIG. 3   The Army Pershing system contains hundreds of thousands of vital parts, and each has to be 100 percent defect-free.

the buyer, the failure of consumer products is not unusual nor unexpected. In fact, producers of these products are spending billions of dollars annually in an effort to keep these service charges at a minimum. The only real difference between the consumer and defense markets is that in the former a relatively inexperienced inspector (the buyer) is responsible for the acceptance test; in defense, the government has a professional and well-organized inspection operation. And it is dangerous to assume that defects in consumer products do not have the dire consequences usually attached to defects in defense work. A mislabeled drug product, an imperfect tire wall, or a badly wired appliance can produce results as disastrous as a rifle that misfires.

DISCOVERY

Whenever the subject of Zero Defects comes up, it invariably prompts the question: "Exactly how did it all start?"* The fact that it did start in the defense industry on an Army-Martin missile system is testimony to the dedication of a relatively small group of people. This same group, given a similar environment, would probably have used the same approach to the production of any product, consumer or defense. Nevertheless, it was a basic quality discovery on this project that changed the thinking of thousands of people within the following years.

In 1961, Martin was conducting the most successful missile flight-test program ever performed at Cape Kennedy (then Cape Canaveral). Pershing's first six flights were complete successes, and the first thirty-three saw only four partial failures. Here was a case history of success—but at what cost? Martin was well aware of the fact that this enviable record stemmed in high degree from the efforts of the inspectors and testers at the company's Orlando and Canaveral divisions. Only by scrupulous and laborious examination of

* Precise historical documentation on the evolution of the program at Martin is unavailable. Since the widespread program application was not anticipated at the time, no journals were kept. The material in this chapter is based on the author's recollections supported by such documentation as does exist.

each system's 25,000 parts were they able to avoid the disasters often associated with the early flights of such complex programs.

Even though Martin's record for workmanship in delivered goods was well above industry standards, these men continued to detect discrepancies in each missile, many of which could bring about flight failure if undetected. For those not familiar with the missile industry, missile failures at Cape Kennedy have been caused by anything from a loose $1.50 valve to a solder splash no bigger than a pinhead (see Figure 4). These are the parameters under which the inspection crew was working. Dr. Robert Gilruth, director of the Manned Spacecraft Center of NASA, reported that the outstanding success of the Telstar satellite was the result of the examination of over 58,000 "acceptable" solid-state devices and the selection of the 2,500 eventually flown into orbit.

What was the solution to this tremendously costly inspection, rework, reinspect, and retest cycle? In the interest of national economy, the industry had to find the answer or else price such programs out of existence.

THE FIRST STEP

Martin spent considerable time looking for a new, fresh approach. Some of the established quality techniques were reviewed and various adaptions made in an effort to cut the costly cycle. Early effort was directed by management and supervision to make all employees more quality-conscious. Special programs were devised to present product quality in relationship to the costs involved. Army personnel stationed at the Martin-Orlando facility joined the drive by offering a special award to any group reducing its rate of defects 50 percent below the acceptable quality level (AQL) for a six-month period. This initial effort resulted in a measurable improvement.

FIG. 4   Missile destruct (failure) at Cape Kennedy. Costly failures such as this have been caused by the malfunction of a $2 part.

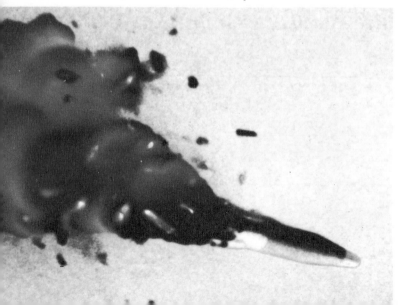

However, at the Cape, the Army-Martin team still maintained its successful flight record by detecting and reworking discrepant hardware. The number of discrepancies was reduced, and most were minor; but occasionally a significant error—one that could cause certain failure—was uncovered. Though the performance was well above the state of the art for the period (and by today's standards also), the results still presented a challenge. Martin, with one of the finest quality-assurance systems in the nation, was forced to rely on the eyeballs of last-minute defect detectors, all capable of the same shortcomings as the people who produced the product. Still searching for the magic answer, Martin followed the obvious course of inspecting and testing more thoroughly and more often—a very costly answer to a very basic problem.

Finally, on December 21, 1961, the effort paid off. A Pershing was delivered to the Cape with zero discrepancies. Now the Army-Martin team knew it could be accomplished. They knew it could be repeated with some degree of consistency, but the solution still lay in very costly detection and prevention techniques.

NECESSITY BRINGS A SOLUTION

Shortly after this achievement, Brig. Gen. R. W. Hurst, then deputy commander of the United States Army Missile Command, telephoned Tom Willey, Martin-Orlando's general manager. His request was urgent. Timely deployment of the Pershing missile system demanded delivery of the first field unit one month earlier in 1962 (February, rather than the contract date in March). Never one to ignore a challenge, Mr. Willey replied with a far-reaching *yes!* And not satisfied with the acceptance of a partial challenge, he added: ". . . and a perfect missile system at that!"

As Mr. Willey reasoned later to the author of this book, "You can't meet a schedule by delivering a nonquality product." This challenge was transmitted to the Pershing team, and the next day, their answer came back in writing:

1. Pershing Artillery Set Number 7 would be delivered in February
2. With zero hardware discrepancies
3. With zero documentation discrepancies
4. And with equipment set up and fully operable ten days after delivery. (Comparable systems had required ninety days or more.)

The exact techniques undertaken to meet this goal are probably no longer known to any one individual. One thing is certain: a complete re-evaluation of past methods was required. In building a system of this size, certain things cannot be omitted. For instance, it takes a certain number of hours to assemble a certain number of parts. It takes time to check out each part and subsystem. It takes a certain amount of engineering effort to make changes and adjustments called out by the customer from knowledge gained on previous flight

IN REPLY, REFER TO   18 MAY 196
ORDEA-Q-O

MR. G. T. WILLEY, VICE PRESIDENT AND GENERAL MANAGER
MARTIN MARIETTA CORPORATION
POST OFFICE BOX 5837
ORLANDO, FLORIDA

DEAR MR. WILLEY:

THE INFORMATION CONCERNING THE SUCCESSFUL OPERATION OF ARTILLERY
SET NO. 8 AT FORT SILL, OKLAHOMA THIS WEEK IS CERTAINLY GRATIFYING AND,
I BELIEVE, CALLS FOR SPECIAL MENTION.

SINCE JULY 1961 WHEN I FIRST BECAME ASSOCIATED WITH THE MARTIN
COMPANY AS THE ARMY CONTRACTING OFFICER, I HAVE FELT A SENSE OF SECURITY
IN THE QUALITY AREA AS A RESULT OF THE CAPABLE AND SINCERE ATTENTION
GIVEN TO THIS FACET BY MR. JAMES HALPIN, YOUR DIRECTOR OF QUALITY. IN
MY MIND THERE IS NO QUESTION THAT MR. HALPIN'S LEADERSHIP AND ABILITY
TO MANAGE SUCCESSFULLY THE MANY QUALITY ENGINEERS INVOLVED IN PLACING A
WEAPON SYSTEM INTO THE HANDS OF THE GOVERNMENT WITH MINIMUM OR NO DEFECTS,
WERE THE PRIME REASONS WHY THE MARTIN COMPANY CAN BOAST ABOUT ARTY SET
NO. 8 BEING ON THE AIR AND OPERATING IN $23\frac{1}{2}$ HOURS WITH ZERO DEFECTS
AFTER BEING AIR TRANSPORTED A CONSIDERABLE DISTANCE.

I WOULD LIKE TO ALSO OFFER MY APPRECIATION TO THOSE QUALITY
PERSONNEL DIRECTLY ASSOCIATED WITH PERSHING UNDER MR. PHIL CROSBY SINCE
I HAVE PERSONAL KNOWLEDGE OF THEIR SINCERE EFFORTS TO DELIVER A PERFECT
SYSTEM.

SINCERELY YOURS,

FERD R. AUMILLER
LT COL, ORD CORPS
COMMANDING

FIG. 5   A copy of the original acceptance letter noting Martin's early success with the Pershing system.

tests. It takes a specified amount of time to complete documentation of the system. The only thing left to cut was the cushion for rework, reinspection, and retest.

The director of the program and his quality manager made this requirement known to every individual associated with the product. Every individual was asked to do his part to eliminate time-consuming errors. And make the effort they did. The results are on record. The Pershing system was delivered to Fort Sill in February, 1962. There were *zero* discrepancies in hardware and documentation (see Figure 5). The missile system was operable in less than twenty-four hours.

This was a significant achievement. Though rework and retest remained factors, these elements had been reduced to the point where an almost impossible delivery requirement was met. Martin quality management analyzed the recent successes at Fort Sill and the Cape. The answer was there, but no one could put his finger on it. Suddenly, one afternoon, the one variable that hadn't been taken into account was brought into the discussion. Management had never questioned its own attitude toward the problem of defects. The reason behind the lack of perfection was simply that perfection had not been expected. The one time management demanded perfection, it happened!

Like everyone else in the world, management had accepted as fact the theory that mistakes are inevitable. By its very actions—setting acceptable quality levels and trying to keep rework costs *down* to a preset level—management was saying: "We expect a few defects now and then, just as long as they are kept within reasonable limits." Actually, the very emphasis on extensive inspection led many workers to reason: "If I miss it, the inspector will catch it. That's what he's paid for."

THE SOLUTION

The actual solution was now close at hand. Management had conveyed its strong interest in perfection to the inspectors at the Cape and, in one case, to an entire program group with astonishing results. Why not carry the same message to every employee in the organization, regardless of task or project? It was obvious that the employee would try to work to levels set by management. When management showed the individual it was interested in high performance, the individual responded accordingly. If every employee reacted as this experience had shown, the rework-retest cycle would be slashed—maybe completely broken.

This was not to say that by one simple move, individual error would disappear from the scene. But by setting examples and making the worker aware of the importance of the individual task, management could instill in each and every employee a constant, conscious desire to do every job right the first time. Once this desire for perfection was evident in both management and employee attitudes, the company would be well on its way to solving one of its most baffling problems.

ACTION

The next step was to put this attack on employee and management attitudes on an organized basis. A team was set up to study the problem and develop a plan of action. The moves made and the action taken are covered, for the most part, in the first half of this book (Parts 2 to 4). After these early steps, the program assumed the position of a day-to-day working tool for both management and the individual employee. This phase is covered in the latter sections of the book. The overall program, as the reader now knows, was pridefully and symbolically called "Zero Defects."

PROGRAM EXPANSION

During the first two years of Zero Defects, many organizations became aware of the program through magazine articles, through visits to the company, and by word of mouth. During this period the author received over 3,000 letters requesting information about Zero Defects, and over 1,000 people visited the plant specifically for firsthand discussions about the program.

Some of the first organizations to implement their own programs were the Small Engine Department of General Electric and divisions of Litton Industries, Thiokol, Westinghouse, and Bendix. The former added a new and important element to the program which became known as the "Error Cause Removal" phase. Almost every one of the early organizations, in fact, had a hand in molding and developing the Zero Defects approach to quality awareness.

During this period, the Army had been observing the program with deep interest. It had been in on the program from the start, and as the results came rolling in, it took the program up the line to the Department of Defense. After a thorough evaluation, the Department of Defense endorsed Zero Defects at two seminars held for key executives of the top 1,000 corporations in the United States. From this point on, the spread of the program was virtually unlimited. At present, there are over 2,500 firms with either planned or implemented Zero Defects programs. These firms are involved in a cross section of American industry and are not limited to defense alone. The programs range from shops with 25 employees to large industrial concerns with over 25,000 workers.

RESULTS

When asked for actual results of all this effort, most ZD Administrators hesitate to give the information because these results are frequently so outstanding that they are hard to believe. This was the problem faced by Martin when the government asked for such a figure. Wanting to be completely accurate, Martin released only those figures dealing with deliverable hardware under government audit. The first two years' 54 percent drop in defects was measured against a modest $14 per defect. When the cost of defect rework, retest, and documentation is considered, this is a fairly low figure for most industrial concerns; for an electronics firm, it is very conservative. When the computers finished their job, the results were an impressive $1,650,000 savings in manufactured hardware alone. This was a real, audited figure, covering the efforts of about one-third of Martin-Orlando's 10,000 employees.

Martin was not alone in receiving such exceptional results. General Electric had a 2-million-dollar drop in rework and scrap costs during the first two years of the program. RCA reports that, in one division, over 75 percent of the departments are meeting or exceeding their ZD goals. Sperry, Utah, reports a one-year overall drop in defects of 54 percent.

Group Achievement

Perhaps some of these large industrial examples are too extensive and all-inclusive to relate to every organization. The true value of the program is seen through the specific accomplishments of the smaller units within these and other large corporations. For instance, Lockheed, Georgia, reported a pre-liminary-design-error drop of 41 percent the first year. This company also realized a 54 percent drop in documentation errors in its accounts payable department. Errors in shipping and receiving were lowered 47 percent. Defects in its motion picture and photographic departments were reduced 60 and 80 percent, respectively. Other companies report the following group achievements: Error Cause Removal savings of over $250,000; downtime on production and test equipment reduced 85 percent; 72 percent reduction in spare-parts faults; a 98 percent improvement in delivery and shipping actions; an 83 percent reduction in drafting error; a two-year reduction of 67 percent in technical manual errors—and so the list goes on.

Individual Accomplishment

The numbers game is interesting and has much merit, but what about the real heart of the program—the individual employee? It is in this area that the "impossible" has really been accomplished. Though some of the results mentioned earlier could have been accomplished by costly procedures changes, automation, and highly intensified inspection, the following achievements can be attributed only to worker attitude—the meat of the entire ZD effort. Take, for example, the forklift driver who has moved over 15 million pounds of delicate electronic hardware without a single incident of damage and at this printing still has a record of Zero Defects; the solderer who made almost one-half million connections without error; the assembler making over 50,000 difficult, complex, defect-free plug assemblies during a six-month period; or a finance clerk who makes hundreds of thousands of payroll computations without error.

These are not "freak" or rare instances. Martin-Orlando recognized hundreds of such achievers in the first three years of the program. It is not unusual to find four or five performers of this caliber in a small work group. And this type of achievement is not restricted to the production of data-processing elements of the ZD organization. Many secretaries carry records of thousands of pages typed without error. There are shipping and mail clerks who have not lost or delayed a single item for two- and three-year periods. There are drivers who have not only gone hundreds of thousands of miles without accident, but who have not had a single incident of damaged or misplaced goods during the same period. There are draftsmen with records of hundreds of thousands of entries without error.

Results like these make the whole effort worthwhile. The fear that the craftsman has left the American scene is now dispelled. He is here; he has always been here. All that was needed was for management to take a positive step to redefine the important role of the craftsman in industry today. Once aware of this role, the individual will rise to the challenge and surpass even his own wildest expectations.

RESULTS OF THE RESULTS

Needless to say, when the first ZD program was started, Martin management not only didn't expect such outstanding short-term results, but also had absolutely no thought that the idea would spread throughout industry. Today, companies and government organizations in every field of endeavor have embraced the program. A partial list of the types of industries, businesses, and organizations involved will give the reader a general idea of the program's wide application:

Air conditioning	Engineering
Airplanes	Explosives
Aluminum fabrication	Film
Aluminum products	Food processing
Appliances	Foundries
Ball bearings	Fuel
Batteries	Garments
Brakes	Gears
Buses	Glass
Business machines	Guidance
Cables	Guns
Ceramics	Helicopters
Chemicals	Iron and steel
Computers	Jet engines
Connectors	Laboratories
Department stores	Mail order
Design	Metal products
Drugs	Missiles
Education	Munitions
Electronics	Nuclear products

Optics	Rubber products
Packaging	Semiconductors
Paints	Sewing machines
Paper products	Test equipment
Plastics	Textiles
Power tools	Tires
Propellants	Trucks
Public transportation	Utilities
Radar	Watches
Radios	Welding equipment
Research	Wood products

If the reader's product or service is not listed, it is probably owing to an oversight on the author's part rather than lack of ZD coverage in that area. To date, almost every task in every commercial and government area has come under the ZD banner. The complete list reads from soup (Campbell Soup Company) to nuts (Standard Locknut, Inc.). With over 2 million people involved in the program by 1965, it is reasonable to assume that almost every task and product has been touched by the program.

User Comments

Measurable results are obviously responsible for this acceptance. Firsthand review of any ZD organization's accomplishments and activities makes a believer out of the most hardened cynic. Today's business executive is not prone to rush into any new program or technique without first carefully analyzing every aspect of the new step. Thus, the praise for Zero Defects was not given lightly; it was earned the hard way. One of the most impressive of such comments was made by Frank Nixon, the quality manager of Rolls-Royce, Ltd:

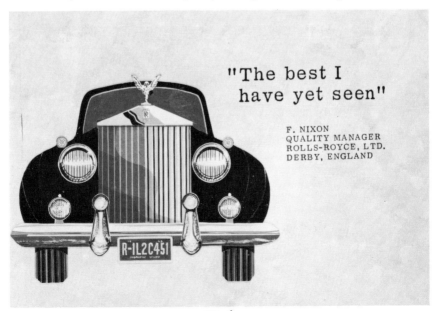

"The best I have yet seen"

F. NIXON
QUALITY MANAGER
ROLLS-ROYCE, LTD.
DERBY, ENGLAND

FIG. 6

"The Zero Defects Programme is the best I have yet seen." That, from the man who is responsible for maintaining the quality standard of one of the world's quality symbols, is worth deep consideration.

The President of the United States has said: "The Zero Defects Program offers timely support for the objectives of our determined effort to eliminate waste wherever it occurs. . . ." The *Wall Street Journal* reported: "Evidence is piling up that ZD can indeed give the tax payer more bang for his defense buck." *Time* magazine commented: "This uniquely simple system is part common sense, part snow job, and wholly successful." But perhaps the most significant statement about the Zero Defects program has come from the head of the second company to implement the program. Ken Bush, manufacturing manager of General Electric's Small Engine Division, said: "Zero Defects has given quality a new dimension. . . ." Thus the title of this book: *Zero Defects: A New Dimension in Quality Assurance.*

The First Steps
of Program Implementation

> *It is important that you understand the plan's philosophy and believe in it before you make an attempt to install a Zero Defects program. You're the one who will have to sell the program right down the line. In order to do this, you must sell yourself first.*
> G. T. WILLEY, VICE PRESIDENT, MARTIN COMPANY

Zero Defects
and Company Organization

This bit of advice, offered to major corporation executives at a national ZD seminar, is one of the soundest pieces of logic ever associated with the Zero Defects program. Before anything moves at all, the Senior Executive and top management must be convinced of the value of the program. Without their wholehearted support, the program cannot even begin to move.

The Zero Defects concept is based on a chain reaction indoctrination/ motivation cycle. That is to say, the Senior Executive must accept the program and, in turn, indoctrinate and motivate top management; top management assumes the same role for mid-management; mid-management for the supervisor; and finally, the supervisor indoctrinates and motivates the individual employee. It is difficult to bypass any of these steps, but you can't even begin the task without the acceptance of the Senior Executive. This man will add the prestige to get your program moving. He is the only person in your organization who has something in common with every department and section, and since ZD is an across-the-board program, it will need this unifying force. He is the one man in the organization to whom *everyone* looks for direction.

TOP-LEVEL PROGRAM PRESENTATION

If the Senior Executive of your organization is the man who has focused his attention on the program or has suggested that the program be "looked into," then the selling aspect of your initial presentation is much easier. If you, the reader, are in fact the Senior Executive of your organization, so much the better. But for those who face the task of presenting the program to a man who has never heard about Zero Defects or who has not been informed about the scope and value of the program, certain steps should be taken to assure understanding.

There are several things your Senior Executive will want to know before he makes his decision:

- Where has it been used before?
- How successful has it been?
- Are my competitors using it?
- Are my customers using it?
- How much will it cost?
- What will I (the company) get out of it?

The answers to the first and second questions are found in the first and second chapters of this book. A small amount of research and a few phone calls will answer the next two. The cost question will require a little more effort on your part.

Funding

Figures provided by key Zero Defects organizations around the country indicate that first-year cost of the program is about $1.50 to $2.50 per person. This includes promotional costs, pins, forms, training aids, rallies, and other indoctrination materials, but it does not include the salary of the ZD Administrator. In large organizations (over 5,000 people) a full-time Administrator may be needed. Smaller organizations may delegate this work on a part-time basis. Thus, if there are 1,000 workers in your company, the program will probably cost about $1,500.

It must be remembered that the true cost of a program is relative. For instance, experience has shown us that Zero Defects does work. In almost every case the defect rates have dropped 25 percent or more. To put the true cost in proper perspective, tally up last year's scrap and rework costs and balance only 10 percent of this figure against the estimated cost of the program (see Figure 7*a*). Or assume that because of the program every worker will make at least one less error next year (surely not an unreasonable assumption); place an estimated, across-the-board price on that defect, and multiply this figure by the number of people in your organization (see Figure 7*b*). In this day of costly reject, rework, reinspection, and corrective action, the total will certainly overshadow anything you may plan to invest in the actual mechanics

COMPARISON OF PROGRAM AND MANUFACTURING DEFECT* COSTS
(in thousands of dollars)

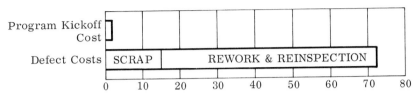

*Based on Previous 6 mo. Audit of Manuf. Dept. only

FIG. 7*a* This comparison was made for an early management presentation in a medium-sized industrial firm. The availability of past scrap and rework costs enabled them to show the extreme differences between the costs of the "sickness" and the "cure" (ZD).

PROGRAM KICKOFF FUNDING

Posters (30 ea. of 3) . . . . $	150. 00
Pledge Cards (1, 000)	25. 00
Supervisors' Handbooks (200).	145. 00
Pins (1, 000)	750. 00
Misc. Printed Mtl.	200. 00
Misc. Admin. Costs	200. 00
Total Cost for 1, 000-man Program . . . . $	1, 470. 00
Cost of 1, 000 Defects ($10. ea. est.) . . .	10, 000. 00

FIG. 7*b* A typical program-kickoff funding chart. The two base figures are emphasized to put over the point that if each worker makes one less mistake, the venture will more than pay for itself.

of the program. Both of these figures will not only answer the question of cost but will also answer the question of what's in it for your company—more profit and a stronger competitive position.

Selling the Program

If this information is presented to the Senior Executive, he will have all the tools necessary for making a final decision. If he still needs assurance, investigate and discover which of his friends and associates belong to ZD organizations and suggest that he ask them for their opinions of the program. As R. F. Hurt, president of Lockheed Propulsion Company, said of G. T. Willey, vice president of Martin:

Zero Defects to me used to be just a catchy term which appeared occasionally in trade journals. . . . There must be more to it than just a slogan or Tom Willey would not have spent his time on it. I have known Mr. Willey for thirteen years. . . . After hearing Mr. Willey's fine presentation and the tangible results he cited, my interest in Zero Defects grew rapidly.

This executive's little "confession" that he accepted a competitor's advice was made to an audience of over 500 of Mr. Hurt's peers at another ZD seminar. The key point here is that you should bring in outside help if you feel you need it.

THE DECISION TO IMPLEMENT

This decision, as was said before, can be made by only one man. It is a step not to be taken lightly. Once committed, the Senior Executive should be ready to go all the way. He must set an example for the whole organization. He must be willing to back his Zero Defects administration with every available resource. He must weld the program into a unifying force throughout his entire organization. He, more than any other single person, will symbolize the program.

Once the decision has been made, the Senior Executive will have to take several actions. The first will be finding a "home" in his organization for the program's administration.

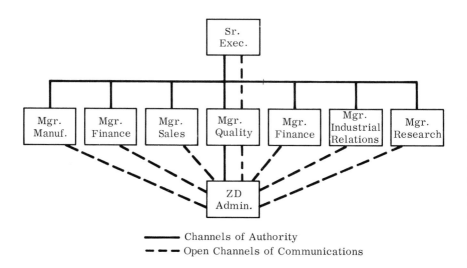

———— Channels of Authority

– – – Open Channels of Communications

FIG. 8 Typical ZD organization chart. Though the ZD administration's home is a step away from top management, the Administrator's lines of communications with this important management area are open and direct.

PLACING THE ZD ADMINISTRATION

Though the actual location will vary from organization to organization, there is one basic rule to follow in placing the ZD administration: the site selected should present the Administrator with open communication lines to the highest management levels (see Figure 8). In theory, the greatest emphasis can be applied to the program by having the ZD function report directly to the Senior Executive. While it is recognized that in many circumstances this will not be feasible, it must be emphasized that the more direct the avenue of communications between the two, the more effective the program.

Further, operated as an organization-wide program, the Zero Defects administration will need all the strength and prestige it can muster. If the program is lost somewhere far down in the organizational structure, it may be construed as an indication that the Senior Executive does not attach much importance to it. In many cases the program has been assigned as a function of the quality department (this is probably the result of its origination in Martin's Quality Division). In these cases, particularly when the quality organization has been strong, the programs have been very effective. To an appreciable degree, this can be attributed to the fact that defect detection and corrective action are inherent functions of such organizations.

Another natural selection would be the industrial relations department since it is active within all other areas of the organization. The easiest technique for selection is to find the department or division that has the most contact and influence with the other departments within the implementing organization.

SELECTING THE ADMINISTRATOR

The selection of a Zero Defects Administrator quite obviously will have tremendous impact on the eventual outcome of your program. Because of the key role he must play, this man should be selected as carefully as any major department head, and his actual position should have the stature of that level in order that he may effectively direct the program. The criteria for selection should include the following:

- He must believe in the program philosophy.
- He must feel that the program goals are attainable.
- He must have the respect of management and worker alike or be able to command such respect once he is appointed.
- He must have a thorough knowledge of the organization, its policies, its politics, and its people.
- He must have the intestinal fortitude, or guts if you will, to drive toward these goals regardless of any roadblocks set before him.

To this list can be added any of your own management criteria to assure you and your organization that the man chosen will do the job.

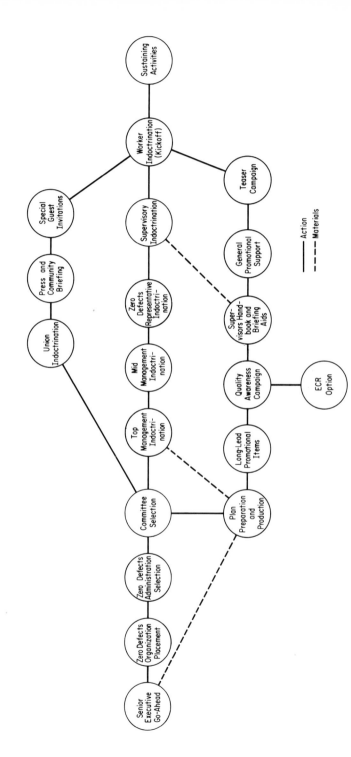

FIG. 9 Typical Zero Defects implementation plan.

——— Action

- - - - - Materials

Final selection of the ZD Administrator should be made by the Senior Executive or the staff member responsible for the program's administrative home. If at all possible, the offer of the assignment to the Administrator should be made by, or in the presence of, the Senior Executive. You will note the term "offer." The position of ZD Administrator is a challenge, just as the program is, and should be presented as such. After the man has been briefed on the scope of the program and his specific responsibilities, he should be allowed time to think about it. If he decides to accept this challenge, he will, in fact, be the first employee to pledge himself to Zero Defects.

It is rare that a company has to go outside for a new hire to fill this position. To meet the criteria, he would almost have to come from within the organization. Almost every ZD organization to date has found the right man in its own backyard.

To properly implement the program, the Administrator will need certain basic facilities; he should be provided all the tools necessary to do the job well. In very large operations, this could mean even a temporary staff. Usually, an office, a phone, a desk, and a few file cabinets will suffice. If the Administrator is doing his job properly, he probably won't spend more than a few hours in his office during the first three months of the program.

A PLAN OF ACTION

First, the Zero Defects Administrator will formulate a plan of action. For this task he will need help. He will have to call upon key people throughout the organization for advice in formulating the master Zero Defects implementation plan. The importance of the administration placement becomes evident with this first task.

To accomplish this planning mission the Administrator will probably call upon people from industrial relations and finance, presentations experts (public relations, advertising, or sales promotion, as the case may be), a planning specialist, and representatives from major divisions within the organization. These men will make up his ZD action committee. Each will advise the Administrator as to actions affecting his particular area. The planning specialist will place all of the steps on a master plan.

At this time, the Administrator will collect facts about the numbers and types of employees to be indoctrinated, available facilities, and promotional costs and production schedules and information on the availability of key personnel and the possibility of conflicting plans or events. By plotting all proposed events on a scheduling chart the committee should be able to fix dates for every step of the indoctrination program and the first year's activities (see Figure 9).

Once this package is complete, it should be presented to the Senior Executive. This is the last go-no-go point in the program. With the scope of the entire kickoff program and sustaining effort for the first year before him, he will be able to pass final judgement. Once approved, this plan becomes the Administrator's "bible." He will have to live with the plan, covering every step in the proposed program for the next year. Minor adjustments can of course be made during the year.

TOP-MANAGEMENT INVOLVEMENT

The program is now ready to be presented to the organization's executive staff. A special meeting of the staff should be called for this purpose to emphasize the importance of the program. Attending will be those members of top management that report directly to the Senior Executive. It might even be feasible to issue formal invitations for this program unveiling.

Top-management Presentation

The meeting should be opened by the Senior Executive. He will explain the purpose of the meeting and give his complete endorsement to the program. The new Zero Defects Administrator should then be introduced, and he in turn will present the actual program plans. He will carefully explain just how the program will affect the operations represented and will make his requests for assistance from each of the attendees at this time. Ample time should be allowed for this key management team to ask questions about the program and the company policy surrounding it. Every element of the concept, philosophy, and program activities should be covered. A copy of the master plan should be provided to each attendee. By the end of this session, very few questions should be unanswered.

If the organization is very large or has widely separated elements, the Administrator can request a part-time Zero Defects representative from each of these men. Basically, the task of the representative is to help the Administrator reach the greatest number of people in the shortest time. (The role of this representative is covered in depth in the next chapter.)

At this time, the ZD Administrator should begin laying groundwork for mid-management indoctrination. He may now make appointments with top management to attend their staff meetings for the next step in the indoctrination cycle. If this and other activities involving top management can be ironed out at this one meeting, the indoctrination cycle can begin the very next day. Careful planning prior to this meeting will provide a big payoff in the end. Once top management accepts the program, all other avenues of motivation and indoctrination are open.

Special Situations

You will rarely find open skepticism at a top-management briefing. This is obviously due to the influence of the Senior Executive's endorsement and the

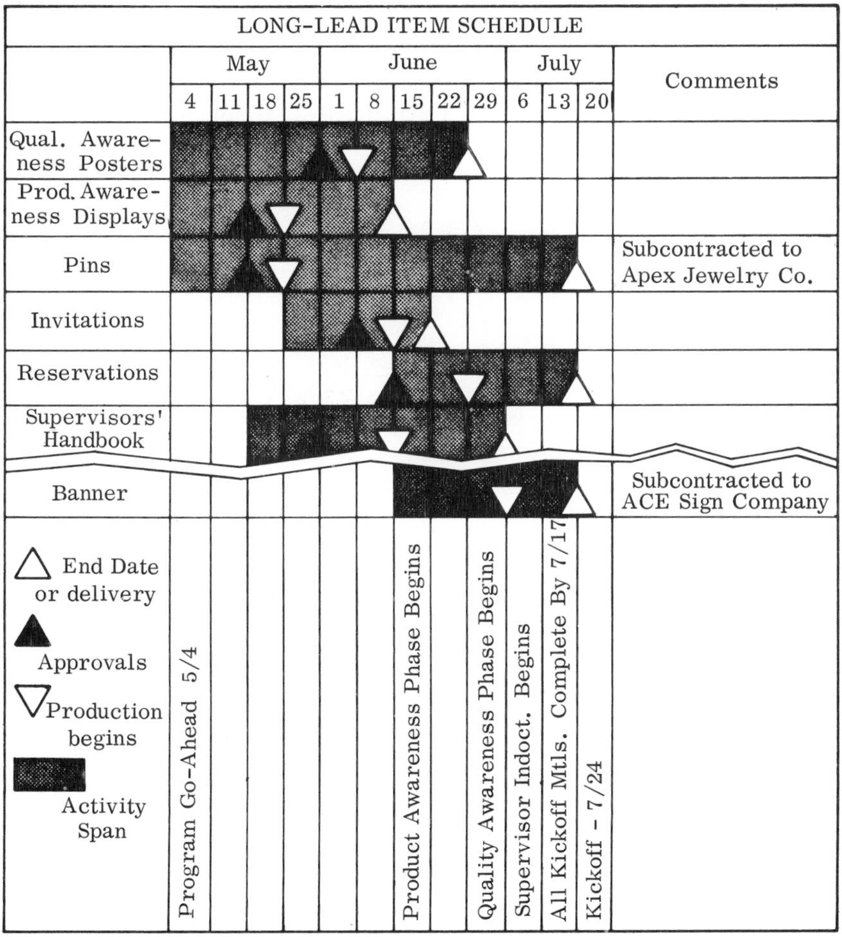

LONG-LEAD ITEM SCHEDULE												
	May				June					July			Comments
	4	11	18	25	1	8	15	22	29	6	13	20	
Qual. Awareness Posters													
Prod. Awareness Displays													
Pins													Subcontracted to Apex Jewelry Co.
Invitations													
Reservations													
Supervisors' Handbook													
Banner													Subcontracted to ACE Sign Company

△ End Date or delivery

▲ Approvals

▽ Production begins

■ Activity Span

Program Go-Ahead 5/4

Product Awareness Phase Begins

Quality Awareness Phase Begins

Supervisor Indoct. Begins

All Kickoff Mtls. Complete By 7/17

Kickoff – 7/24

FIG. 10   The planning member of the Administrator's committee should make every effort to identify and schedule for long-lead items early in the planning stage in order to avoid any last-minute delays.

common-sense, good-management approach of the basic program concept. But, at this point, it is absolutely necessary that any member of top management with reservations about the program be immediately identified. Since it is unlikely that a member of management not in complete accord with the program will challenge the Senior Executive in public, it is up to the Administrator to identify such individuals and make every effort to put them on the team.

The most effective means of accomplishing this identification is to conclude the question and answer part of the top-management presentation with the following offer: "In order to conserve time for the entire group, are there any of you gentlemen who would like to sit down with me privately at a later date to discuss specific applications and problem areas?" This will give those members of top management with reservations about the program the opportunity to voice their opinions and give the Administrator the opportunity to iron out any possible difficulties. The Administrator should make it a point to follow up on these requests as soon as possible and come to such meetings prepared to answer questions with specific advantages of a ZD program in the manager's area. Complete acceptance by and cooperation of the top-management pyramid is absolutely essential to the organization-wide indoctrination cycle.

Once the basic steps outlined in this chapter have been completed, the Administrator is ready to get down to the job of organizing, indoctrinating, and motivating for the kickoff of the program. He now has management's blessing and wholehearted support. He has an approved plan and an action committee to help him carry out the plan. He is ready to do battle with the organization's defect problems.

The various members of his committee should move at once on long-lead items. The presentations specialist should begin the design and production of promotional material. The planner should keep the plan current and report on any critical scheduling problems (see Figure 10). The industrial relations member should begin arrangements for union indoctrination (see next chapter). The Administrator should be setting up mid-management indoctrination sessions. The entire team should move ahead with all speed since proper timing of events is essential to the success of the program.

In the midst of all of this activity, do not overlook one basic fact: this is a Zero Defects program! As such, it demands essentially defect-free performance. If the actions of the committee, the Administrator, and top management are less than 100 percent perfect, the program will lack accordingly.

4

Expanding the ZD Team

In addition to his major task of indoctrinating the organization's work force (see Chapter 3), the Administrator will discover other elements both within and outside of the organization that need highly specialized types of indoctrination. Some of the people involved will have a direct bearing on the build-up of the ZD program, and some will have only indirect influence on it. Regardless, experience has proven that none of these important elements should be missed. They include: union officers; local, state, and federal government officials; special ZD representatives; and all others who may be asked to participate in the program.

UNIONS

Union involvement in a Zero Defects program is usually a source of concern for any organization in the process of implementing the program. It need not be. From its earliest days, Zero Defects has had its staunchest support from American labor. The basic Zero Defects concept of a nondiscriminatory program has come into play in this area. ZD belongs to the union just as much as to management. Before an implementing organization gets too far down the line in its indoctrination series, it is absolutely necessary that the unions be asked to join the ZD team. This is best done early in the program, before union members and officers begin to pick up half-truths or inaccurate information about the program. Most organizations bring their unions in on the program at about the same time general management is being indoctrinated.

Though situations may vary, the tried and proven Zero Defects motivation techniques can accomplish the job with ease. This same technique has given excellent results in plants with highly stable single-union shops as well as in complex multiunion situations where there has been a history not only of union-management difficulty but of continual jurisdictional disputes between the unions themselves. In all cases, Zero Defects has risen above existing labor-management differences and has received universal acceptance from all parties concerned. In several cases, the program has proved a stabilizing influence in overall labor relations.

There is a basic reason for this wide acceptance: the Zero Defects philosophy. What is closer to labor's heart than craftsmanship, the dignity and importance of the individual, and the theory that American labor is capable of producing the best possible products in the world today? Like motherhood, apple pie, and John Wayne, Zero Defects just cannot be denied.

When ZD is presented in a manner that brings out these key points, union officers will almost always offer wholehearted support to the program. Union endorsements such as the following by Wise W. Stone (see Figure 11), assistant director of the UAW, can give added impact to your presentation:

> It is always a pleasant experience for labor to participate jointly with management in a program which emphasizes the dignity and appreciation of individual accomplishment. This, in our way of thinking, is the primary strength of this Zero Defects program. Accomplishments by individuals joined collectively in

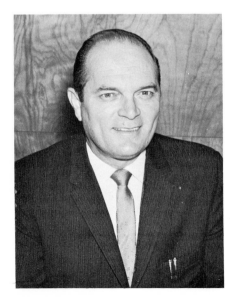

FIG. 11   Wise W. Stone, assistant director of the UAW: " . . . a program that emphasizes the dignity and appreciation of the individual."

an environment for improvement are, and must always be, the goal of organized labor. There is no company in any industry that can succeed without the talents of its workers from the top executive to the least skilled. Nor is there any company in industry that can succeed without a true appreciation of individual needs for job security and recognition of accomplishments.

He goes on to state:

I have discussed the program with union leaders both at the local, executive and international levels and I can assure you of the UAW's support of the program. Further, the program is attractive to our union because of the emphasis on the individual and his attainments. The Zero Defects program creates a strong identity between the individual and the product or service with which he works. The very fact that management and labor are closely associated in the development and manufacture of the finest products possible by joint effort, creates confidence in the defense and consumer market which lends economic stability to our nation. In a world of increasing competition, it becomes mandatory that management and labor continually strive toward maintaining our industrial leadership.

Mr. Stone does issue one warning:

. . . a word of caution about the Zero Defects program. The basic philosophy as expressed by industry management, that management does not harass employees or use Zero Defects as a club, is vitally important. I have been assured by many local executives of the unions at the Martin Company, Hayes International, North American Aviation, and many of the other companies having Zero Defects programs that one of the primary reasons for the success of the program in their plants is based on the concept of rewarding employees through public recognition of superior accomplishments and not harassing them for their mistakes. This is the positive as opposed to the negative approach.

This conclusion echoes a vital point that must be made clear in any union indoctrination: ZD *never* punishes; it recognizes achievement. (This does not mean that management should discontinue necessary worker reprimands. Just don't use ZD as the reprimand "club.") Union officers must be assured that the pledge made by all workers—to strive toward a goal of Zero Defects—is not something that will be held up to them at a later date if errors are made. Where pledge cards are used and unions are involved, many companies have allowed the union to review the pledge prior to printing or distribution. It is also a wise move to allow the union officers to be the first to sign up for the program. In itself, this will almost assure universal union membership acceptance on kickoff day.

Union officers should also be asked to indoctrinate shop stewards, much in the same way management indoctrinates its supervisory staff. Stewards, like supervisors, work closely with rank-and-file employees who probably will come to them for advice when ZD is initially presented. Your Zero Defects Administrator should offer his services in planning and conducting the in-

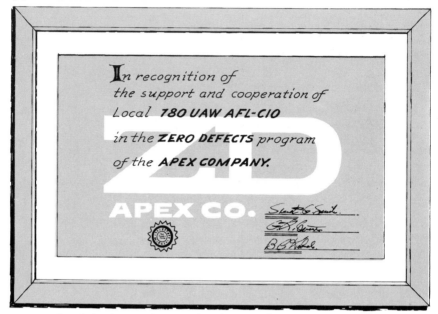

In recognition of
the support and cooperation of
Local **780 UAW AFL-CIO**
in the **ZERO DEFECTS** program
of the **APEX COMPANY.**

FIG. 12   A typical union award presented to the union for program support during the implementation period.

doctrination session. Management should give union officials time off for this important meeting. In a follow-up effort, to assure complete coverage, the Administrator also should check whether any stewards or union officers missed the initial meeting.

After the program has been kicked off, the union should be encouraged to continue its participation. Union officials should play a significant part in every important event. The Administrator should also consider some form of special recognition for union achievement and effort (see Figure 12). Both local and national editions of the union newspaper will welcome releases on union members and their achievements.

Don't sell the union short. Its participation on the ZD team makes the Administrator's task 100 percent easier. Without the cooperation of union officials, involvement of the union membership is unnecessarily difficult.

ZERO DEFECTS REPRESENTATIVES AND COMMITTEES

In larger organizations, complete administrative coverage is almost impossible with a one-man ZD staff. To aid the Administrator and to take some of the burden off management and supervision, many companies have appointed part-time divisional and departmental Zero Defects representatives (see Figure 13). In extremely large groups, these men have established committees representing subgroups. Though the tasks of these representatives and committees are relatively small, the service they provide is a key to the success of ZD in their areas.

The ZD Administrator usually suggests that each member of a large operation, such as a manufacturing or administrative department, assign one individual as a clearing house for all ZD activity. This man checks all ZD information coming into the department and all recognition information leaving the department. He acts as a contact between supervisors and Administrator on defect problem areas and suggests services which the ZD organization may provide. He will also be in a position to answer all questions on policy, procedure, and techniques. If appointed early enough, he can contribute to the supervisor-indoctrination sessions.

This may all seem very time-consuming; yet in organizations where this technique has been used, representatives spend less than eight hours a month on ZD assignments. There is one catch: to do their jobs properly and efficiently, representatives must be thoroughly versed in ZD procedure, philosophy, and technique, almost to the same degree as the Administrator. Otherwise, they will have to take every problem to the Administrator and will thus defeat the purpose of having such representatives.

The indoctrination procedure for these important members of the ZD team must include all the elements of management, supervisor, union, and worker indoctrinations. Not only must each representative's initial training be extensive, but he must be kept up to date on changes and new techniques. This can be accomplished easily through short monthly meetings or by a regularly distributed information sheet mailed from the Administrator's office.

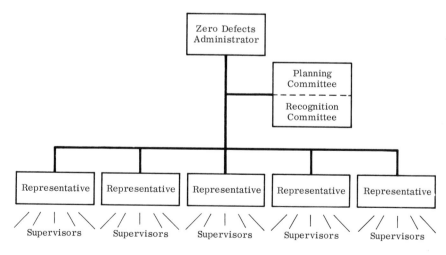

FIG. 13 Zero Defects organization. This type of organization would be used in a medium-to-large operation where the Administrator would have to rely on representative support for supervisor indoctrination and contact.

Since these representatives will be helping ZD by helping others attain their goals, it is important that the Administrator take special pains to assure representatives are recognized for their efforts. In order to motivate, one must be motivated himself. If the Administrator simply turns these men loose and sits back waiting for results, results will soon disappear. This philosophy of motivation is true for anyone on the ZD team.

Under certain conditions, representatives may wish to start small departmental ZD programs within their own organizations. After first coordinating all plans through the Administrator, a representative may appoint a departmental ZD council. This council can be made up of people in every area of the department, including secretaries, clerks, production workers, and supervisors. The council's task usually is to ferret out any defect problems and try to rectify the situations at the department level. It often suggests special citations for workers and work areas that may not quite qualify for company-wide recognition but nevertheless have made notable contributions or shown improvement trends. It is a good idea to rotate membership on the council so that more workers get a chance to participate and contribute.

Representatives are only as valuable as their training and motivation make them. As a member of the Administrator's ZD team, the representative is in a position to speak and act for the program. His words and actions must reflect the program concept. It is up to the Administrator to make sure this is the case.

COMMUNITY INVOLVEMENT

Where the organization implementing a Zero Defects program is in a small community or where it has a large impact on the economy of the surrounding area, an effort may be made to extend the program into the rest of the community. This has been done by several ZD organizations with highly rewarding results.

When General Electric kicked off the program at the Lynn, Massachusetts, organization, the entire community participated. Not only did the mayor and his staff attend all of the activities, but they renamed the town Turbotown for the day (General Electric manufactures turbine engines in this plant). When workers returned from the kickoff rally, they found local stores featuring such things as ZD haircuts and Zero Defects dinners. Local press, radio, and TV were brought in on the program, with the net result that everyone in the town knew what General Electric was attempting. In addition, almost everyone in town considered himself a part of that effort.

One word of caution about local publicity. If the activities of your company are of considerable interest to local news media, it is best to brief them early in the program. Adverse publicity or inaccurate information can harm the impact and understanding of your program. When provided with all the facts, the media people will almost certainly cooperate.

SPECIAL GUESTS

The Zero Defects concept is so widely accepted today that you may wish to go outside your immediate community for additional support. Many organizations have featured state and national leaders in their kickoff programs. Senators, governors, members of the House of Representatives, and even the Vice President of the United States have participated in Zero Defects programs. Since scheduling is an important requirement in engaging these people, it is well to make your plans well in advance. It is also a good idea to provide them with complete information on your particular program. More than once, this same information has been read into the *Congressional Record* or has appeared later in the texts of speeches by these nationally prominent people.

People brought in from the outside to help with ZD program orientation or the actual kickoff should be selected carefully and briefed fully prior to their contact with management or employees. ZD Administrators often invite management members from other successful ZD organizations to help with executive and mid-management indoctrination. There is nothing like a personal testimonial to get the success of any program across. But every program has its own "personality." Every ZD program has special techniques and methods unique to that particular organization. If an invited speaker were to start discussing one of these techniques—say, one foreign to the implementing organization's program—he would confuse and mislead his audience.

This is not to say that the exchange of ideas is not worthwhile. It is simply a case of good organization and planning to present a single story upon introduction of your ZD program. For instance, you may be planning an Error Cause Removal phase six months after kickoff. If a guest at your kickoff spends fifteen minutes talking about ECR while you are simply trying to convey the basic concept and philosophy of Zero Defects, the results can prove damaging.

On the positive side, make full use of your guest. Don't simply prop him up behind a lectern for a short speech and rush him home again. This man has gone out of his way to help you, and he should be given full opportunity to do just that. If he was deemed worthy of addressing a gathering of your employees, he certainly can have greater impact talking directly to individual workers on your production lines or in your offices. A capable ZD Administrator will exploit these visits for every possible value and arrange a complete day of activities for such visitors.

Visits by astronauts, test pilots, Medal of Honor winners, and ranking officers have had tremendous impact on workers in the defense industry (see Figure 14). Actually meeting a man whose very life depends on your craftsmanship can be an impressive experience. Martin-Orlando was gratified to discover that workers also enjoyed talking about Zero Defects and their products with enlisted men from units using these products in the field. Thus the guest need not be a nationally known figure to secure desired results. All that is needed is a common interest in defect-free performance of the product or service your organization offers.

You need not be in the defense business to make use of visiting speakers or guests, however. A cosmetic firm might well invite a famous model or a well-known Hollywood makeup man; a drug company could invite a nationally known medical figure or an officer of the American Pharmaceutical Association; a tire manufacturer could invite a famous racing driver or aircraft pilot. Whatever the product, there is a user; and every user has a strong personal interest in the quality of workmanship your employees exhibit. In an age where mass-production techniques have moved workers farther and farther from the end product, you have to bring the customer back into focus in the eyes of your worker before you can really sell the need for craftsmanship. There is nothing better than carefully planned and directed customer contact to accomplish this end.

SUMMING UP

Regardless of who the person is or how long or extensive his contact with your organization, any spokesman reflects directly on your ZD program. Care-

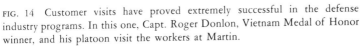

FIG. 14 Customer visits have proved extremely successful in the defense industry programs. In this one, Capt. Roger Donlon, Vietnam Medal of Honor winner, and his platoon visit the workers at Martin.

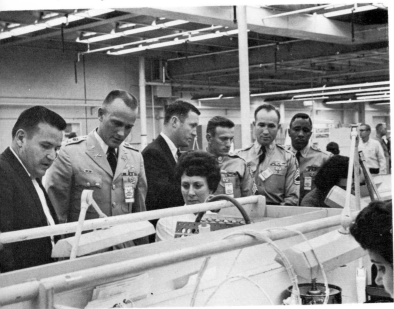

ful indoctrination of everyone involved in your program administration or presentation is mandatory. The two words to remember are "Zero Defects." Not only does the program try to convince others that perfection is possible, but to be effective, it must also demand a defect-free standard of itself. A disorganized, confused presentation of the program cannot have effective impact on an audience. A well-planned, carefully conducted program presentation which features a continuity of message, emphasis, and direction can and will succeed.

5

Management and Motivation

MOTIVATIONAL IMPACT

A successful Zero Defects program involves top and mid-management in two motivational aspects: first, motivating of the managers themselves; and second, management's motivational impact on supervisors and employees. Both activities are important, and both present difficulties in analysis and evaluation. The effects of motivation can be measured easily, but the actual process of employee motivation virtually defies concurrent critical analysis. It is almost a case of not knowing how successful you have been until it is too late to do anything about it. As H. J. Eysenck, head of the psychology department at University of London's Post Graduate Medical School, wrote:*

> Without motivation the work of the world would never get done and the history of man would be a blank tablet. Yet no aspect of human behavior has proved more resistant to analysis and measurement. The effort of psychologists to grapple with drive and motivation has evoked a remarkable variety of unsatisfactory solutions, ranging from purely semantic exercises to pseudo-mathematical treatment of non-existent data. As a result there is still no generally accepted method of measuring the degree of motivation under which a person is working at any particular time.

Whether or not motivation can be measured scientifically should not deter successful managers from their duties. Armed with the knowledge that this elusive element called "employee motivation" does exist, management can be assured that workers will respond with better craftsmanship, better productivity, and an overall superior attitude toward their assigned tasks. One thing experience has shown: motivation goes hand in hand with effective, sustained, two-way communication.

One of the attributes of a good manager is that he can "feel" the degree of motivation exhibited by his colleagues and subordinates and channel this force in the right direction. When this force is absent, the good manager takes steps to correct the situation through time-tested management techniques. One of these techniques is Zero Defects.

MOTIVATIONAL FACTORS

Much valid work has been done in determining factors which affect motivation. Professor Frederick Herzberg, chairman of the psychology department at Western Reserve University, has directed a six-year motivation study at Texas Instruments, Inc. The major conclusions of this study have been reported by M. Scott Myers in the *Harvard Business Review*.

Myers' report states employees are motivated to work effectively by "a challenging job which allows the feeling of achievement, responsibility, growth, advancement, enjoyment of the work itself, and earned recognition." Workers are dissatisfied in most instances with peripheral work factors: ". . . work rules, coffee breaks, titles, seniority rights, wages, fringe benefits, and the like." Workers become dissatisfied "when opportunities for meaningful achievement are eliminated and they become sensitized to their environment and begin to find fault." Thus, the absence of positive motivational factors causes the worker to strike out at an entirely different set of peripheral factors—usually those involving company policy, rules, and regulations.

POSITIVE APPROACH

A successful Zero Defects program is based on the positive factors that tend to increase employee motivation. Zero Defects makes every task interesting simply by offering the challenge of doing things right the first time. This program lets the employee know that his management, regardless of the level, is aware of his effort and provides him assurance of proper evaluation and chance for advancement. Through the Zero Defects emphasis on pride in performance and craftsmanship, the employee actually enjoys his work more. And above all, Zero Defects provides an avenue for public recognition of significant individual accomplishments.

Most experienced managers try to provide all these things in their employee work atmosphere. What Zero Defects does is give management a natural avenue for such activity. At the same time, Zero Defects offers employees the assurance management will not slip up and lose track of a single deserving individual.

Once a manager understands that Zero Defects can be his most effective employee relations tool, he will support the program freely and without reservation. Each manager must be persuaded not only to include Zero Defects in his day-to-day activities but to make the program a part of every one of his activities. By doing so, he will probably be able to eliminate many of his most difficult tasks and problem areas. When presented properly with the program, management cannot help but conclude that it should be given a chance. Past Zero Defects history indicates that a logical, understandable presentation of the basis and potential of the program almost ensures complete management support.

Challenge

This support may not come overnight, however. There is always the man who says: "I don't care if it has worked in every company in the industry. Our organization is different. It won't work in my area!" This man—and fortunately there are few ranking managers with such narrow views today—will have to be convinced by seeing the program in action in the areas surrounding him. Once he sees others making considerable gains through Zero Defects, he will probably become a staunch supporter. These are the advantages of Zero Defects: it makes sense, it works, and the record indicates that it will not let you down.

MOTIVATIONAL METHODS

The motivational techniques used in indoctrinating management on all levels are basic to the entire program. Once your Senior Executive has decided to go with the program and a plan of action has been formulated (see Chapter 4), the step-by-step procedure for getting the message down to the individual employee begins. The Senior Executive presents the program to top management (see Chapter 3). Top management should then make the presentation of the program to middle management. Where the actual presentation is not made by top management, this important management level should at least be present to convey openly its unequivocal endorsement of the entire concept. Though the actual nuts-and-bolts briefing may be handled by your ZD Administrator, there should be no doubt in anyone's mind that top management is behind the program 100 percent.

Management Briefings

If the implementing organization has a large middle-management team, the briefings should be split into small meetings. Every manager should have the opportunity to ask questions and get answers that remove all doubts about the program and its aims. He should also be free to ask top management specific questions about the organization's stand on certain aspects of the program. Though the program must be entirely voluntary, every effort should be made to bring every member of this important segment of your organization on board. One nonresponsive manager can isolate hundreds of employees from the communications chain necessary for total effectiveness.

It is logical to assume that, regardless of the voluntary aspect of the program, other management levels will feel obligated to follow suit once Zero Defects is endorsed by top management; but this is not enough. In the next indoctrination step, it will be these same managers who must convince first-line supervisors to join the program. These supervisors will be quick to note an attitude of "I'm only doing this because the old man says we have to." If the Administrator senses that one or more managers are not really convinced of the program's value, he should act at once to dispel all doubts.

Negative Attitudes

There are several effective ways to correct negative attitudes. The Administrator can put the manager in touch with a man in another, similar organization that has enjoyed success through the ZD program. Industry and government results should be presented in such a way that he can see how others are making use of this important management tool. A simple information packet on the program concept, its goals, and its results can be presented to each member of mid-management during these early briefings. If a manager believes the program is too time-consuming, then the Administrator should offer to help him with some activities. A reluctant manager can be shown how a Zero Defects representative can ease this work load and provide more complete coverage within the manager's area of responsibility. It is also a good policy to invite experienced ZD administrators from other organizations to participate in initial meetings designed to sell management.

SUPERVISOR INDOCTRINATION

Most Zero Defects Administrators find their task relatively simple when it comes to indoctrinating and motivating management, but generally the problems increase when they move to the next step—management's indoctrination and motivation of first-line supervisors. These difficulties are encountered because of the nature of both the indoctrinated and the indoctrinator. In the earlier management sessions, it was a case of a highly motivated expert speaking to a select audience of senior management. We can't reasonably expect *every* member of management to be able to convey the same knowledge or enthusiasm that the Administrator conveyed when they carry the message down to the next level. Yet, supervisors are, in fact, the key to the entire ZD program. In cases where supervisor indoctrination and motivation has been conducted properly, Zero Defects has been universally successful. In other cases where this important phase was not given proper care and attention, programs have achieved only limited success. After all, it is the supervisor who has day-to-day contact with each worker. The supervisor assigns his work, answers his questions, praises or corrects him, and directs his every activity. If the supervisor believes in the program and knows enough about it to convey both concept and challenge to the worker, then almost all workers will accept Zero Defects as a part of their lives.

Indoctrination Methods

The supervisor motivation and indoctrination technique varies little from that employed at other organizational levels. If the basic rules are followed, the motivational goals will be accomplished. Here it is mid-management rather than top management which endorses Zero Defects. In many cases, depending on the size of the organization and the availability of the ZD Administrator, mid-management will also conduct the actual supervisor briefings. It is obvious why complete mid-management indoctrination is so important.

The actual briefing of supervisors is best conducted during the managers' regular staff meetings. This helps put across the point that Zero Defects is an important part of the organization's normal business structure. A special meeting may be called for this purpose, but mass supervisor indoctrinations should be avoided. Like managers, supervisors must have the opportunity to ask

FIG. 15 Supervisors' handbooks. These valuable program tools are used in almost every industry, and though they take a wide variety of shapes and sizes, the intent is always the same: to help the supervisor become a more knowledgeable and productive member of the ZD team.

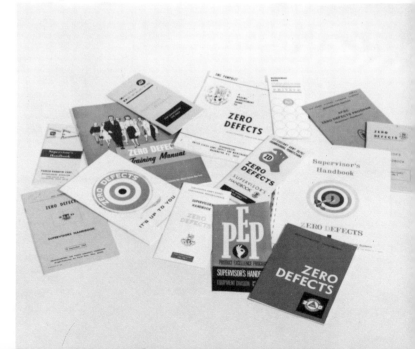

questions about the program and management's policy in support of it. Also like managers, nonresponsive supervisors must be identified and convinced. The basic truths of the program concept, if properly handled and coupled with an obvious show of endorsement by middle and senior management, will bring the supervisory staff willingly into line behind the program.

Supervisor Briefing

Since supervisors must fully understand the detailed applications of the program in order to answer all workers' questions, their indoctrination generally takes longer than middle-management briefings. In this instance, the Administrator or the manager must show not only how the program will help the supervisor in his job but how to present the program to his subordinate workers. To aid in this briefing and fill any gaps, a special supervisor's handbook (see Figure 15 and Appendix D) may be prepared. This document usually is pocket size and includes the basic concept of the program, the supervisor's role in the program, the supervisor's role in the recognition phase, and the answers to questions expected from the workers on kickoff day.

The major points to get across at a supervisors' meeting are:
- The philosophy of Zero Defects
- The goals of the program
- That the program has been a success in every aspect of the American economy (stress facts and figures from similar and competitive industrial organizations)
- That management is solidly and actively behind Zero Defects
- That Zero Defects is in the organization to stay
- That everything possible will be done to make the supervisor's ZD efforts pay off
- The obvious advantages to the supervisor, the company, and the worker
- That management is counting on supervisory cooperation and will recognize the supervisor's efforts
- That the ZD Administrator is always there to help the supervisor

Timing

The best time to begin motivation and indoctrination of your supervisory levels is as close to the organizational kickoff date as possible. One word of warning: Allow yourself extra time to fill in any supervisors who missed the regular and special briefings (see Figure 16). Some of these important members of your team may be on sick leave, on vacation, or unable to attend for some other pressing reason. If these men do not have the right answers for their workers on kickoff day, those workers will fail to receive the total impact of the kickoff presentation. It is much more difficult to recoup after an omission has been made than to avoid the omission in the first place. Complete supervisor indoctrination records should be kept to assure all concerned that no one has been missed.

BRIEFING SCHEDULE – SUPERVISORY

Division	Department	7/6	7/7	7/8	7/9	7/10	7/13	7/14	7/15	7/16	7/17	7/20	7/21	7/22	7/23	7/24	Location	Responsibility
Manufacturing	1 – 5	10:30															Room 101	R. Jones
Manufacturing	6 – 13	2:30															Room 101	Admin.
Manufacturing	14		11:00														Room 101	R. Jones
Manufacturing	15 – 17			3:00													Room 101	R. Jones
Manufacturing	18		9:30														Main Aud.	R. Jones
Manufacturing	Makeup					3:00											Room 101	Admin.
Finance	Administrative	9:00															Room 82	L. Smith
Finance	Bookkeeping		3:00														Room 88	L. Smith
Finance	Makeup			10:00												KICKOFF	Room 80	Smith & Admin.
Personnel	General					10:00											Room 202	Walsh & Admin.
Personnel	Makeup						3:00										Room 202	Walsh
Engineering	Design	1:00															Main Aud.	Edwards
Engineering	Systems		1:00														Main Aud.	Edwards
Engineering	Reliability			1:00													Main Aud.	Edwards
Engineering	Laboratories							9:00									Room 15A	Admin.
Engineering	Makeup									10:30							Room 17A	Admin.
Plant-Wide	Makeup										10:30	2:30					Main Aud.	Admin.

FIG. 16 The Administrator is encouraged to keep tight control over supervisor briefings to assure that no one is missed. This type of schedule will serve this purpose well.

Supervisor Rejection

The problem of supervisor rejection is very slight if the program is properly presented by management. The supervisor's most common objection will be that he does not have time to take on another program. Supervisors seem to be continually involved in one program or another. Just as soon as a new problem arises, management comes up with a supervisory technique to answer it. In truth, Zero Defects is not *another* job for supervision. It is a revitalization of a long-established assignment—that of being aware of the workers' problems and trying to motivate them to do a better job.

Often, the many demands placed on a supervisor make him feel that he is the middleman in a management tug-of-war. It sometimes seems that the various company-sponsored programs are at cross-purposes with each other. The difference with Zero Defects is the complete organization-wide approach. The chief executive, every manager, every supervisor, and every employee— all pull in the same direction in pursuit of a common goal. As soon as the supervisor is made aware of this, he will realize that the Zero Defects program is tailor-made for him. He will gain from every action taken. Every effort on behalf of Zero Defects will be an effort in support of his regularly assigned responsibilities. Every man in the organization is a member of his own personal team.

Follow-up

So far in this chapter we have stressed management motivation and indoctrination problems and techniques prior to program kickoff. Employee-motivation effort does not stop with program introduction; actually, it is intensified. Supervisors must continue to encourage employees, and management must stay on top of supervisor activities and must support the supervisor actively and openly in his day-to-day dealings with the rank and file. Management must also maintain a continuous line of communications with the worker. This does not mean that the manager should suddenly become "one of the boys" and invite all his workers home to dinner. It does mean the manager should let the worker know what is expected of him and that management is aware of his achievements and failures.

Personal Contact

The task of conveying management's desires to subordinates is not so easy as it sounds. Naturally, most workers respond to some extent to almost any reasonable request made by their supervisors. But the manner of making these requests and the requests themselves must be given careful consideration. As Finley, Sartan, and Tate in *Human Behavior in Industry* conclude:

> Management can never get superior performance from workers if it is interested only in performance. It must be interested in workers as ends in them-

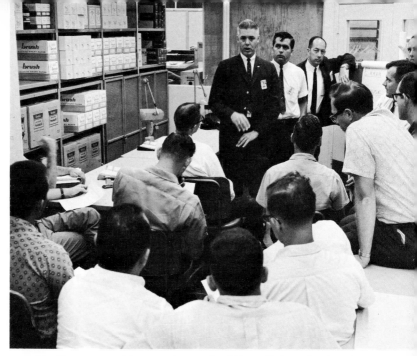

FIG. 17 Management visits to work areas should be well planned and made as productive as possible. Individual or group talks can go a long way to promote the feeling that management is really interested in the goals and achievements of the work force.

selves and not merely as means to an end. In a word, if management is to get the best from workers, it must respect them enough to be interested in what they can do, even if one pays very well for their work.

The means by which management members contact employees personally determines the success of this undertaking. Higher management, in particular, should not be patronizing toward employees. In many organizations ranking management members make regular tours of employee work areas. On these occasions many managers practice the technique of greeting workers by name and asking personal questions about home life, the progress of children, and such matters. This approach generally does more to put the manager at ease than it does to convey any real feeling of "togetherness" to the worker.

Yes, management should show interest in employees as people—but primarily as working people. If conducted with sincerity and honesty, mutual discussions of working conditions, work itself, work accomplishments, and other business matters will do much to advance productivity and general employee/management relations (see Figure 17). Zero Defects presents an outstanding opportunity for such discussions, and the subject of work comes up automatically as a topic of major importance to both management and worker. Since Zero Defects is nonselective, it is common to all levels of any organization. Thus, the program assists in the difficult communication task of bridging the gap between management and workers and, at the same time, channels this communication into the most important subject in any organization—productivity or work accomplishment.

REVIEW

The entire management approach to Zero Defects can be summed up in four basic actions.

First, management should study its own organization in the light of this new technique. What are the organization's major failures in product quality? What are the critical areas in each manager's own department? What group contributes the most to these failures? How does this group differ from that with the least defects? What specific part or service is causing the group the most trouble? These questions and others like them will reveal the elements which can be improved through Zero Defects. Actually, these elements are the "why" of Zero Defects and will form the basis of management's ZD plan of attack.

Second, management must establish broad, general goals which can be met by establishing ZD consciousness in individual groups. Experience has shown that a well-run ZD organization can expect anywhere from a 25 percent to 50 percent decrease in defects the first year the program operates. This gives some indication of the results management may expect and, hence, the goals that might be set. Specific group goals and measurement techniques will be developed later in the program, but an overall aim is necessary from the start.

The third management action in support of Zero Defects is the constant maintenance of a dynamic personal role. Managers must be, and must appear to be, enthusiastic in their support of the program. This continued enthusiasm will provide the spark needed to maintain a successful program. The worker will only do as management does.

The fourth and final requirement for successful management involvement in a Zero Defects program is the recognition of outstanding effort wherever it occurs. Prompt action of this type not only assures the worker that management appreciates his effort, but it tells the individual that management is aware of his task and considers it an important part of the end product or service.

Initially, a ZD program may appear to be an additional responsibility to already overburdened members of management. Actual practice has shown, however, that the implementation and continuation of a Zero Defects program generally assists management and supervision in the performance of their normal duties. A successful ZD program eliminates many of the problems which normally take up a large amount of supervisory time. It will be the duty of management to see to it that the levels below him understand that ZD helps not only the overall organization but that it will help each individual perform his own duties more effectively.

Thus management has the primary burden of spreading a complete under-standing of the Zero Defects concept throughout all levels of the organization. Management must be willing to set the example for others to follow. Wherever a program lag has been discovered, it has always been traced to some member of management who wasn't doing his job properly.

6

> *One of the tragedies of modern industry is that so many workers do not have the sense of making a genuine contribution. The craftsman of an earlier period had it, and also the farmer, the professional man, and others. But today, many jobs have been broken down into small parts, and each part is given to a worker as his whole job. The result is that many people have little idea of what they are doing from the standpoint of real relation to the finished product or to the social order as a whole. Under these circumstances, of course, many people work almost entirely for money—and are unhappy no matter how much they get—because they see nothing else to work for.* FINLEY, SAR-TAN, AND TATE, *Human Behavior in Industry.*

Employee Motivation

The short passage above puts the entire employee motivational challenge in a nutshell. The basic job of any serious Zero Defects organization is to convince the worker that his efforts are important—to himself, the company, the customer, and society in general. Every technique, method, and action in your program should be directed toward this goal. The indoctrination period is aimed at convincing the employee to be proud of his efforts and to try to do everything in the best possible way. He will be convinced through the Error Cause Removal phase (see Chapter 8) that management places enough importance on his task and knowledge to solicit his advice. The measurement and reporting phases are simply to point out facts and figures in support of important achievements in excellence. And the recognition phase repeats the message that management is aware of the worker's efforts and thinks enough of his accomplishments to do something about it.

TECHNIQUE

ZD does not congratulate or pat the backs of the employees just to make the employees feel good. These actions are taken to accentuate management interest. Simply telling a worker that his job is important and that you appreciate his efforts is not going to get the worker to change the strong mind-sets noted in the first chapter of this book (everyone makes a mistake once in a while; to err is human; etc.). The worker must be shown and convinced by actions and examples that his job—any job—is worth doing well. Only then will he see any reason to make the effort that ZD performance requires.

For example, when, in the course of an employee/supervisor meeting, the boss says, "You're doing a fine job. Keep up the good work," does this tell the worker anything about the status or importance of his job? No, it simply tells him that the meeting is over and that he should go back to his bench.

How *do* you get the program message across? The answer is a combination of well-chosen words backed up by management action. The Zero Defects motivation process makes this combination pay off. It presents the worker with an entirely new picture of his job, his product, and the importance of his very being in the organization.

There are several obvious (to the worker) things going for you when Zero Defects is properly introduced to the rank and file. The amount of work and effort put into a ZD kickoff is impressive. The fact that the program is operation-wide is impressive. The fact that management is doing something it has never done before is impressive. These three facts alone show the worker the emphasis that management places on the program.

PRODUCT AWARENESS

The first step is to get the program down to the specific—the individual. This is done by making sure the individual knows the reason for his existence in your organization in the first place. The important relationship of his task to the end product should be driven home before any further program steps occur. You can't ask a man to do a good job on something if he's not quite sure what it is, why it is, and what will happen if he does it wrong.

This problem is not as farfetched as it sounds. For instance, how many automobile manufacturers' secretaries relate a memo to the sale of a convertible in a showroom in Seattle? How many air conditioner production workers relate a solder joint to a possible hospital installation in Miami? How many checkers on a line producing rubber washers relate their task to a man spraying his lawn in Phoenix? Though the answer to these questions is probably "none," there is a simple answer to the problem itself. The main reason these people have so little idea about the outcome of their efforts is that no one has ever bothered to explain it to them. It is easy to say, "Sure, our workers know we make cars," but there you have used the word "we," meaning *"management"*—not "he," meaning the "individual." Individuals don't make cars anymore. They haven't for about sixty years. Individuals make brake assemblies, they install engines, and they conduct finishing processes on fenders and bodies.

Pride in performance is a personal thing. To be effective in your product awareness campaign, you must relate back to the individual task. Every task is important or the task shouldn't be there in the first place. Thus, when you speak to the worker of the end product, relate it not only to the user but back to the individual tasks that went into making the product. What if your company does not have a formal end product? What if your company deals in a service or in small components? The job is even easier. You have every product of every customer to choose from. The world of commerce is your end-product oyster.

Since it is rare that a company or organization will have only a single product or service, the ZD potential of each must be given careful consideration. The Administrator should ask himself the following questions:

1. Is every employee involved in every product or service the organization offers?

2. Is there one large product or service that overshadows all the rest?

3. Do the workers tend to associate with one product or service?

4. Are there natural organizational divisions or workers involved in specific products?

5. How many workers have ever seen our end product or service in action? How many have seen it at all?

6. How many have used our product or service?

Once the Administrator has the answers to questions like these, he can move on a plan of action for product awareness. Depending on the product or service, the Administrator's task may be anything from routine to highly complex. The farther his workers are removed from the end product, the more difficult his job will be.

The company that produces a popular consumer product has probably already established a certain degree of product awareness through the day-to-day use of the product by the employee. In most cases, he or she tends to buy the product either out of desire to support company sales (job security) or because of an extra degree of confidence in the item ("I have seen it made and I know it's OK"). Company outlets where the product is sold to workers at discounts also increase employee use. Whatever the reason, this interest could probably be stepped up. It is natural to assume that the worker will take more interest in something that affects him personally, as is pointed out in the basic Zero Defects philosophy.

Where the organization's product or service is one that the employee would never use or would rarely have a personal consumer interest in, the task requires deeper study and consideration. But by a careful review of the situation, the Administrator will discover dozens of ways to get the point across. Some suggested actions are found in Chapter 9, but it will be up to the Administrator to tailor this phase to meet his own organization's particular needs.

QUALITY AWARENESS

Concurrently with the product awareness phase, a strong drive toward a goal of quality awareness should be conducted. Before asking anything of the workers, take a good look at the quality-management operation of your organization. Consider at least these basic ingredients:

- Do you have an obviously active, organized quality-assurance program?
- Have you, or are you prepared to, set quality standards at least for your production areas?
- Do you, or are you prepared to, measure performance against these standards and report the results accordingly?
- Do you have an organized procedure for reporting customer complaints and rejects?

Don't just answer these questions with a quick "of course." Consider all of these factors and make sure. If you find any basic quality elements missing, start to rectify the problem at once. You can't expect your workers to become aware of quality when it is obvious to everyone that management policy has serious quality gaps.

After you have cleaned your own house, then turn to the individual worker. Here again, the supervisor and management should go all out to stress the importance of quality. The various in-plant communications media can be used as backup, but the basic message can really be put only in firsthand management talks (see Figure 18). Here the effects upon the competitive position of the company and the inherent effects upon the security of the individual will be emphasized.

Error Cause Removal

During this period many companies initiate the Error Cause Removal (ECR) phase of Zero Defects to back up quality emphasis with management action. ECR has proven highly effective as a quality awareness technique because it allows the worker himself to actively participate in the quality housecleaning program. It shows the worker that management is really serious about quality awareness and is willing to back up its talk with solid action—to "put its money where its mouth is."

The ECR technique, developed by the General Electric Company as part of its ZD program, simply offers every worker a tool by which he or she can identify any real or potential cause of error. Though the ECR mechanics will be covered in Chapter 9, the procedure is as follows:

1. All workers are provided with a form with which to identify any existing or potential causes of error. They do not have to suggest corrective action but they are welcome to do so.

2. The form is turned into the supervisor who takes immediate action to

correct the situation if at all possible. Experience has shown that the supervisor can provide the solution in 90 percent of the cases.

3. If the supervisor can't handle the problem within his own department, the ZD Administrator or representative takes on the task of bringing together the elements within the plant that can straighten out the situation.

4. Every effort is made to get a reply to the employee in the shortest possible time. You never want to give him cause to think that by submitting a form he is really dropping it into a bottomless pit of red tape.

5. If, after serious consideration, the supervisor finds that the error cause is imagined or for some reason can't be corrected at that time, he carefully explains why to the worker.

6. Regardless of the outcome, the worker realizes that management has given his Error Cause Identification serious consideration and has taken the time to make sure that any possible cause of error is checked out thoroughly.

Now, this may seem like giving the worker a license to steal. Many people expect the worker to ask for extensive facility changes, new machines, completely new procedures, and so on. The truth is quite the opposite. Out of over 3,000 Error Cause Identifications submitted by workers in the first month of ECR at General Electric, almost all were resolved within thirty days and over 90 percent were acted upon by the first-line supervisor himself. They usually were problems like a poorly placed lamp, a machine set up for a right-handed man with a left-handed operator, or a phone on the wrong side of a

FIG. 18   Supervisor-led product and quality awareness sessions help the individual to understand his place and the importance of his task in the overall scheme of things.

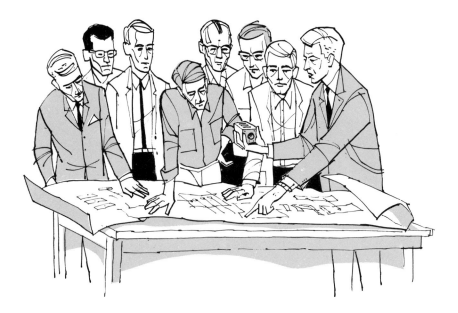

desk. They turned out to be the little things that get under a worker's skin but are never quite important enough to make him come to management for a change. Once ECR opened up this avenue of communication, the workers were eager to use it.

Of course, the program places a burden on management and supervision, but it is a burden of care and not one of money. The only thing expected of the supervisor is that he act swiftly and occasionally take time to explain a fact or two to a receptive worker. In reality, the worker is helping management do its own job since management should be on the lookout for potential causes of error and poor workmanship in any event.

Posting Quality Ratings

The last and perhaps most far-reaching form of quality awareness is the act of letting the worker know where he stands. This is best accomplished by letting the worker see where the record of his group stands in relation to other groups and to the established standards of performance. During the buildup period, prior to kickoff, the Administrator, the various departments, or the data staff should post defect-rate charts in as many areas as possible. It is a good idea to begin with those already under audit and later go into the process of determining measurement techniques for those not covered. The fifth section of this volume covers many of these techniques.

To raise the competitive spirit between groups, the Administrator can set up a group award for any section that stays a certain percentage below a predetermined level of error rate for three months or more. Or he can have a traveling award for the lowest rate and the most improved rate each month.

Though the full significance of the charts will not be appreciated until after kickoff, this type of information will go far in making the employee aware of the quality of performance expected by management. In most cases, all that has been done was to take some records from a book on the manager's desk and post them on a board. By this simple act, management has transferred much of the quality-assurance burden from the shoulders of the inspector to the hands and minds of the worker where it belongs.

ZERO DEFECTS INDOCTRINATION

If the previous steps have been properly executed, the Administrator and the supervisor are now ready to begin talking about Zero Defects per se. And what about the worker? Whether you realize it or not, he is in a sensitive position. Through your product/quality awareness campaigns, including ECR, you have left him without a defense against your challenge of Zero Defects. He knows the product story. He knows his own contribution to your product or service. His quality charts tell him where his group stands. He has the proper training. And every detected cause of error has been removed (at his request) by management. If he makes an error now, it can only be because he simply doesn't care, he is unable to understand all that came before, or the error was unavoidable.

At this moment, with your workers in a receptive frame of mind, the kickoff should take place. Though your workers will realize something new is coming up and some may know it is Zero Defects, almost none will be prepared for the scope of the proposal to be made by management. Though workers will be impressed by posters, speeches, rallies, and other activities that convey management's position and determination, it still will require face-to-face communication between management and worker to put the ZD story completely across. If properly indoctrinated and motivated themselves, your managers and supervisors will handle this job with ease.

Supervisor Responsibility

Before the first employee asks the first question about the program, each supervisor should bring his workers together for a ZD briefing. If he supervises a union area in the shop, he should have the indoctrinated steward at his side. He should then briefly outline the challenge to the workers (even if it has been done previously at a rally or other gathering) and answer their questions about the program. He should be the first in his group to sign the pledge, and he should do this in front of the workers. He should then give them the opportunity to go back to their work areas and think about the program. As soon as the workers sign up for the program, he should thank them and make every effort to see that they get a recognition pin (if one is to be used) as soon as possible. If some of his workers do not sign up immediately, he should not "hound" them. Remember, ZD is strictly voluntary. In almost every case, the worker will soon come around to pledging himself to the program aims. The desire to excel will push the slower ones along.

What about the man who refuses to sign? This situation will have to be played by ear by the supervisor. If the worker openly opposes the program, then the supervisor may best ignore the man and work hard on those around him. The program has obviously gotten to this person, and he will try twice as hard as the others to prove that he didn't need to sign a pledge to do good work. The man the supervisor really has to watch out for is the individual who doesn't respond one way or the other. This man has missed the entire message. Patience and special care will probably bring him actively into the program.

Postkickoff Effort

Just because a supervisor has a 100 percent sign-up doesn't mean his work is done. With the aid of management visits, group meetings, and individual contacts, the supervisor must now convince the worker that ZD is not a one-shot program. Though the ZD Administrator will direct messages at the worker on an organization-wide basis, it will be up to the supervisor to keep the program active on the group level.

Since recognition measurement can't begin prior to your implementation date, there is usually a certain lapse of time between the kickoff and the first official achievement recognitions. During this period the supervisor should continue to point out the challenge of the group record of defects or rejects. He should never miss a chance to recognize drops in defect trends. He should continue to encourage participation in ECR. He should keep his own eyes open for possible error causes and any upward trends in defect rates.

Sustaining Effort

Though this effort is covered in detail in the last section of this book, a few points should be made at this time. The Administrator should make a continuing effort to remain close to the supervisor and his problems. It is not enough to indoctrinate the supervisor once and then turn him loose for the life of the program. The supervisor's problems are the Administrator's. In many cases, a supervisor will not wish to go to his manager with a defect problem for fear of appearing to be unable to handle his own section. Working on these problems with the ZD Administrator or his divisional ZD representative usually seems like a more positive, do-it-yourself approach to things. When the Administrator loses touch with the supervisor, he is in fact losing touch with the reason for the program—the individual.

Just as in the case of the supervisor and the Administrator, top and middle management also have a continuing responsibility. Managers must constantly be on the alert for evidence of outstanding supervisor effort. The supervisor is an individual, too. His effort should not go unrewarded. Managers should discuss the program and its application in staff meetings. They should also continue to take the time to talk to the workers themselves in an effort to maintain the image that management cares.

Once your recognition and sustaining programs are under way, the program will take care of itself. If management and the ZD team take that small amount of time, once or twice a month, to assure the worker he is important and his task is worthwhile, the program will certainly prove successful. When management makes it a habit to care, the workers will make it a habit to care and the workers will make it a habit to excel in everything they attempt. Management —it's up to you!

7

Put Your Suppliers on the Team

As has been noted in the earlier chapters. Zero Defects is nondiscriminatory. It must be an across-the-board program to work. If you have suppliers contributing to your end product (and most organizations have), these people also should be given the opportunity to join the ZD team. The acceptance of the Zero Defects concept by your suppliers will not only help their organizations, but it will give a measurable boost to your own program.

SUPPLIER RESPONSIBILITY

For instance, you can hardly preach care in assembly of an item when your assemblers know the part they are attaching has a good chance of failing the final test or check-out. It is difficult to convince a solderer to take extreme care on a job when he knows that a certain amount of his work will end up scrapped due to bad components. And extra effort won't seem worthwhile to a secretary who realizes that, because of improper servicing, her typewriter couldn't possibly cut a decent stencil.

It should be obvious that, after making all this effort to assure that your own people have quality/product awareness, you should not turn your back on the components and services from outside sources that go into your product.

Before the Administrator can consider the possibilities and activities for extending the program to the supplier team, he must first review his supplier-team members. Most organizations are serviced and supplied by a wide variety of companies, some very large and some quite small. The size relationship (to the implementing organization) is the key to the direction the supplier ZD program will take.

If the implementing organization is a medium-sized industrial firm and the supplier in question is a multibillion-dollar electronics firm, then it is not reasonable to expect the giant supplier to shuffle its entire organization to adjust to the smaller customer's ZD program. In most cases this would not be necessary because the major company probably already has a ZD program under way. At the time of this printing, 50 percent of the top 100 industrial corporations have planned or implemented a Zero Defects–type program.

This chapter is directed toward the ZD organization's supporting activities with smaller suppliers—those that do not necessarily have the ways or means of implementing a program on their own. It is to these suppliers that the implementing organization has a certain degree of obligation. As the customer, the ZD organization will be asked and expected to offer leadership. This aid need not be expensive or time-consuming. For the most part, it can be channeled through already existing customer/supplier avenues of communication.

Zero Defects is presented to a supplier in much the same manner that you offer it to your workers. The program, to be effective at all, must be voluntary. It is pointless to direct your vendors to become ZD organizations. The same careful procedures of indoctrination, motivation, and recognition hold true throughout the program.

Though many companies wait until the program is well established within their own operations to make this move, it is advisable to bring the suppliers in as early as possible. This will not only make them feel more involved with your end product, but it will also assure you of help in total product or service coverage after kickoff day.

The best way to offer the challenge of Zero Defects to the supplier is in a personal, face-to-face presentation. If you have only a few suppliers, management can call them in or, better, go to each organization to present the program. The presentation should be handled the same as any management briefing on the program (see Chapter 5). If, like most organizations, you have dozens, hundreds, or even thousands of suppliers, individual presentations are usually impractical.

SUPPLIER SEMINARS

Under the latter conditions, your first step (as with your own internal program) is to present Zero Defects to the supplier's management. This is best done by organizing a management seminar for your suppliers during relatively the same time frame in which your own management is being indoctrinated. If most of your suppliers are located in your section of the country, simply invite representatives of their management to your home office for this indoctrination. If, on the other hand, your suppliers are spread throughout the country, it may be advantageous to hold several briefings at your regional offices.

This program need not be complex or expensive to execute. To conduct such a meeting, all you will need is a modified version of your management information package (see Figure 19) and the presence of several of your key management people. The presentation will inform the suppliers of your own plans and suggest ways they can coordinate their programs with your own. It will naturally include the basic philosophy and techniques of the program.

Naturally, your procurement chief, your supplier-quality chief, and any other member of management whose people deal with the supplier should be present. Their presence shows supplier management that your organization means business and is willing to back its words with action all the way down the line. The ZD Administrator and concerned management should try to attend all such sessions.

The meeting itself should be planned along the same lines as the top-management briefing described in Chapter 5. A member of top management should welcome the guests and make the keynote address to the group. The ZD Administrator should explain the program, its philosophy, its techniques, and its history of success throughout the industry. Then each of the involved managers or directors should explain how the program will affect his particular area of supplier contact. If a supplier attendee represents a company that already has such a program, give him the opportunity to tell of his organization's Zero Defects experiences. This alone will do much to dispel any apprehension that you, the customer, are trying to force a program down your supplier's throats.

Once the briefings are over, it is desirable to have a break or a luncheon to give the attendees a chance to mull over what has been presented and to collect their thoughts on the subject. After the break, all the speakers should sit as a panel and allow the suppliers to question any phase of the program they wish. It might be advisable in large presentations to provide question cards at the start of the meeting to be turned in before the panel discussion. In this way, you will be able to consolidate similar questions and to determine what areas are of greatest interest to the attendees. Even if cards are used, you should still offer them the opportunity for floor questions since the answer to one query will probably elicit five more.

At the end of the meeting, positive action and assistance should be offered to any supplier who wishes to accept the ZD challenge. It is not enough simply to inform them about the basic program and then turn them loose to struggle along by themselves. Any company that is willing to make the extra effort should be given all the encouragement and assistance your organization can muster. One of the most helpful things your organization can do for the participating suppliers is to hold a workshop for its supplier ZD Administrators (see Figure 20).

ADMINISTRATOR WORKSHOP

Since many of your suppliers will not have a large staff or the services available to promote the program on the same level as your own organization, they should be given the opportunity to share in your Zero Defects indoctrination plans. If you have few suppliers, this will simply involve inviting the new supplier Administrators to visit your Administrator. If, on the other hand, a large number of suppliers decide to adopt the program, it will be necessary to arrange more formal activities.

An Administrator workshop can be arranged in much the same manner as the management seminar. The actual invitations should be issued at the earlier seminar. This will motivate the suppliers to begin selection of Administrators as soon as they return to their organizations.

The workshop presentation, though not necessarily time-consuming or costly in itself, does require planning and coordination. To assure that the workshop is a profitable venture for all concerned, the Administrator will have to take great care in scheduling events. One of the Administrator's major tasks is the formulation of a meaningful lesson plan for the workshop. This

FIG. 19   A supplier packet can be made up with samples of the smaller items used in the kickoff program with a short, explanatory cover letter.

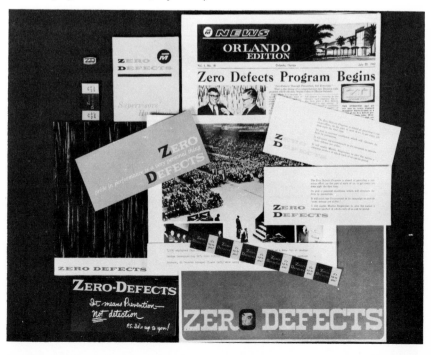

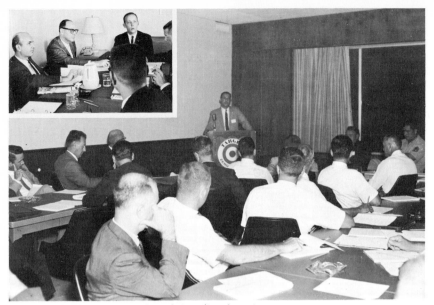

FIG. 20   Supplier seminar and workshop (inset) sessions.

will assure him that none of the key program points are overlooked. The
actual outline may be bound in loose-leaf notebooks with blank pages left
for notes. A copy of the supplier-management package may also be inserted
in the notebook, along with any other materials available from your own operation or other ZD organizations around the country. Each attendee should
receive one of these packages at the start of the workshop. There is absolutely
no need to prepare special brochures or costly presentations kits. Assuming
these men are coming to the workshop to learn and naturally assuming that
as ZD Administrators they are already sold on the program, your basic job
will be to help and direct, not to indoctrinate as you would a worker in your
own shop.

It is also a good move to list names, addresses, and phone numbers of attendees in the back of the workbook. This will allow them to contact each
other at a later date and share information and promotional techniques.

Basically, the program would be conducted as follows:

1. A member of management welcomes the guests and presents the customer's (your organization's) view of the program. This short talk will assure
the attendees that their customer is 100 percent behind the program.

2. The customer Administrator briefly outlines the program philosophy and
goals in case some of your supplier management did not cover all the facts
with their Administrators. There may be times when a supplier Administrator
does not know what his duties are or why he is at the workshop. This man
will probably have to go back and start from scratch with his own management to get the program moving. Though these cases are rare, your own
Administrator should be on the lookout for them and plan special assistance
for the supplier Administrator involved.

3. The Administrator should then go over the various planning steps for the program and show examples of his own schedule, indoctrination cycle, promotional production and funding plans, and all other elements that go into the program.

4. The next step should be a discussion of the actual promotional material and paperwork that support the indoctrination phase. The Administrator should present the plans and material he will use in his own kickoff. He should provide, when available, copies of all these things for each attendee. The supplier Administrators should be urged to use any of these readily available supplies in their own programs. Though the host company should not be expected to produce volume runs of this material for each supplier, the supplier should be allowed to "buy into" runs or borrow poster art and print mechanicals for production in their own shops. They should also be made aware of the fact that almost every ZD organization in the country is happy to lend such material. Where products or services have been held in common, this technique has been used to great advantage by hundreds of companies, big and small.

5. Some coverage should be given at this time to the measurement and recognition areas of the program. Since it is unlikely that you will all be together again until well after your respective kickoffs, a discussion of the sustaining phases will be of value to the attendees. This is a good time to announce some sort of a supplier-award program sponsored by your organization. The details of this program will be covered later in this chapter.

The supplier Administrators should be encouraged to begin their own internal recognition programs shortly after kickoff. Since you are involved in the same end product, certain aspects of your measurement techniques will have much in common. By telling them your plans and proposed methods of evaluation and criteria setting, you will more than likely be laying the groundwork for their own recognition programs. The most intense attendee discussion will probably occur during this portion of the workshop. Remember to take the time to answer their questions.

If the attendees seem to be preoccupied with the question of measurement, try to show them that their prime task is the indoctrination of the rank-and-file employee. Once this is accomplished, the question of measurement appreciably takes care of itself.

If any of your suppliers do not have existing methods of quality inspection or defect reporting, this is a larger problem than can be solved at one workshop. ZD needs a base to build on, and without a fundamental quality program, few companies can accomplish much through a Zero Defects program. ZD provides its best benefits where an active quality control organization is in operation.

6. The attendees should be given the opportunity to assimilate the information they have received and ask questions of the Administrator and the other

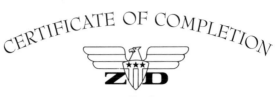

CERTIFICATE OF COMPLETION

Col. Richard P. Davidson, CE

OF THE

U.S. Army Missile Service Command

COMPLETED THE ARMY MATERIEL COMMAND

ZERO DEFECTS WORKSHOP

TRAINING PROGRAM ON
6, 7 May 19

W. T. ANDERSON
ZERO DEFECTS WORKSHOP
PROGRAM ADMINISTRATOR

JOHN M. CONE
MAJOR GENERAL, USA
DIRECTOR, QUALITY & RELIABILITY DIRECTORATE
ARMY MATERIEL COMMAND

FIG. 21   Administrator's workshop-completion certificate, presented to all supplier administrators attending the sponsoring organization's training workshop. This is a copy of an actual
certificate used in one of the earlier ZD workshop series (sponsored by the Army Materiel
Command).

speakers. If possible, because of the large amount of information to be absorbed, plans should call for a two-day affair. The first day would be spent in
covering all aspects of the program; the second day would be left open for
general discussion and panel sessions.

Large Workshops

In cases of workshops involving over twenty participants, it is suggested
that more than one instructor be used. In such situations, the Administrator
may ask his action committee members to help out (or his ZD representatives
if his organization has them). Regardless, the persons selected must have a
firm grasp of the entire program and be able to convey the scope and responsibilities of Zero Defects administration to the attendees. Where several groups
are being trained at one time, it is essential that the entire workshop be
brought together for an exchange of ideas at the end of the program. This is
usually done through the question-and-answer panel session prior to the close
of the workshop.

Attendee Recognition

Just as you recognize a worker for extra effort, the supplier Administrators
should be recognized for taking the time to attend the workshop. This recog-

nition usually consists of a certificate (see Figure 21) stating that the supplier Administrator has completed the workshop course. Though this simple act may not seem impressive, experience has proven that it goes a long way to build both the supplier Administrator's and his management's confidence in their ability to handle the program.

Area Workshops

As mentioned earlier, when large supplier forces are spread throughout the country, the Administrator may wish to hold regional workshops. This can be accomplished at very little additional expense or effort by simply indoctrinating quality and sales field representatives as Zero Defects experts (see Chapter 4). Once properly indoctrinated, these men will be able to convey the Zero Defects program story to all of your far-flung team members. They can use either the regional-workshop system or personal, individual contact with supplier, management, and Administrators.

Workshop Follow-up

After the supplier-workshop phase has been completed, the Administrator has a continuing duty to the attendees. After all, they are as much members of his ZD team as is, for example, the section head in Department 813. He should arrange to follow-up on the progress made by each and then offer his services accordingly. This could be accomplished by sending each Administrator a questionnaire fifteen to twenty days after the workshop. On this, he could request information about problem areas or areas where the supplier Administrators feel they need assistance. If, through the returned information, the Administrator discovers prevalent problems or problem patterns, he and/or his field representatives should move at once to remedy the situation.

A monthly newsletter or a special information sheet could easily be included in supplier mailings to keep the supplier Administrator informed of new techniques and to provide answers to old problems (see Figure 22). The main point to be remembered here is, after you have gone to all the trouble to indoctrinate supplier management and to train their Administrators, don't let it all go to waste for the lack of a little follow-up.

SUPPLIER-RECOGNITION PROGRAMS

It is only natural, in following the Zero Defects philosophy, to recognize the supplier for his accomplishments in much the same way that you recognize your own workers. This is usually the least complicated, yet one of the most rewarding parts of your recognition phase.

Since most organizations have a quality-acceptance or incoming-materials check system already in operation, it takes little effort to review the existing

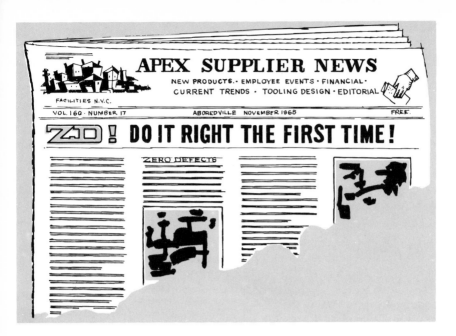

FIG. 22 If the implementing organization does not have a regularly scheduled, formal supplier publication, the implementation of a Zero Defects program is a good reason to start one. Not only can it be used to convey program information, but it will also provide management with a vehicle for other supplier information as well.

data for signs of supplier achievement. If your organization does not have such a system, it is advisable to set one up, not only as part of your ZD program, but just as good business practice. A company that does not care what sort of materials comes into its plant can't be serious about Zero Defects.

The actual procedure is simply to review your acceptance data to find which supplier is maintaining the lowest defect rate over a set period. When you discover the company, recognize it. Usually, a top-management representative presents the supplier's Senior Executive with some sort of an award (see Figure 23). Most companies use a scroll or plaque for this purpose. The next step is to follow up the presentation with promotion through advertising, your vendor newsletter, a supplier honor roll in your lobby, and any other form of promotion at your disposal. The supplier himself may wish to publicize the fact that you have given him this well-deserved honor. Many suppliers have used such endorsement in ads and other forms of promotion to win new business (see Figure 24). What you are giving him, in effect, is a "satisfied customer" letter on a rather grand scale. Every company thrives on such praise.

The Administrator should also offer to participate in the supplier's worker-recognition programs. Suppliers should be encouraged to send their outstanding workers to your company to see the end product or service in operation. This not only serves as a special form of recognition, but it tends to bring the supplier's work force into a new product and quality awareness.

VENDOR REJECTION

There are times when the Administrator will run into outright vendor rejection of the program. Though this rarely happens when a well-planned vendor-indoctrination program is carried out, the fact is, there are some people who refuse to try anything new. If the supplier in question is delivering defect-free parts or services to your organization, then you may assume that he is accomplishing this through an efficient quality-assurance and awareness program. It will suffice to make him aware of your ZD program and to offer him the opportunity to join the team. Since, in one way or another, he is already attaining the ZD goals, he should not be pressured or cajoled.

When you meet rejection from a supplier who is making below-par deliveries to your operation, the solution is simple. This supplier is already walking on thin ice and probably knows it. His rejection of the ZD challenge is probably made in defense of an established bad record. It is a case of basic good business to give a supplier of this type a prescribed time limit to bring his work up to the acceptance level. Extra effort should be made to show the supplier that ZD is a most economical method of reaching this objective.

ANNUAL WORKSHOPS

After any Zero Defects workshop, the question asked most often by attendees is: "When are we going to get together again?" An annual Administrators' workshop might be set up for the sharing of ideas and the discussion

FIG. 23 Supplier awards need not be expensive or overly ornate. Just as with the individual award in the in-house program, it's the management message that counts.

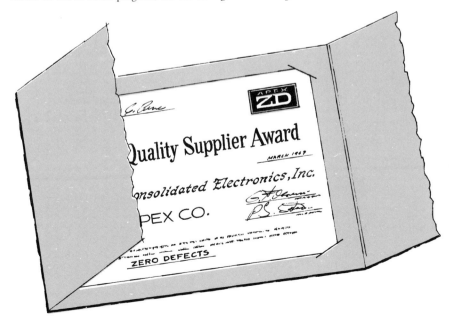

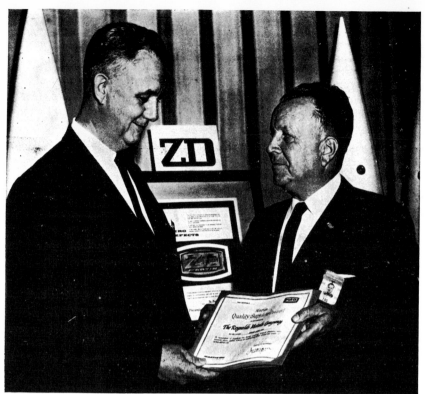

Reynolds Vice President-Operations, W. Monroe Wells (left) accepting Zero Defects
Award from G. T. Willey, Vice President and General Manager Martin-Orlando Division.

Reynolds Quality Honored by Martin

**Reynolds Metals Company receives the Martin
Company's first Zero Defects Award given to a
materials supplier.**

Zero Defects—at the Martin Company's Orlando
Division—is practically a way of life. It's Martin's
rigid, sweeping quality program that controls everything that goes out of this aerospace firm, including
the Pershing and Bullpup missiles. It means absolutely no mistakes, no deviations from specifications.
It means getting the job done right the first time.

Now Martin is applying the Zero Defects standards to its suppliers as well as to its own production.
And Reynolds Metals Company is naturally proud

to be among the first suppliers Martin has recognized for quality performance.

Reynolds quality control program is working for
Martin and for the entire metalworking industry.
Our goal—to supply the highest quality aluminum
products. Whatever your aluminum requirements—
ingot, sheet, plate, extrusions, tubing, wire, rod, or
bar—look to Reynolds for quality. *Reynolds Metals
Company, P.O. Box 2346-TJ, Richmond, Va. 23218.*

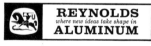

REYNOLDS
where new ideas take shape in
ALUMINUM

Watch the Richard Boone **Reynolds Aluminum Show,** Tuesday nights NBC-TV

FIG. 24   A supplier makes sales mileage through an ad featuring the receipt of a ZD award.

of new techniques and problems. This event can be a part of the parent organization's ZD anniversary program (see Part 4).

The main difference between this meeting and the earlier workshop is that
the annual sessions are for the sharing of ideas while the first was for learning
the basic facts about the program. These follow-on workshops are usually
conducted in the following manner:

1. The group is welcomed by the supplier-management team who go over the accomplishments of the past year and cite the award-winning members of the supplier team for their accomplishments.

2. The customer's Administrator assigns teams and task leaders to work on specific problem areas of interest to the entire group. It is a good idea to select task leaders prior to the meeting and to give the attendees the opportunity to volunteer to serve on specific teams.

3. The teams retire to meeting rooms to consider problems and to prepare reports on the various subjects.

4. The task leader of each team makes his report before the entire group, leaving time available for floor discussion.

5. The decisions reached by the teams plus the support information offered from the floor should be prepared in report form and mailed to each attendee as a follow-up to the workshop.

The Administrators should be encouraged to bring all promotional materials and information on new measurement and recognition techniques to these sessions. Sharing such ideas and materials will not only improve the effectiveness of all ZD programs concerned, but will reduce program operational costs by cutting down on promotional and research expenses.

TEAMWORK

It has been shown that the supplier is an important member of your organization's ZD team. Just how effective and contributing a member he is will depend largely on the success of your own program and the efforts of your Administrator. A tightly knit supplier team coupled with a well-organized internal program is the eventual goal of any Zero Defects administration. By accomplishing this goal, the Administrator has not only improved the competitive position of his own organization and that of his suppliers, but he has, in fact, done a real service to the thousands of workers and members of management involved. In other words, we should never overlook the first obligation of any ZD administration to the individuals and their own personal needs and aims.

PART **4**

Zero Defects in Action

The "How-to" of ZD Implementation

8

Techniques of
Product and Quality Awareness

Going back to the basic ZD philosophy, it must be remembered that the Administrator is dealing with a deeply rooted mind-set—one of the oldest alibis known to man—*everyone makes a mistake once in a while*. The primary goal of all prekickoff activities and the kickoff itself is to upset this mind-set.

The method used must be more than a blare of trumpets followed by an announcement over the public-address system. To be successful, the kickoff must be backed up with an extensive, well-organized, hard-hitting readiness cycle. It involves not only the efforts of the Administrator and his immediate ZD team, but also the active support of every member of the organization's management. Without this extra effort, the most elaborate and dynamic kickoff program will be seriously impaired.

In fact, every step of the readiness cycle demands the precise care, extensive coverage, and management support which surrounds the Zero Defects implementation itself. This chapter and the next cover the actual mechanical steps for implementation of the program. It must be remembered that the examples presented are only suggested actions; the Administrator and his staff will have to adapt each step to the organization's specific needs.

The theory behind most of these steps was presented in Part 3. It will now be up to the Administrator to give this theory solid application as it is transformed into a wide variety of activities on the working floor of your organization. When motivating workers toward an attitude of error-free performance, deeds—more than words—provide the impact necessary for a successful campaign.

PRODUCT AWARENESS PHASE

As pointed out in Chapter 6, employees often lose sight of the goal or end product that incorporates their individual tasks. Before a worker can see any reason behind his search for perfection, he must equate his actions to some service goal or end product; thus, Zero Defects readiness includes a product awareness phase. This phase will probably be carried out concurrently with the quality awareness phase; but for our purposes, it is best to consider them separately.

There are several techniques for accomplishing the task of product awareness; any one of them or a combination of several will probably serve your purpose. The important note here is to tailor the phase to the organization's specific needs.

Media Review

The first step is to review existing media. By collecting product information and passing it on through bulletin-board notices, the company publication, posters, and other information devices, a great deal of information can be presented in a relatively short period of time. A quick check of past issues will reveal how much product information the company paper carries. If the publication lacks such information, the Administrator should work the problem out with the editor to assure that such vital information gets prominent placement. For example: Martha Kirby enjoys reading that she won the sack race at the company picnic; but wouldn't she and her fellow employees find it just as interesting and more informative to read that the company has just landed a big contract to produce a new product that directly affects their job security and opportunities? The fact is, employees are always receptive to product news; so why not give it to them? And while you inform them about the product, insert a little information about *their* role and responsibilities in making the product a success. Subjects such as new contracts, new products, key deliveries, development breakthroughs, and customer information, all tend to drive home your product story.

Supervisor and Management Discussion

As with any promotional display of information, the message must be coordinated with management and supervisor support. The simplest and most rewarding method is simply to have first-line supervisors convey product information during regular worker meetings. For instance: A food company introduces a new, unique line of dehydrated baby-food products, and the company, through an accelerated information program, tells the workers about the new product and its importance to the market position of the company. The workers on the packaging line are now aware that the new product exists and probably understand that its success will mean additional job security for everyone concerned. But does this motivate them to take any positive action? It does not—unless the new product is related to their day-to-day tasks. The supervisor and a member of the sales force could speak to the workers about the problems of new-product, first-purchase merchandising, letting the workers on the line know that, regardless of the original product demand, it will be almost impossible to hold onto the market if housewives have trouble opening the boxes; the packages leak in the boxes; the boxes fall apart; or any other packaging failures attributable to sloppy workmanship occur. Armed with this information, the packaging-line workers will take a new, sharper interest in the product. They now have a responsibility for the end item. It is a real product with a real user, not just another item on a shipping invoice. All of them can now associate their tasks with product use in the field. The supervisor has bridged the gap between the product and the individual.

Customer Contact

Another technique, mentioned in Chapter 6, is the customer visit. Such visits have proved effective where the product is defense-oriented and any

FIG. 25 Small displays can be used to great advantage in work areas to show the individual where his task fits into the overall product picture. These displays can also be used as demonstrators for first-hand-supervisor talks on product awareness. The above display and demonstration show the importance of a single-tube assembly to a TV set's operation.

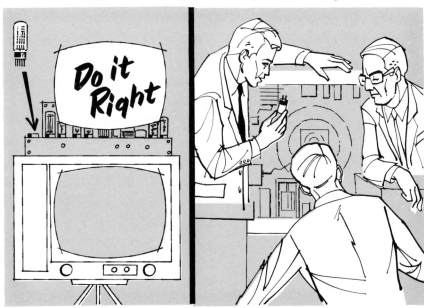

failure can mean disaster to the user. Employees of companies in hard-goods businesses or those providing industrial or government services, rarely meet the customer. Hearing about the product, its actual uses, and the needs of the customer—from the customer—tends to emphasize to the individual the importance of the most menial task. Now our baby-food company shouldn't be expected to bring a baby out on the line, but a representative from the Food and Drug Administration or a famous baby doctor would really get the necessary message across.

Product Displays and Demonstrations

Bringing the finished product into areas where earlier assembly steps are made gives the worker the opportunity to see where his task fits into the whole product picture. Small portable displays featuring your product, photos of it in use, customer statements about the product, and other items of interest can be used effectively in almost any area in your organization (see Figure 25). If the organization has more than one end product or service, prepare several displays and circulate them around the shop. If you have no real end product, work something out with the customers who buy components or services from your organization. Incidentally, if the display contains a product model or the actual end-product hardware, be sure the display is sturdy enough to stand a certain amount of handling. A "Don't Touch" sign on the display defeats your purpose.

Never take it for granted that your workers know where they fit into the overall product picture. Though they may see the end product in your plant from time to time or may even buy it for home consumption, they can only align the product to the task if it is displayed in their own work area. The supervisor should use the displays or models in his talks with the workers.

FIG. 26   Quality awareness posters.

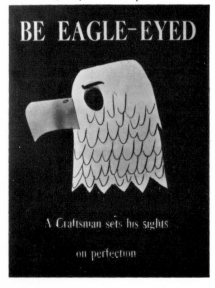

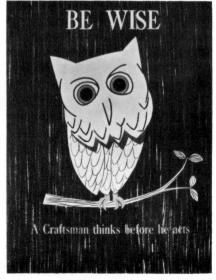

For instance: A purchasing clerk or a secretary may handle the documentation on "Part Number BX-97-722, Rubber Gasket, set of two," for years without knowing what the items do or if they have any real importance to the product at all. Provided with a model or a product display, the supervisor would need but a moment to point out the importance of this item and its function. Such action sheds new light on what previously was just a number on a piece of paper.

Regardless of the techniques selected, the Administrator should try to see that every worker in his organization understands the final product or service and, especially, that he understands his own personal contribution to that product or service.

QUALITY AWARENESS PHASE

In Chapter 6 it was stressed that before you emphasize quality performance to the worker, you should first assure yourself that management has made every effort to support your message with a strong quality apparatus of its own. Without such action, there is really nothing for the worker to become aware of.

Actions Rather than Words

The real employee sell in the quality awareness phase is what has come to be known as "soft sell." The best method to use in achieving the goal of quality awareness is for management to set examples, and let the workers sell themselves. The product awareness phase will do some of this work for the Administrator. The fact that the supervisor has taken time to talk to him about the product and the fact that management has obviously gone out of its way to present the product story to him, proves to the worker that management does care about the product. Management feels that individual craftsmanship in turning out the product is a worthwhile goal.

Quality Information

The Administrator will probably use the regular lines of employee communications to present the quality awareness story (see Figure 26), but, as has been pointed out before, the general message must be brought down to the level of the individual task. The posting of group quality rates is a good example of this method (see Figure 27). Group quality data should be conspicuously posted on walls or hung from the ceiling. Charts should have titles such as "Quality Standing," with the section name or number below. The chart simply shows the percent of defective work for each group by week and month. It is a good idea to place an upper limit on the chart to warn the workers when their area is getting out of control. The supervisor must empha-

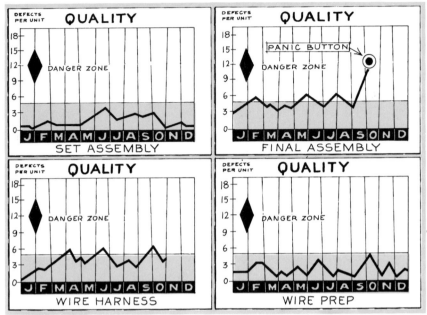

FIG. 27   Group-quality-level charts. These charts are usually posted during the quality awareness phase, with a Zero Defects goal, or "objective," line added once the program is kicked
off. A "panic button" or some other device should be used to highlight problem areas.

size that this line is not just something to stay below, but something to shun.

Two notes of caution regarding such charts: First, never chart the *individual*
workers. This causes ridicule of the poorer worker—a thing that Zero Defects
never does. Second, do not try to chart every area in your organization at
once. Take those that are already under quality audit first and, later in the
program, hit the hard-to-measure groups.

The competitive awards, mentioned earlier in the book, should be traveling
awards, and every posted group should be able to win one. Two large trophies
or large signs, reading "Best Quality Record of the Month" and "Most Improved Quality Record of the Month," should do the job quite well. Award
of the plaques or signs should be made on the floor with management representatives present. It is wise to remove the award from the previously recognized area the night before the award is made so that the loss is not openly
emphasized. The workers will be aware of it and will strive to get it back. If
loss of the award means public ridicule, no one will want it in the first place.

ECR AS A QUALITY AWARENESS FACTOR

The Error Cause Removal phase (see Chapter 6) of the Zero Defects program is a quality housecleaning effort aimed at the removal of all existing or

potential causes of error. It is the most positive action taken by management in the quality awareness campaign. As such, it will leave the strongest impression of any of the quality awareness activities.

Planning

The Administrator's first task will be to decide when to introduce ECR into his program. He may include it in the quality awareness portion of his program or use it as a sustaining factor after kickoff. Regardless of when it is used, the decision to go with an ECR phase should not be taken lightly. Even though it is a part of the overall program, it must be presented, sold, and initiated in much the same way, and with about the same effort, as the basic program itself. At the least, it will take a month to work out the details and prepare the material for this phase. Management involvement is just as great with ECR as it is with the program kickoff. The demands on supervision are higher than those of the regular program. But the rewards are so great that no company should do without ECR.

ECR Technique

So that the Administrator may fully understand the scope of this project, the following list of implementation steps is presented for his consideration.

1. *Management Review:* As with anything else in your organization, management makes ECR a reality. If ECR is to be implemented prior to kickoff, it will have to be presented in the Senior Executive briefing as a major program task. The same treatment will have to be given to the phase in top-management and mid-management briefings. Since ECR is a management action technique, all management and supervision must be willing to take the extra effort to make it work.

2. *Key Management Assistance:* The Administrator will find that one or two in-plant functions will be more involved with the program than others. Although over 90 percent of the ECRs acted on are corrected from within the originating department, the other 5 or 10 percent will require some outside support. This support usually involves facilities, maintenance, and other service functions. Since speed of action is one of the key prerequisites of a successful ECR phase, these people must be willing to move rapidly on any request made by the Administrator. Unfortunately, in most organizations, these same service groups are already overworked and usually find it difficult to meet existing requirements. It will be up to the Administrator to convince these groups that ECR is important enough to receive the extra effort the phase requires. If ECR has already won the support of top management, this task should prove much easier.

3. *Supervisor Indoctrination and Motivation:* Since the first-line supervisor is the true key to the success of this phase (he will be doing most of the work), he must be given detailed indoctrination into the philosophy, techniques, and

rewards of ECR. You cannot expect to accomplish this feat in the same meeting used to introduce the basic program. A special staff meeting should be called by the manager who in turn will endorse this phase to his supervisors. The Administrator or area representative will then brief the supervisors on the phase. He will show them how ECR can make it easier to sell the ZD concept. He will also show the supervisor how ECR will improve his (the supervisor's) image with his people and management and stress the extra effort necessary to assure quality of product. Last, but not least, he will show the supervisor how and why workers will have greater respect for the supervisor who has the individual's interests at heart.

Again, this task will seem like "one more thing on my overworked shoulders" to the supervisor. For this reason, the Administrator and management should make every effort to point out any and every personal advantage the supervisor will receive from ECR. Since, by this time, ECR will be a policy fact of life, the supervisor will not have the opportunity to accept or reject it; but he can certainly defeat its purpose if he does not give the phase his complete support.

To help the supervisor in his day-to-day ECR tasks, the Administrator should prepare an ECR supervisors' handbook. This need not be an expensive production, but rather a small booklet showing how to fill out the forms, how to act on a worker request, how to say no and still retain the worker's

FIG. 28   Promotion sheet showing the "why" and the "how" of the Error Cause Removal phase.

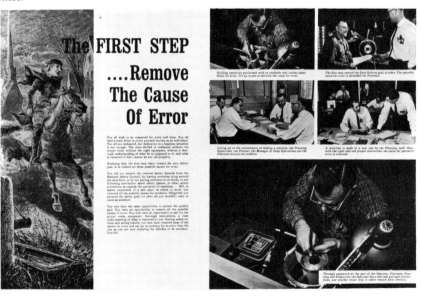

support and enthusiasm, and other details of the program. The handbook will also eliminate confusion between ECR and other employee suggestion programs. The "suggestion" forms available to the worker must be fully covered. (A copy of such a handbook is found in Appendix D of this book.)

4. *Employee Indoctrination:* The phase should be presented to the workers by the supervisor. Whenever possible, management and the Administrator or one of his representatives should be present. After hearing about the program from the supervisor, the individual workers should be presented with a copy of the ECR form and a brief information sheet. This information should be backed up by other information media: articles in company publications, bulletin-board notices, and posters (see Figure 28). Regardless of the extent of this type of support, never allow your communications media to take the place of face-to-face supervisor/worker contact.

5. *Form Use:* The basic ECR form, or Error Cause Identification (ECI), is usually a numbered, three-part, snap-out form (see Appendix C). The forms are made available to the worker from the supervisor or in conveniently located racks (see Figure 29). The worker fills in the first page of the ECI and submits it to his supervisor, who then checks over the entries to be sure the individual has provided all the necessary information. If the form is complete, the supervisor tears off the last sheet which contains the number of the form and a note from the ZD Administrator thanking the worker for taking the time to identify a cause of error. This is the worker's record, which can be used for follow-up later if needed.

6. *Supervisor Action:* If the supervisor can remedy the situation at section level, he should do this at once and report his solution on the back of the form. He then calls in the worker and informs him of the action to be taken. The employee signs the ECI stating whether or not he is satisfied with the findings (they almost always are). The worker receives one copy of the form as evidence that management has acted upon his request; the other copy goes back to the Administrator (see Figure 30).

7. *Special Action:* There will be a few cases—not many—in which the supervisor can't handle the Error Cause Identification within his own section or through the normal operational avenues open to him. In these cases he first checks with his manager to see if the latter can resolve the problem. If the error cause can't be corrected within the department, the supervisor notes this fact on the back of the ECI, along with any suggestions of his own, and passes the form along to the ZD Administrator or representative. The key management assistance (noted in step 2) now comes into play. The Administrator reviews the form and through his offices resolves the ECI in one way or another. The form is then returned to the supervisor for presentation to the worker.

8. *Negative Replies:* If the supervisor has thoroughly explained the purpose of the ECR phase and the method of using this valuable tool, there will be

few cases where negative replies are necessary. When one occurs (and it will), he should take extra time and use tact in passing the decision on to the worker. Such replies may be occasioned by: confusion with pure cost-effectiveness situations, imagined or unreal cause identifications, or ECIs that do not deal with error cause at all. An example of the last case would be a worker reporting that a certain work procedure should be changed because it is causing him to make errors. The supervisor checks and finds that the worker doesn't understand the procedure and explains it carefully, showing him how the procedure, properly used, actually helps prevent errors. The result is no change in procedure but a better-satisfied and more productive worker. Another case would be a worker who states that he feels that all workers having over three years service should get three weeks vacation per year. He does not equate this statement at all with error or error prevention, except to say that workers would work "better" if they had more time off. Here the supervisor must use tact in explaining that the ECR form is for identification of specific causes of error to be changed so that the individual can do his job right the first time. The ECI is not a company-policy complaint sheet or a suggestion-box item. From this point on the supervisor should handle the problem in the manner he feels suits the individual. He should try to stimulate the employee's thinking in the right direction by giving him some examples of real causes of error identified by his fellow workers.

FIG. 29 Error Cause Identification blanks should be placed in convenient locations in all work areas or be made readily available through the supervisor.

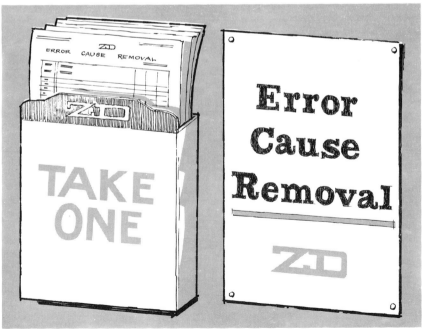

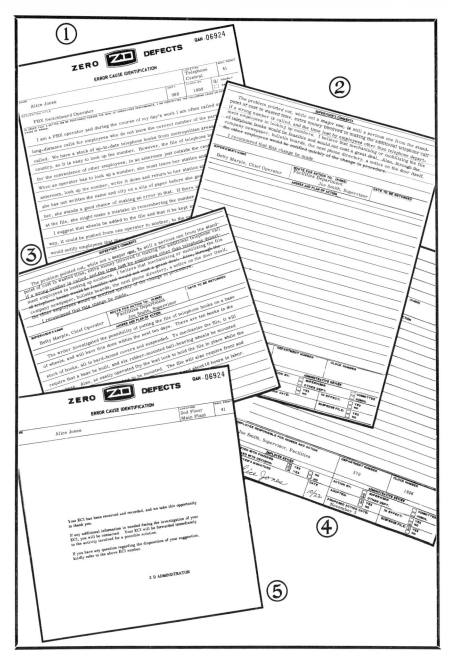

FIG. 30 ECR-form procedure. The employee fills out the ECI identifying a possible cause for error and makes a suggestion for correcting the situation (1). She gives the form to her supervisor and receives the Administrator's acknowledgment sheet (5) with reference number in the upper left-hand corner. The supervisor investigates the ECI, finds it valid, and sends it on to the facilities department for action (2). The facilities representative investigates further and decides to follow the suggestion on the ECI (3). The supervisor presents the findings to the employee, and the latter signs off as being satisfied with the action taken (4).

9. *Administrator Review:* The Administrator reviews the forms to see if the error-cause identifications and their solutions have applications in other areas of the company. Where they do, he passes the information along to the managers or representatives in those areas. When he finds an outstanding case of supervisory action or a case that could be of interest to the entire operation, he passes it along to the company publication or other appropriate media for its obvious publicity value (see Figure 31).

Once a month, the Administrator should issue a list of actions by the various department supervisors. This list along with copies of the forms noting outstanding actions are sent to each department manager, thus assuring the supervisor that his efforts will not go unnoticed.

If upon review of the completed forms, the Administrator notes a surge of "no action" entries coming from a particular area or supervisor, he should follow up accordingly. Occasionally, one supervisor will say no to everything without trying to discover if the suggestion has merit. In such a case, the Administrator should also check the forms for the content of the negative replies. "We can't do it" is not enough of a reply for the worker. The answer must indicate serious consideration of the ECI.

To review: The ECR phase will be only as successful as the degree of extra effort by supervision allows it to be. The supervisor will cooperate only when

FIG. 31 A simple, typed information sheet can be used to distribute information about error-cause discoveries with organization-wide application. This same vehicle can also be used to recognize groups and individuals submitting ECIs.

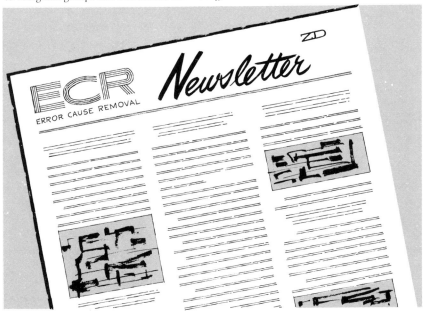

ECR PHASE PLAN

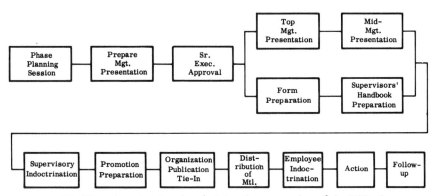

FIG. 32   Flow chart showing the administrative sequencing of the ECR phase.

he is assured that management will recognize his effort and that management feels the phase is worthwhile. Management will not endorse the phase until the Administrator has shown that the ECR concept is of value and that valuable supervisory time or effort will not be wasted. And the Administrator can't give this assurance without the backing of the Senior Executive and several key members of his staff (see Figure 32). Although it may seem like a vicious circle, a well-run ECR phase is one of the most rewarding systems ever found for the betterment of management/employee relations.

General Quality-promotion Techniques

To complement the ECR activities, management emphasis, and communication-media stress on quality awareness, the Administrator may wish to carry out a specialized poster campaign for added impact. This may consist of a pre-printed poster format having a quality message with room for the addition of specific quality-achievement information. Thus, when a group or the whole organization are involved in key product deliveries, receive customer praise, or earn any other quality achievement, the information can be quickly and inexpensively added to the specific poster areas concerned. Small table tents can be used for the same purpose. The prime aim of such action is to let the individual know that management appreciates quality achievement. These posters can also be used to highlight ECR suggestions which have application in several sectors of the organization.

OVERALL TIMING

The product and quality awareness phases, including ECR, provide the necessary foundation on which the Administrator builds his Zero Defects program. The events and activities during this period should be scheduled to increase gradually in tempo as the kickoff date approaches. By that time the workers will be well aware that something is going to happen and will be anticipating the next move. That move—the kickoff—is discussed in the next chapter.

Up to this point, the term Zero Defects has not been mentioned to the rank-and-file employee. Only management is aware of the full impact and the depth of the entire program. Once the kickoff or turning point is reached, terms such as "product awareness" and "quality awareness" should be replaced by "Zero Defects products" and "defect-free performance." The message remains the same, only the names have been changed. The techniques used in the readiness portion of the program should not be discarded. They continue to be part of the whole program and, as such, should even be accelerated after kickoff day.

9

Kickoff Readiness

The kickoff phase of Zero Defects is primarily a management communications program. This is not to say that it is an advertising campaign. As was pointed out earlier, the real program sell will be accomplished through face-to-face manager/worker contact. All promotional aspects of the program must support such contact. This chapter deals with the promotional and administrative tools that support the kickoff and the various activities surrounding this important day.

Care

Zero Defects communications differ very little from other worthwhile management/employee communications except that they must meet one special criterion—they must be defect-free. For instance: A general manager speaking before hundreds of workers can't carry out a Zero Defects theme if his audio system goes dead in the middle of his talk; a poster won't motivate workers when the copy reads "Zero Defcts. It's up to you!"; a pledge card doesn't have much meaning when half the message is smeared in printing. Defect-free communication tools require a little more effort and cost a little more money, but, in this case, the end result can influence the success or failure of your kickoff. This requirement for perfection extends to everything from a memo to a company-wide rally. The media, whether oral, printed, or filmed, speak for the program, and the program speaks for management.

KICKOFF-TECHNIQUE SELECTION

There are three basic impressions of the program that planners should try to get across during its introduction: (1) its challenge, (2) management support, and (3) its importance to the individual and his role in it. There are dozens of techniques for presenting this message. Selection of the best method will be up to the planning committee of each implementing organization. The two most common techniques are built around a carefully planned system of supervisory indoctrination, coupled with either an operation-wide rally or smaller departmental meetings and management visits. The most successful approach is a combination of both—a large, impressive rally followed by smaller departmental meetings. This, in turn, gives the program impact as well as the personal management touch.

The advantage of the rally is that it provides a central location for distribution of material and presents an impressive show of management endorsement for the workers (see Figure 33). It gives the implementing organization a time and place for everything. Its shortcomings include the logistic problems of getting all of the workers to one spot at one time; the impersonal aspect of a large rally (where no personal follow-up is planned); and the fact that an error in presentation could possibly be made before the entire organization.

Smaller meetings have the advantage of being more personal; they disrupt the work schedule less than the rally; and they eliminate the need for moving large groups of people from one place to another (see Figure 34). The disadvantages of the smaller meetings include increased material-distribution problems; difficult scheduling of management and worker meetings; and the simple fact that the Administrator has more elements to control.

Both techniques require extensive presentation preparations. The small-meeting technique will require more coverage by all available media. It is fairly simple to decorate a hall and provide backup audio equipment for one pedestal. When meetings are being held throughout the organization, it will be necessary to blanket your plant with promotional material to provide a backdrop wherever a manager, supervisor, or company officer is speaking. In many cases, these men will also need special equipment to support their talks.

PROGRAM PROMOTION

Promotional material supporting the program usually falls into four categories: backdrop or poster presentations; brochures, advertisements and newspaper and magazine articles; training aids; and special support items. All must, in some way, convey the basic challenge of the program, and all should be of the quality and caliber to convince the employee that management really means business. A factor that always works in the program's favor is that, even though companies spend millions of dollars and thousands of man-hours talking to their customers, rarely is even a limited promotional campaign ever directed toward the employee. About the only thing he ever sees is a conglomeration of safety, security, and union-news sheets tacked to a congested board behind the water cooler. Thus, a simple show of posters, signs, booklets,

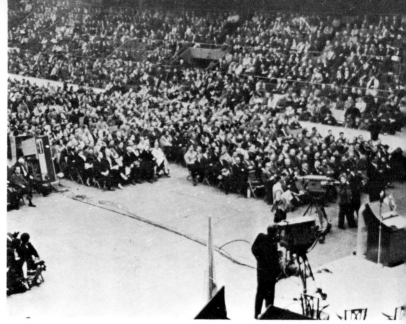

FIG. 33   A large rally—in this case, the Boston Gardens kickoff of GE's Small Aircraft Engine Department (7,000).

and pins makes the employee stand up and take notice. Of course, the more *meaningful* the promotion is, the heavier the initial impact and the greater the show of management interest.

Media Review

As in the earlier phases, the first step in promotional technique selection is a review of existing media. Since most organizations have bulletin boards, poster frames or easels, an organization newspaper, and other forms of day-to-day employee communications, all of these can be used to great advantage if properly woven into your overall communications package. A key factor to remember is that, when ZD is introduced, it should not share the spotlight with any other program. It deserves its own exclusive showcase.

In-house Program Planning

For the first two or three weeks, the ZD message should stand alone. Many organizations have extended this single-message technique to all of their in-house activities. For instance, rather than keeping up a steady flow of ZD promotion, the program is promoted on a regular schedule, alternating with other in-house campaigns such as safety, security, bond drives, etc. The people involved in the other activities are usually cooperative and welcome the opportunity for more effective use of employee communications tools.

Sharing

Though a certain amount of ZD promotion must be tailored to the implementing organization, a wealth of existing material in industry and

95

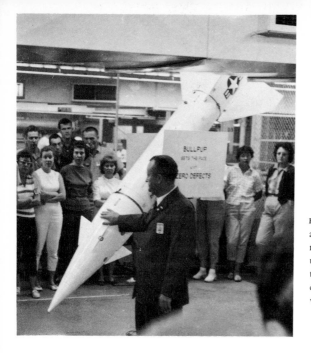

FIG. 34 A department kickoff, where an organization-wide presentation was not feasible. When this technique is used, it is advisable to complete all of the small kickoff programs on a single day in order to maintain organization-wide impact.

government, general enough to be used anywhere, is available. It will pay the Administrator to review this material and to arrange with other ZD Administrators to copy or use this ready-to-go promotional support. Very little of the existing Zero Defects promotional material has been copyrighted. Administrators generally welcome the opportunity to share promotion material (as well as measurement techniques, recognition methods, etc.) with other ZD organizations. It may even be advisable to leave the originator's logo or identification on the piece, thus letting the worker know that his organization is not alone in this venture. In most cases, implementing organizations are willing to lend print mechanicals or negatives, cutting your production costs greatly.

PROMOTIONAL TOOLS

The actual promotional tools selected by the Administrator and his staff will naturally vary with the organization. But the quality of such material and the extent of the coverage should always be the very best the organization can muster. The following list of promotional devices have won wide acceptance in major program kickoffs. The starred items are considered necessary to the success of any Zero Defects operation. The unstarred items are offered as suggestions, but, as noted before, final selection will depend on the needs of the particular organization. Do not let this list limit you, but rather, be creative. Try to devise several original items for your own program.

Backdrop or Poster-type Presentations (See Figures 35a and 35b).

Teaser Posters: generally used the week before kickoff. This poster technique will add to the suspense or anticipation of the program. Most posters of this type are designed around a build-up technique, revealing a bit more information about the program each day and disclosing "Zero Defects" on the kickoff day. One method of design consists of making a jigsaw out of the poster and adding a key piece each day. Other companies have used a certain character who, after kickoff, becomes the trademark of the program. These characters have included everything from a Zorro-type caricature to a cartooned astronaut.

Kickoff Posters: usually announce the program kickoff and contain some program message such as "Do it right the first time" or "Prevention, not detection." Do not try to put too much information on these early posters. If you can get the program name across and impart some meaning to that name, the poster has done its job. The final poster in the teaser series will also serve as a kickoff-day backdrop poster.

Banners: used in areas where poster presentation is difficult. They can be hung on the walls in cafeterias, high-bay areas, or on outside walls. The message should be coordinated with the kickoff poster.

Gate Signs: highly effective in multibuilding plants. Outdoor signs placed at key traffic areas with messages facing both incoming and outgoing traffic will help to assure complete employee coverage.

Bus Cards: simply a variation of the posters, placed in or on all company vehicles.

Flags: can be hung below the American flag or on a special mast in a conspicuous location.

Table Tents: used mainly in clerical, management, and other office areas, where poster or banner placements are impractical. They may also be used in congested shop areas.

Stickers: usually placed on high-use items, such as pencil sharpeners, time clocks, water coolers, or glass doors.

Portal Signs: hung over entrances and exits of the plant or office. The message usually informs the reader that he is entering or leaving a Zero Defects organization.

Brochures, Ads, and Articles

General Information Booklet: handed out the morning of, or the evening before, the kickoff. This need not be an elaborate production, but, as with the other material, the copy and production should be defect-free. The booklet will inform the employee about the program, its philosophy, and its challenge.

Paycheck Inserts: inserted into paycheck envelopes. If this technique is used, try to arrange the kickoff so that it falls on payday. To give the item secondary use, some organizations have printed a wallet-size ZD calendar on one side of the insert.

Tie-in Advertising: to be used in the company and in the local press. One technique is to print in-plant teaser posters in the same daily sequence as

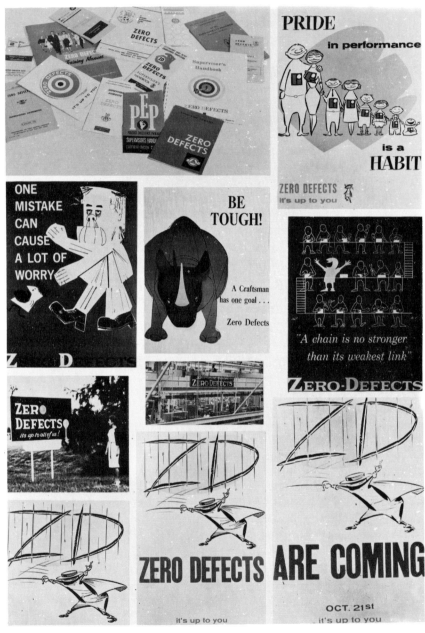

FIG. 35a   Assortment of kickoff aids and promotional pieces. The series of posters in the bottom row was used as "teasers," building up to kickoff day when the center poster identified the program.

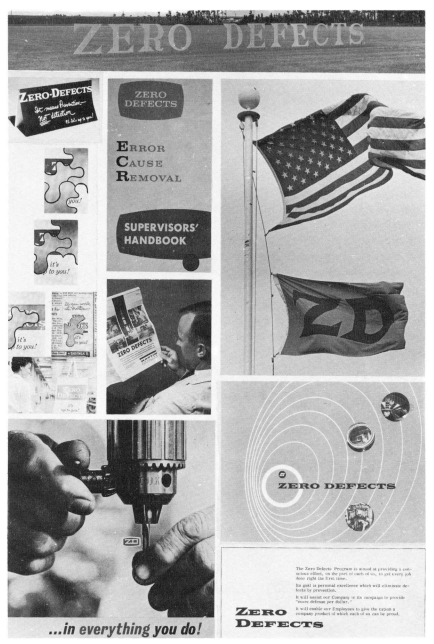

FIG. 35*b* More kickoff promotion. Another teaser series is at left center. The item on the right with the circular pattern is an employee-information brochure of the type distributed by many of the larger organizations on the evening prior to kickoff.

advertisements placed in the local press. If the budget allows, this can also be carried on TV. On kickoff day, local press coverage can be supported by reproducing a kickoff poster in the paper. This technique is recommended where the implementing organization is of major importance to the community.

*Company Publications:** The kickoff should be coordinated with the publication of the company's paper or internal news medium. The entire issue, or as much of it as possible, should be devoted to the program. Additionally, a special ZD issue should be planned, to feature follow-up articles and broad photo coverage of the events of kickoff day.

Training Aids

*Supervisors' Handbook:** prepared early in the program for supervisor indoctrination (see Appendix D). This book will be a valuable tool for the supervisor during his employee-indoctrination sessions.

Training Films: may be borrowed or specifically prepared, depending on budget limitations. Many such films are available throughout government and industry and can be used in earlier management-indoctrination sessions as well as on kickoff day. They are particularly effective as indoor-rally support items.

Charts and Slides: used in smaller indoctrination sessions at the discretion of the person doing the briefing. The Administrator should review all such material to assure that these visual aids meet program standards—that they do, in fact, present the Zero Defects concept and philosophy in the best possible light.

Special Support Items

*Pledge Cards:** used by almost every ZD organization to date. This card has a brief explanation of the program on one side and a formal pledge for the employee's signature on the other (see Appendix A). Some organizations have included a wallet-size tear-off for the employee to keep. Many organizations have a counter-signature line for the supervisor's acknowledgement of the employee pledge. There are two basic things to remember here: (1) be sure the wording states the employee will constantly "strive" toward perfection—he is not pledging never to make a mistake again; (2) devise some way of following up and tabulating the number of employees signing. To ensure the latter, many companies have printed pledge cards on punch cards so that fast tallies can be made on their business machines. Knowing the number of people signing the pledge will give the Administrator a good idea of the general acceptance of the program and will highlight potential problem areas.

*Sign-up Recognition Pins:** used by management to recognize workers who accept the Zero Defects challenge (see Figure 36). This is a case of "do it well or don't do it at all." To be effective, the pin or badge must be of such quality that the employee will wish to wear it. It must be durable enough to stand long-term use. Most employees wear their pins daily and continue to

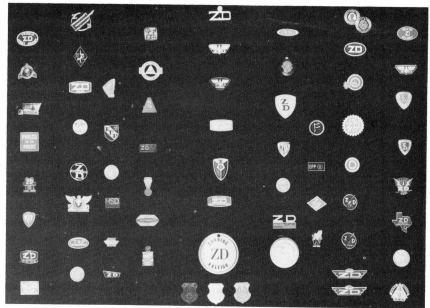

FIG. 36   A selection of industry and government ZD pins.

wear them several years after kickoff. Since the pin will be the largest single program expenditure, great care should be used in design and style. Many organizations plan to use the same design later in the program in an achievement-recognition pin (see Chapter 14). This is done by casting the same pin in a different metal or using different color enamels on subsequent pins. Either technique saves extra design and die costs later in the program. Another cost-reduction technique in pin selection is the use of an existing ZD pin design. There are now hundreds of designs to choose from, and many carry no company identification. Other ZD Administrators will be happy to pass on the name of their supplier and give permission for additional runs on their dies. Most pins in use today cost from 20 to 30 cents each on orders of 1,000 or more. When ordering, be sure to allow for new hires and possible pin losses during the first program year.

Luncheon Specials: Where the organization has its own cafeteria, arrangements can be made for a special ZD luncheon on kickoff day. This consists of a specially priced meal available to anyone wearing a ZD pin.

Giveaways: A wide variety of giveaway or premium items have been used by ZD organizations. To be effective, these items should be restricted to useful items that actually help the employee perform his day-to-day tasks, for instance: slide rules that call out parts selections, pocket-size conversion tables, or soldering brushes. Imprinted standard items, such as combs, key chains, etc., are costly and not as effective.

A final reminder: Do not use this list as the final promotional word.

Improve on it, add to it, or make deletions from it as your organizational needs dictate.

THE INTRODUCTORY MESSAGE

At kickoff, the Zero Defects message should be presented as simply as possible. Posters and other forms of "one glance" promotion should stick to the standard, meaningful ZD slogans: "ZD means prevention, not detection" or "Zero Defects—do it right the first time." Wherever these slogans or messages can be tied to the product, do so. This is certainly no time to let up on product awareness.

Other media such as the company publications, booklets, or management talks will present the full story. On kickoff day, the prime message is that it is possible *and rewarding* to strive constantly to do everything right the first time. To get this point across, the kickoff will obviously need more than a few slogans.

A common technique in both speech and copy is to make comparisons between the worker's personal life and his job. Some of the elements from the ZD philosophy (see Chapter 1) can be used to this end, for instance: "How many times a week do you wear one black and one brown shoe to work?" or "How often do you get short-changed in cashing your paycheck?" Faced with such obvious "never" answer questions, the employee is ready to be asked: "If you can accomplish perfection in one thing, then why not in another—your job?" The double standard can also be exposed by questioning the worker in this manner: "You certainly don't expect your doctor or dentist or automobile mechanic to make mistakes. Why do you condone error in your day-to-day job?"

The main point in all kickoff communications is to bring the message to the level of the individual worker. If Zero Defects is just something for management or "the company," the worker will be less than receptive. When he can relate it to his own personal life, he will be more likely to accept it.

LAST-MINUTE CHECKS

During the last few days prior to kickoff, the Administrator and his staff should review every piece of promotion, every activity, and every support item that has anything to do with the kickoff. A slipup at this time could be disastrous. To discover that a key element is missing on kickoff day could seriously impair the overall effectiveness of the entire program introduction.

Rallies

If a large employee rally is planned, every item connected with the affair should be checked and double-checked. All audio and visual systems should have at least one backup. Speakers' commitments should be verified. All protocol should be worked out. An escort should be assigned to each visitor to assure that he gets to the program on time. All management schedules should be reviewed, and basic speech outlines prepared if requested. Every participant should be allowed to make a dry run of his speech and to review the program. Where worker transportation is necessary, all arrangements should be reviewed and special traffic assignments made.

It is also imperative to have an after-the-rally plan. The day's activities do not end with a "thank you and good-bye" at the close of the rally. Management and guest visits to work areas should continue throughout the day.

Departmental Kickoffs

If the management of each department is handling its own kickoff, support problems increase. Where necessary, a specific time should be scheduled for such activities. Audio equipment should be scheduled accordingly. Special props, such as product models and lecture cards, should be placed in the areas well ahead of time. Visits by the Senior Executive and his staff should be planned to coincide with departmental activities. The ZD committee's scheduling expert will really earn his salary in this type of kickoff.

Media Distribution

Since promotional materials will probably be distributed the night before kickoff, key distribution points should be set up well in advance. A special team should have specific assignments concerning the location and setup procedure for all such material. Since actual setup will have to take place in a short time (in order that the workers do not become aware of the preparation), this team will have to be exceptionally well organized.

Pin and Pledge-card Distribution

Both of these items must be available on kickoff morning. If the cards are to be passed out at a rally, the logistics problem is easier. If the supervisors distribute the cards (the suggested way) and present the pins, then every supervisor will have to know ahead of time the location of such material. If at all possible, arrangements should be made for a team to deliver these items to the supervisors on the morning of the kickoff.

Pledge Tabulation

Some technique for rapid tabulation of sign-up should be arranged. A card-pickup and pledge-count system should go into effect the morning following kickoff. This count will enable the Administrator to inform the workers of the extent of the program sign-up.

Troubleshooting Service

On kickoff day, one or more special telephone numbers should be set aside for emergency calls. Either the Administrator, one of his representatives, or

104 ZERO DEFECTS IN ACTION

one of his committee members should be on hand at all times to answer any calls. All management, supervisors, union officials, and anyone else concerned with the kickoff activities should be provided with a card listing these numbers. This way, such problems as shortages of pledge cards or pins, missing speakers, special audio-equipment needs, and other potential hazards and defects can be rapidly overcome and solved.

SUMMING UP

Once again, the key point to remember is that this is a Zero Defects program. If the Administrator and his management team act accordingly, the kickoff will be an outstanding success.

10

Program Kickoff

The complete scope of a well-organized program kickoff can best be realized by considering the actual activities surrounding the event. This chapter will take you through the program-kickoff activities for a medium-sized industrial organization. Though every event and technique discussed may not be applicable to your organization's needs, it is best to consider each carefully to comprehend the planning and coordination techniques behind the overall program. The kickoff discussed here never actually took place; it is a composite of several successful program plans and of the experiences of the hundreds of individuals administratively involved.

SETTING THE STAGE

The kickoff you are about to study is being held in a city of about 200,000 people. The company is a medium-sized division of a large appliance company. The 4,000 employees represent almost all of the trades and professions usually found in such an organization—production, engineering, research, administration, sales, marketing, shipping, and maintenance. A month of extensive ECR activity and a product and quality awareness campaign have just been completed. The kickoff will take place this Friday.

TEAM REVIEW

Midweek, the Administrator calls his team together for an assignment review and for reports on preparations. This group includes his original planning committee, his department representatives, and the other special staff members assigned to this particular project.

The promotion committee member reviews all the materials and media to be used during the kickoff. He shows examples of each so that all attendees are familiar with them. He then reviews distribution plans for all items and locations of special stockpiles in case shortages occur on kickoff day. He also discusses promotion setup plans and informs the Administrator where extra help will be needed in readying the plant and offices. He also covers the rally-support preparations, including setup and rehearsal times. He provides every attendee with a copy of his schedule and a list of material-pickup locations.

The Administrator next reviews the techniques for providing supervisor tools and assistance. It is planned to hold brief supervisor meetings in each department on Thursday, during which the ZD representatives will brief the supervisors and provide them with pins and pledge cards for each worker in their groups. The promotion representative affirms that the supervisors' kits are ready for pickup at a certain location. Each of the representatives reports that he has a backup ready in case of sickness, etc. All are cautioned to check out each supervisor in the department to assure that none is missed.

The rally chairman (in this case, the employee relations committee member) reports on rally plans and procedures. He runs through special-guest-escort assignments and confirms the fact that key management is available for the program. All key management members and special guests have been pre-briefed on the program earlier in the week. A rundown of audio-visual equipment and its backup is made, and the actual program is reviewed. Seating and protocol questions are then ironed out, and a rehearsal schedule is set. A team is assigned to set up the hall (in this case, a large warehouse next to the main plant), and seating capacities are reviewed.

A representative from the plant security force reviews the exit and return time schedules and reports on critical traffic areas. Several changes are made in the overall evacuation plan, and an alternate plan is made in case of inclement weather. An awning has been provided for the most heavily traveled route in case of rain.

The Administrator then checks his master list of assignments and points out potential problem areas. He emphasizes the importance of rapid reporting of employee sign-up and the need for tight coordination in case of unexpected problems. He presents each attendee with a card listing numbers to call for special equipment needs, emergency management or union action, and administrative advice. He reminds each of the importance of error-free performance and offers to answer any last-minute questions.

KICKOFF EVE

On Thursday morning, the department managers and ZD representatives brief the supervisors. Each supervisor is given an envelope containing pins, pledge cards, and a kickoff schedule of events program. Times are announced for special departmental ZD meetings, and the supervisors are reminded not to discuss the program with employees before kickoff. Extra copies of the supervisors' handbook are made available to any who have misplaced their books.

Later, the promotion representative distributes posters, banners, tent cards, signs, and other material to the special setup locations. Folding chairs have been moved into the rally area, and an audio-visual team has installed and checked out all systems. The hall decorations have been delivered but are not yet put up since employees must move through the area during the day.

Promotion Setup

As each employee leaves the plant on Thursday night, he receives a small brochure explaining the basic concept and philosophy of Zero Defects. This is the first time the rank and file have heard the name used. The fact that the brochure is handed out the night before kickoff will not lessen the impact. It will, in fact, increase it. The brochure will develop more curiosity since it does not go into program details but centers its attention on philosophy and concept.

As soon as the workers have left the plant, the setup team moves into unoccupied areas and begins preparations for the next day. A group is assigned to each floor in each building to expedite the work. Another group takes care of the hall decorations. When they finish, several of the speakers go through dry runs on their talks and film and slide presentations are test-run. A special crew of maintenance men (prebriefed on the program) help set up heavier promotional items, such as parking-lot signs, large letters spelling out Zero Defects on the front lawn, and large banners hanging in the manufacturing areas.

Administrator Review

Once setup is complete, all workers report to the Administrator so that he can check off the specific areas. (If well organized, the work can be done in a few hours, even in a large installation.) The Administrator tours all areas to assure complete coverage and rally readiness. He takes along a small crew on this tour to help him in case an area has been missed or changes are necessary. Only after the Administrator is completely satisfied with every part of the setup should he call it a day. Kickoff morning is not the time to make repairs or changes.

KICKOFF DAY

In the morning, the Administrator and his team arrive on the scene ahead of the rank and file. As the employees arrive, they see a ZD message wherever they turn. Since they have read the folder given them the previous evening, they know the reason for this coverage, but they are not quite sure of the full impact of the program. By the time they reach their work areas, there is no doubt in their minds that management is "really up to something." The first person the employee turns to for information is his supervisor. The supervisor informs them that the full significance of the program will be explained at a big rally at nine o'clock that morning. He answers some of their questions about the program but asks them to wait until after the rally for the more specific ones.

Rally Arrangements

During this time, the guest speakers have been escorted to the rally area. They are all given a final briefing and are shown where they will sit during the affair. All management speakers and the Senior Executive attend this session and then move to their places as the time approaches for the rally to begin. At this time, the public relations representative is giving the final briefing to the local press, TV, and radio people. He provides them with press kits containing information on the kickoff and future plans.

At a prearranged signal, in this case a series of blasts from the plant alarm systems, supervisors bring their employees to the rally (see Figures 37 and 38). As they are being seated, a slide presentation of poster art, slogans, and other ZD information is shown on the screen. Once they are all in their seats, the Senior Executive opens the rally.

The Rally

The Senior Executive welcomes everyone present and introduces nonspeaking guests, including the mayor of the city, state congressmen, and local dignitaries. He delivers the keynote address of the program, discussing the importance of individual achievement to the company, the product, the customer, and, of course, the employees themselves. This is followed by a film of interviews with customers—each speaking about the product and what he or she expects from it. The film also points out a few of the disastrous effects of serious errors that could possibly cause harm or discomfort to the user.

The Senior Executive then introduces the ZD Administrator who explains just what Zero Defects can do to assure the company and the customer of the best possible product at the lowest possible price. The Administrator discusses the key points of the program and offers the ZD challenge not only to each employee in the audience but to management, the union, the guests, and the Senior Executive. An oversized, symbolic pledge card has been provided for

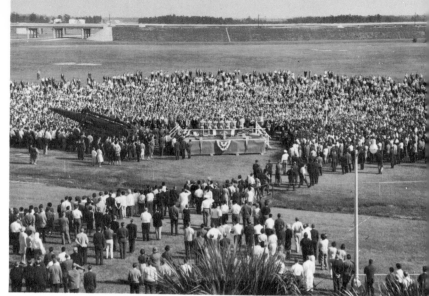

FIG. 37   The logistics problems of a rally are extensive, but the end result is usually impressive. This is an 8,000-worker outside rally at a large defense plant.

each of the speakers to sign. The Senior Executive explains the pledge and is the first to sign.

The next person to talk is a customer—in this case, the president of the company's largest chain outlet. He endorses the program and tells the workers just how important he, the customer, considers the efforts of each and every one of them. After his talk, the presidents of the local unions address the group. (Though there is no firm protocol, it is best to check with labor relations on the recommended order of appearance.) Each speaker endorses the program to his members and offers some words on craftsmanship and the fact that it is a union worker's obligation to do his best at all times.

The Senior Executive now introduces the guest of honor. In this case it is a United States senator, who speaks of the government's interest in the program. He discusses the value of Zero Defects to the nation's economy and its place in the free world. (This guest can be anyone from the chairman of the board, the inventor of the organization's most successful product, a prominent figure in the national government, or a famous consumer, to the ZD Administrator of another organization.)

The close is handled by the Senior Executive, who wraps up the ZD challenge and asks each worker to go back to his area, to consider the program, and if he is willing, to accept the ZD way of life and sign the pledge. [This wrap-up speaker can be any member of the management team who is (1) a good speaker, and (2) respected and known by the rank and file.]

Supervisor Follow-up

Upon their return to their work areas, the employees are presented pledge cards by the supervisors, who explain the pledge and all of its implications.

109

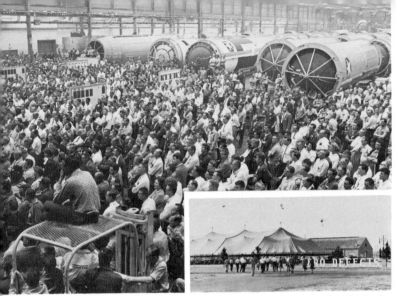

FIG. 38 Two large rallies: the main photograph shows an inside rally in the manufacturing area of a major defense contractor; the inset shows a tent rally used where there was no building available because of the size of the audience.

Pins are presented to those who sign (see Figure 39), and the cards are turned in to the representatives.

Later in the day, department and divisional managers visit the work areas to speak to the employees about their specific tasks (see Figure 40). At these sessions, the supervisor introduces the managers to the employees and the management representatives point out the goals for each specific area and task. Managers with small departments accomplish this briefing by speaking to individuals and small groups. Managers of large departments call group meetings and, with the help of the supervisors, try to personalize the message as much as possible. This is done by picking employee tasks at random and by speaking about a good cross-section of the departmental activities.

Other Activities

During the day, other general employee activities are taking place. A ZD lunch (at a special price) is being offered in the cafeteria (see Figure 41). Since it is Friday (payday), special ZD inserts have been put in pay envelopes. In truth, everything in the organization has been "ZD-ized" for the day. On their way out of offices and factory, employees will be handed a special ZD edition of the company paper. On their way home they will hear ZD messages over their car radios. That night, they will read about their activities in the local paper and will see an ad featuring the pledge and the challenge the organization has taken upon itself.

Administrator Follow-up

During all these activities, the Administrator and his temporary staff have not been idle. They have been seeing that supervisors who need extra pins

110

get them; they have been escorting guests and the local press through the plant for visits and interviews with the employees; they have solved the problem of a union steward who did not attend the rally and asked his workers not to sign the pledge—and so it goes. After the first shift, they begin on the second shift. Since fewer numbers are involved, the task is less complex, but it is nonetheless demanding. The kickoff will not be over until every employee in the plant has been indoctrinated and presented with the challenge of Zero Defects. This may take several weeks, what with vacations, sickness, and out-of-town assignments.

The Days that Follow

The Administrator's next task is to become better informed so that he may inform others. He will now collate all sign-up information and post the results on large cards displayed throughout the organization (see Figure 42). The count must be accurate; the closer it comes to 100 percent, the more obvious the position of the nonsigners becomes. Special bulletin-board releases carry the current count and show photos of kickoff-day activities. All the union leaders and other rally participants are presented with certificates recognizing their contribution to the program. Any department reaching 100 percent sign-up receives a special sign denoting the fact.

The Administrator checks and rechecks the sign-up records and ZD-representative reports to assure complete coverage. A noticeable lack of either from a given area usually indicates some type of organizational breakdown. Any members of management who were out of town or for some reason missed the kickoff-day activities are urged to visit their work areas and speak to the employees on the subject.

Committee Review

A week or ten days after the kickoff, the Administrator calls the ZD committee and key department representatives together for a kickoff-review meet-

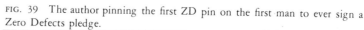

FIG. 39   The author pinning the first ZD pin on the first man to ever sign a Zero Defects pledge.

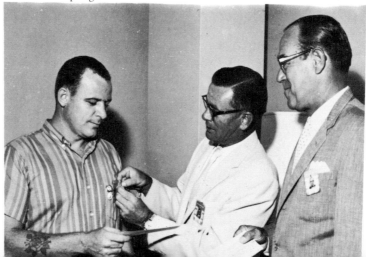

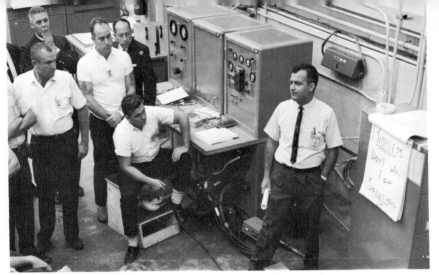

FIG. 40 Supervisor follow-up sessions fill in the gaps and answer important worker questions following the kickoff presentations.

ing. They discuss the reported impact of the program and its reception by the employees. Special areas and activities are pinpointed for more extensive follow-up. Once all reports are in and the Administrator has a firm picture of the overall kickoff effect, a special report should be prepared for the Senior Executive and other members of top management. This report also outlines plans for the coming months. The emphasis here is on measurement and recognition. The Administrator personally presents the reports, taking the opportunity to explain to each member of management his continuing program role. All levels of management are made aware that ZD is not a one-shot program; the real payoff comes only through total management commitment.

RECAP

The kickoff program discussed in this chapter contained all the elements necessary to present the program to the employees. Though the Administrator may wish to vary the activities to suit his own organization, the following results must be obtained:

1. All employees know and understand the challenge of Zero Defects.
2. Each employee understands his own role in the program.
3. The fact that management is 100 percent behind the program is made obvious.
4. Every employee understands the pledge he is making.
5. Management recognizes the individual for accepting the challenge.
6. Management recognizes the supervisor for his support.
7. The worker understands the program scope and the extent of sign-up.
8. All influencing elements (union, press, community leaders) understand and back the program.

9. All management becomes actively and personally involved in the program.

10. Each employee is given the opportunity to join the team, but none is ever coerced by management into accepting Zero Defects.

Regardless of the techniques used, if these results are obtained, the organization's Zero Defects program is well on its way to success.

SUSTAINING

Once the Administrator has completed his indoctrination task, he is ready to turn to the operational aspects of the program. Since achievement measurement and recognition are the keys to this effort, his next step will be to help management set up such procedures. The next three chapters deal with the problem of measurement. There is no reason why many of the measurement activities can't be worked out earlier in the program. Many organizations begin establishing measurement criteria at the same time that management is indoctrinated. Regardless of when this work is begun, most of the organization's work force should be under some type of audit, evaluation, or other form of measurement within a month or two after kickoff. People expect to see results, and ZD is a program that will give quick results if the organization has a way to measure and record them.

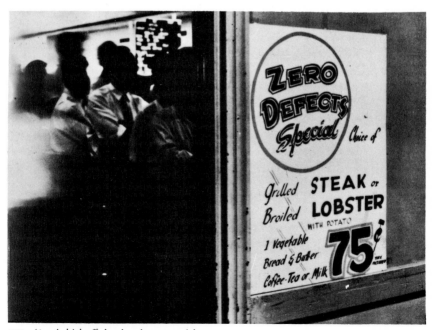

FIG. 41   A kickoff day luncheon special.

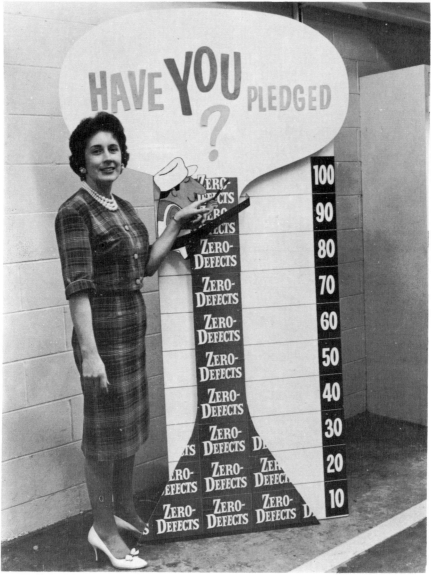

FIG. 42   A pledge-sign-up display showing the percent of organization participation.

The Administrator should plan to begin individual recognition six months after the program's implementation date. To do this and to provide some meaningful data about program trends for top management, he will have to move with all speed in this direction. It must be remembered that the Administrator can only advise and motivate. Management must set goals, direct employee interests, and recognize achievements. From this point on the program becomes, in truth, a management tool. And like any other tool, it must be used properly to give results.

PART 5

Performance Measurement

Measurement Techniques in
Three Basic Areas

11

Production-measurement Techniques

It is not our intent in the following chapters to present a treatise on measurement. This information is available in any good text on quality-control methods. No organization can become really serious about Zero Defects unless it has some sort of organized quality activity. In fact, it would normally be reasonable to assume that any successful business must have adopted certain performance standards to maintain its position in the market. Nevertheless, the question of measurement has come up repeatedly in Zero Defects seminars and workshops from coast to coast. Thus, some discussion of the subject appears to be necessary.

A word of caution: Management and the Administrator should not recklessly establish measurement values and standards throughout the organization at the expense of the basic ZD-program principles and activities. Complicated measurement systems may, to some degree, offset the beneficial results of the rest of the program effort. A frantic attempt to put every little activity in the organization under firm audit could prove twice as costly as the defect and reject expenses that brought about such action in the first place.

THE ROLE OF MEASUREMENT IN ZD

Measurement serves one basic purpose within the structure of the Zero Defects organization: it gives management the criteria upon which to base recognition. There are secondary values (as far as the program is concerned), such as problem-area highlighting, group-accomplishment awareness, and the reporting of the overall program payoff. This is not to deny the value of quality data for corrective action, but such activities fall into the detection area of production and not in the preventive (or ZD) area of employee motivation. In fact, one of the prime goals of ZD is to reduce the need for correction. The sharp reduction in material review board actions noted in Chapter 2 is evidence that the program is meeting such goals.

The reason for all of this concern about measurement can be summed up in one of the key program words—"awareness." Management must have some way of knowing when an individual has made a significant contribution to the program. The individual must be aware of the goals and criteria set by management in order to attempt to meet those goals. And the individual's fellow workers must be made aware of the fact that certain goals are being met by one of their own before they will all be truly convinced that ZD is a real and living program. False recognition or recognition of anything less than outstanding performance tells both the individual receiving such "honor" and the rest of the work force that management isn't really serious about outstanding effort at all. Thus, when management presents Zero Defects recognition to an individual, it must be sure that the action is deserved, that it will be understood by the individual, and that it will be accepted by the rest of the organization.

A New Desire for Measurement

Almost every organization has some form of audit or measurement in certain areas of its operation. This we call "established measurement." There are other areas that are actually under a form of audit, but since the auditing technique is not used for individual-defect information, it isn't apparent. An example would be insurance claims against damaged goods that are checked back against the names of the handlers and shippers involved. This we could call "indirect measurement." Both of these types of measurement or data collection are generally accepted by both worker and management as part of day-to-day operations. Now, with the advent of ZD, the need for measurement is evident in areas that not only do not have existing data systems but which rebel at the thought of such systems being introduced. These are also difficult areas in which to set up formal measurement systems since they usually include nonrepetitive or creative types of endeavor. It is in these areas that the Administrator will note a remarkable concern with measurement as soon as management has begun the recognition phase of the program. Interest is usually weak as long as measurement symbolizes management censure—but when (through Zero Defects) measurement results in management recognition, the entire picture seems to change.

ZD has sparked a change in *attitude*. This is not theory or wishful think-

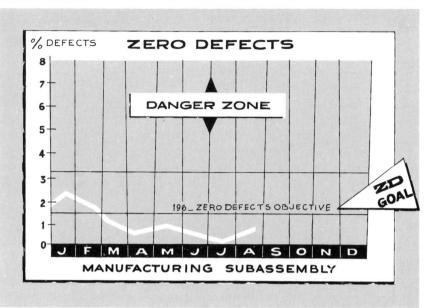

FIG. 43   A ZD objective, or temporary goal, is added to quality-level charts after kickoff.

ing; a new desire for measurement is apparent in hundreds of ZD organizations throughout the country. And for this reason, management should not push measurement too hard at first. If management offers encouragement, suggests criteria, recognizes effort, and offers assistance, the very people who say "we can't be measured" will come up with their own goals and criteria. It is the old case of the tail wagging the dog. If management has done its job in implementing and kicking off the program, the newly "aware" individual will want to know more. He and his supervision will have a very personal need to know just where they stand in the overall scheme of things (see Figure 43). And they will certainly want top management to share this awareness when it comes time for recognition.

Group versus Individual Measurement

The individual is the key to the entire program. ZD is not beamed at an organization or a department or a section; it speaks to, and deals with, the individual. Thus, individual-achievement measurement is necessary in order to pursue a successful program. Group measurement provides a secondary function of awareness. It lets the individual know where his group stands in relation to its goal of Zero Defects. The only area where group measurement serves a recognition function is in evaluating supervisor and manager achievement since, in many cases, the effort of the group reflects the effort of the supervisor. Group measurement can also be used to stimulate team competition, and many organizations use the data collected as the basis for group awards for best record of the month and most improved record of the month, which stimulates interest in the awareness campaign (see Figure 44).

119

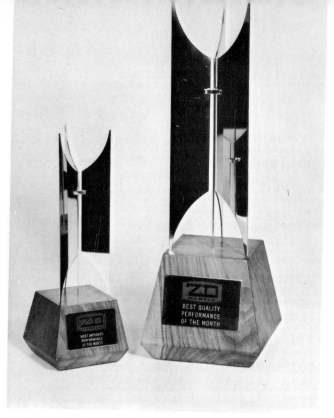

FIG. 44 Traveling group-achievement awards for most improved group and best group of the month.

The reason Zero Defects organizations avoid individual postings is that by publicly identifying the low man on the pole, you, in fact, punish or embarrass him. This ZD never does. Individual-defect records should be kept confidential between the worker and management. The only time they are released is at the moment of recognition.

In the same way, group-measurement data alone should never be used for individual recognition (with the exception of supervisors). Just because a person is a member of a high-achievement group, it does not mean that he is an achiever. That would be as senseless as saying: a greyhound is a dog; all dogs have four legs; therefore, all four-legged dogs are greyhounds. It doesn't work that way! And the individuals concerned will be the first to realize it. If non-achiever Irving is recognized for the efforts of Tom, Dick, and Harry, will any of them respect the recognition? Will that recognition tell them that management is really interested in the individual and cares about his personal efforts and achievement? Will non-achiever Irving work any harder next month to win future recognition? Will Tom, Dick, and Harry continue to make the effort, knowing that management obviously doesn't know or care which of them did a good job and which let the organization down? To all of the questions, the most optimistic answer that can be given is "it's doubtful."

The only exception to this rule is where two or three workers operate the same machine at the same time (see Figure 45). In such a case, it would be almost impossible to determine defect responsibility since the work involves joint effort on a single operation. Here, if measurement indicates outstanding achievement, each man should be recognized as an individual.

Measurement Criteria

From the foregoing, we can see that group measurement is basically for information and motivation purposes—individual measurement is for achievement recognition and personal awareness.

This raises the question: "Do I have to measure each and every person in my organization?" If it's Zero Defects you're after, the answer must be yes! At the same time, it must be understood that ZD measurement means only awareness by the supervisors of individual accomplishment. Everyday, every worker in every factory and office is undergoing some sort of measurement or evaluation. To prove this, the reader need only go to the nearest supervisor and ask. There is not a supervisor who will admit that he does not know what his people are doing and which ones are accomplishing the most and the best. Just ask him how he knows and you are well on your way to establishing formal measurement standards in the most "difficult" areas of your organization.

This leaves you with the supervisor who states that "all" of his workers are top achievers. One ZD Administrator has a standard question for this man: "What if you had to lay off five out of six employees—which one would you keep?" In a "moment of truth" any supervisor can rapidly "discover" criteria to pick out his achievers and non-achievers.

FIG. 45   A program-promotion piece noting an example of team achievement on a two-man welding machine. This type of operation presents the only situation where members of a group should be recognized as individual achievers.

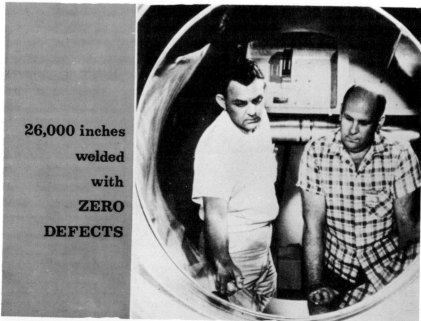

26,000 inches
welded
with
ZERO
DEFECTS

This part of the book has been prepared to provide the Administrator, manager, and supervisor with some suggested guidelines to help them build a solid basis for ZD recognition. There is no magic formula that will provide instant measurement for every individual. In some areas, measurement will depend almost entirely on supervisor observation. In others, the worker's every effort will fall under formal data audit. The majority of the people in most ZD organizations fall into the middle ground, where recognition is based on formal records and supervisor opinion. In these areas the Administrator should concentrate most of his activity.

PRODUCTION MEASUREMENT

Probably the most comprehensive experience in defect measurement has taken place in the manufacturing or production areas of industry. It has almost become a necessity to employ some form of quality control on manufacturing processes in order to survive in today's highly competitive markets. This production measurement usually takes one of the following forms:
1. Actual tally resulting from 100 percent piece and part inspection
2. Sampling tally based on inspection of a predetermined number of units
3. Final end-product inspection by either of the above methods
4. User tally (either by in-house assemblers or by the customer)
In most cases, detected defects can usually be traced to the responsible group. This is done either through material review board actions or through actual group or individual identification stamps and tags on the product. The organization with a detection system but no organized method of finding out why and where is ignoring the most important cause of the inspection or measurement cycle—the reason the error was made in the first place. Simply to find and reject errors is only to assure that most of your mistakes will not reach the customer. To find the source or cause of error is the first step in the corrective-action cycle. Thus, most organizations that have quality controls (and most production operations do) have some method of tracking the source of defects. The key question here is how far back this tracking technique goes. To be an effective ZD tool, it must go back to the individual.

After it has been determined which group is responsible for a fault or defect, it is possible, with a little extra effort, to pinpoint the responsible individual or group of individuals (in cases where a single operation requires the efforts of more than one person).

Low Production Runs

Where an operator handles less than 100 units a day, the commonest technique is to use an operator identification stamp or tag on each item. In operations where this has not been standard practice, some employee apprehension regarding such identification may be encountered. Here again, ZD comes to

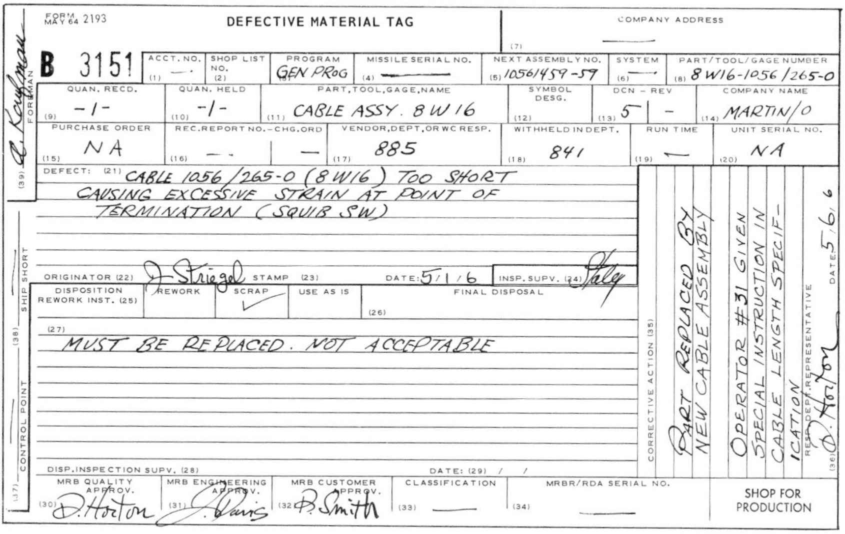
FORM 2193 MAY 64

DEFECTIVE MATERIAL TAG

COMPANY ADDRESS (7)

B 3151

ACCT. NO. (1) — · SHOP LIST NO. (2) PROGRAM GEN PROG MISSILE SERIAL NO. (4) —— NEXT ASSEMBLY NO. (5) 1056/459-57 SYSTEM (6) — PART/TOOL/GAGE NUMBER (8) 8W16-1056/265-0

QUAN. RECD. (9) -1- QUAN. HELD (10) -1- PART, TOOL, GAGE, NAME (11) CABLE ASSY. 8W16 SYMBOL DESG. (12) DCN – REV (13) 5 – COMPANY NAME (14) MARTIN/O

PURCHASE ORDER (15) NA REC. REPORT NO. – CHG. ORD (16) — — VENDOR, DEPT, OR WC RESP. (17) 885 WITHHELD IN DEPT. (18) 841 RUN TIME (19) — UNIT SERIAL NO. (20) NA

DEFECT: (21) CABLE 1056/265-0 (8W16) TOO SHORT CAUSING EXCESSIVE STRAIN AT POINT OF TERMINATION (SQUIB SW)

ORIGINATOR (22) J. Striegel STAMP (23) DATE: 5/1/6 INSP. SUPV. (24) Foley

DISPOSITION REWORK INST. (25) REWORK SCRAP ✓ USE AS IS FINAL DISPOSAL (26)

(27) MUST BE REPLACED. NOT ACCEPTABLE

CORRECTIVE ACTION (35) PART REPLACED BY NEW CABLE ASSEMBLY OPERATOR #31 GIVEN SPECIAL INSTRUCTION IN CABLE LENGTH SPECIFICATION

RESP. DEPT. REPRESENTATIVE (36) D. Horton DATE 5/6/6

(39) FOREMAN R. Kaufman (38) SHIP SHORT (37) CONTROL POINT

DISP. INSPECTION SUPV. (28) DATE: (29) / /

MRB QUALITY APPROV. (30) D. Horton MRB ENGINEERING APPROV. (31) J. Davis MRB CUSTOMER APPROV. (32) B. Smith CLASSIFICATION (33) —— MRBR/RDA SERIAL NO. (34) —— SHOP FOR PRODUCTION

FIG. 46 Typical defect documentation of the type found in defense industry quality operations. The responsible worker is noted in the Corrective Action section in the lower right-hand corner of the tag. Prior to ZD, this information was used primarily for corrective action and was not reviewed to determine which workers did not have such documentation logged against their efforts.

the rescue. When the identifying stamp is treated as a craftsman's hallmark and not simply as a technique for management to catch a defect-producing "offender," the worker usually likes the idea. This approach has proved effective in most new measurement procedures. In every case, measurement should be carefully explained to the individual and the positive approach stressed over the negative or disciplinary approach (see Figure 46).

High Production Runs

In cases of semiautomated or high-rate-production runs, individual-defect identification poses a slightly more difficult problem. But the very device or technique that enables the operator to make daily volume runs usually contains the means for identification—automatic markers and color coders. Where such techniques prove costly or where they do not fit into the existing operating procedures, other criteria should be established. So as not to overburden the supervisor, techniques and criteria should be easy to observe and record. Such techniques would include:

1. The number of minutes "down" per month due to improper feeding or other worker error

2. The amount of raw material used against machine or operator output, signifying the number of self-corrected errors and the number of loading and operating defects

3. Supervisor spot check of operator output on a regular basis
(Note: Though this technique is based on a law-of-averages principle, any long-run sampling method can provide a reliable index to operator achievement.)

Nonrepetitive or Multitask Production

The production-measurement problem becomes more complex when the operator is not involved in a repetitive task. Such assignments would include touch-up and rework of most types, extremely low-production-run items, special test-model fabrication, and servicing and maintenance activities. Though some of these efforts may fall into the regular reporting cycle, many are in the "special assignment" category and, as such, do not come under formal audit. Also, individuals who handle such tasks are usually trained in several production techniques and will, in turn, perform several different tasks in a given work period.

Here, the supervisor will have to find some "common" criteria to cover all the individual's functions and tasks. There are no set formulas to cover all such activities, but a survey of existing criteria will provide guidelines for specific types of activities. Some of these criteria might include:

Service or Maintenance Activities

- A count of the number of "repeat" service or maintenance calls regarding the same problem
- An "action" check of the time lag between service call and response
- A review of service complaints
- A study of the time spent on calls to discover average downtime over a set period
- A review of incomplete or incorrect documentation
- Measurement involving spare- and repair-part accountability
- User-satisfaction-survey-form analysis
- Actual supervisor audit and sampling techniques, involving regularly scheduled reviews of operator activities
- Rework activities (Note: These criteria should be considered in cases where it is impossible or inadvisable to return the product through regular, primary inspection channels.)
- Audit of rework documentation and reports of additional defects discovered by rework operators
- Items salvaged against items scrapped
- Preventive-action suggestions or other creative contributions to defect prevention
- Supervisor sampling of effort on a day-to-day basis with emphasis on defect-free performance rather than on a specific task

- Review of reports from final test and check-out as well as user-complaint reports

Shipping and Handling Activities (Note: In most of these cases, individual responsibility is handled through operator packing slips or identifying stamps on the packages involved.)
- Regular review of breakage and damage reports as well as insurance claims
- User or customer complaints
- Lost-shipment-action review
- A study of late-shipment or delayed-delivery reports
- Standard documentation review
- Shipment-shortage report balanced against supervisor and individual responsibilities
- And once again, actual supervisor sampling and review of on-the-job tasks

Short-run- or Single-item-production Activities
- A review of test results of engineering prototypes (usually conducted by other departments and not included in production-control data)
- Scrap count
- Machine downtime due to worker error
- A review of any of the techniques used on larger runs converted to small-scale implementation

The Supervisor's Role

In all of these cases, the measurement burden is primarily placed on the supervisor. Even where the actual data comes from another source, the supervisor must seek this data out and develop usable recognition criteria from it. If the task is presented as a challenge and as something that will enhance his position, the supervisor will generally come up with more than enough criteria for proper evaluation of all the employees in his group. On the other hand, if he is simply told to "get some figures in" each month, the results will reflect the lack of managerial motivation.

Once the achievers and their supervisors in the regularly measured production areas receive public recognition, the difficult areas will provide a surprisingly large amount of defect documentation in short order. The Administrator should not press the supervisors in these areas too hard for recognition inputs but rather should concentrate his efforts on seeing that the reported achievers get maximum promotion.

Administrator Follow-up

At the same time, the Administrator should always be on the lookout for low input areas. By keeping records of achievement by department and section, long-term omissions can be brought out and acted upon. Just as the Administrator and management should not pressure the supervisor, it is unfair to individuals reporting to the supervisor to allow a six-month gap in recognition go unchecked. Follow-up in these cases usually reveals: (1) that other supervisor problems are either causing a lack of achievement in the section or are causing the supervisor to neglect his ZD responsibilities; or (2) that the supervisor is actually unaware of his responsibilities to the individuals under him and to the program. The latter case is usually caused by a slipup in supervisory indoctrination or a change in supervision.

Through the achievement information the supervisor can conduct his recognition activities as well as have the meat for group reports in determining the overall organization performance. The averages, posted within the work area, give a fair evaluation of the group's position with regard to its current ZD goals.

Support Data

In many cases, actual defect-data or standard-measurement results are not enough on which to base recognition recommendation. For instance, in the case of a worker who makes 100,000 consecutive difficult operations without error during a six-month period, the supervisor has no doubt as to the individual's achievement. But where the individual has been audited by a sampling technique or the production run was not long enough to eliminate the element of "chance" perfection, other criteria must be used to back up the available defect data. These criteria (attitude, program participation, etc.) are covered in the recognition chapter (Chapter 14) and should become a regular part of each supervisor's measurement-evaluation process.

INDIVIDUAL-MEASUREMENT-DATA EVALUATION

Once the supervisor has established measurement criteria and has set up some method of collecting and sorting data, the next step is, obviously, to use the data. This is the point where many ZD measurement systems fail. Almost every case of incomplete achievement documentation or the lack of such documentation at all, can be traced back to the supervisor's simply not knowing what to do with the information he has. It is a case of not seeing the forest for the trees.

To discover his top achiever or achievers, the supervisor need only make a simple chart balancing defects or negative factors against each individual's total output or hours worked. With this information before him, listed in the order of magnitude of achievement, he can readily ascertain the following information:

1. Which employees have achieved Zero Defects goals for the period
2. The average achievement level for the group

3. Those individuals who need special attention to bring their records up to the group's average

4. The cutoff point where an individual moves from the "average" category to a possible "achiever" classification

GROUP DATA

The importance and uses of group data have been covered extensively in the earlier chapters of this book. To date, no single base or formula has been devised to provide a common standard for all groups within an organization. The groups differ among themselves as much as the individuals who make up the groups. Yet, in order to give meaning to group awards and to group competition, some standard should be set.

This standard is usually set in the same manner as acceptance quality levels are established (discussed in Chapter 8). Since workers do need specific goals, supervisors, management, and the Administrator should agree on annual or monthly goals for each section and department. All of these goals should be reasonable, yet challenging, for the individuals involved in the specific group.

The most common formula for determining a group's defective work rate is

$$\frac{\text{Total number of defects}}{\text{Number of people} \times \text{hours per month} \times 0.01} = \text{defects per 100 hours}$$

The total number of defects is determined through the defect-measurement technique selected and is based on criteria common to the group. In many cases, this group criteria will differ greatly from the individual-measurement criteria. This is especially true in groups that contain several types of job classifications and in which a variety of tasks are performed. It is up to management and the supervisors to determine the common ground in such cases.

Setting ZD Goals

Once the group-measurement technique and criteria are established, management can set objectives. Any line drawn on a chart other than the one crossing zero cannot be considered an ultimate goal. At best it can be called a "temporary goal" or better still a "ZD achievement level" (see Figure 47). Going back to the original ZD philosophy, workers will strive to attain the levels set by management. If management expects the individual to be anything less than perfect, the individual will usually accommodate management by being just that. Thus, when these levels are set, the employee must be made to realize that the goals are temporary and are there only to serve as guidelines in his drive toward perfection.

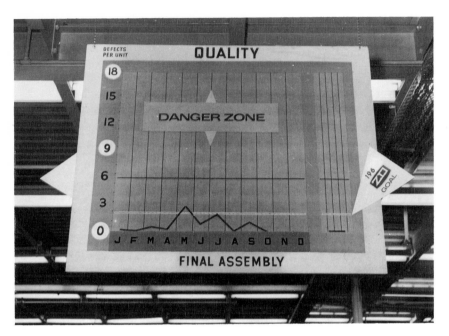

FIG. 47 Quality chart in author's plant showing acceptable quality level (top line) and ZD goal, or objective level (broken line).

As for the levels themselves, a good rule of thumb is to set them from 25 to 50 percent below pre-ZD levels. Once the group reaches the level set, they usually plateau out just under it. After this leveling trend is well established, management should reevaluate the goal and, if reasonable, lower it. This second downward step will, obviously, not be as great as the first. As the group nears zero, the challenge and difficulty in meeting the "goal" become greater. If the supervisor has done his job in explaining the purpose of these levels in the first place, the employees will not be dismayed at seeing the goal move down once more.

A word of caution: in these later steps, management must take great care never to allow the goal to get completely out of reach. The situation is like that of the mule that is enticed to pull the wagon by a carrot dangling in front of his nose; as long as he can smell the carrot and see it clearly, he will try to get it. Move it out of sight and smell and he will sit down in the middle of the road and do nothing. We do not imply that employees are mules, but there is enough "mule" in each one of us that we won't continually strive for a goal that is completely out of reach.

Goal Review

Just as the normal quality-performance levels are reviewed and reevaluated as to changes in operation, changes in numbers of workers and pieces produced, changes in equipment, and any other factor that could have an influence on the group's performance, so should the ZD objectives be revised from time to time. This is especially true in areas showing great fluctuations in workers or output. It must be remembered that ZD is a motivational symbol and not an economically feasible and attainable objective per se. The establishment of the ZD group-achievement level must be given the same care and consideration by the quality statistician (tempered by management judgment) as is exercised in the establishment of regular quality-performance levels.

PRODUCTION-MEASUREMENT REVIEW

It cannot be stressed too strongly that experience has proved that the company without any quality standards or controls can't really be serious about Zero Defects. ZD needs a base to work from, and that base must be a solid awareness by management and the individual employee of the importance of a quality product or service. Without some type of formal quality-assurance program, the implementing organization is almost doomed to failure from the start.

This is especially true when dealing with a production organization. Regardless of the product, some measurement base must be available in key operational areas. Where this base is present, it is simple to extend it to cover every aspect of production from the supply room to final documentation and delivery.

Once measurement techniques have been firmly established in production areas, the Administrator can turn his attention to those areas that usually do not fall under quality audit—the administrative and creative areas. Yet here again, a quality-conscious organization will usually have some methods of performance measurement. They may not be apparent at first glance, but they are there, ready to be used. The next two chapters will uncover some of these existing criteria and make suggestions for their use in individual and group measurement.

12

Clerical- and
Administrative-measurement Criteria

Next to manufacturing operations, the most extensive defect auditing is found in the administrative and clerical areas of an organization. The main difference is that defect information from these auditing systems is a by-product and, prior to ZD, an unused by-product, at least so far as individual-quality-performance measurement was concerned.

For instance, many companies use time cards. These cards are checked and tallied by a clerk, punched out, and fed into a computer for payroll information. The computer itself highlights errors in computation and brings them to the attention of the payroll department. These same errors are rapidly corrected by simply punching a new card and inserting it into the system. Both clerks and machines work long hours checking and reproducing the documentation necessary for a company payroll. Since the errors are merely paper errors, since they are almost always caught by the machine or the clerks themselves, and since the only material thing lost is a small piece of cardboard—why bother to find out who and what is making the errors? The answer is simple. The "bother" is necessary because machine time and man-hours are as much a part of the product cost as a nut, bolt, or semiconductor. In one ZD organization, a supervisor, after much prodding to install measurement, was surprised to learn that during the first six months of the program, one of his employees had made over 100,000 time-card computations without error. When asked why he hadn't looked for this information before, he reported that he had been seeing it every day—he simply had not been relating it to individual performance!

AREAS COMMONLY UNDER AUDIT

In every clerical and administrative operation, whether in government, business, or the professions such as medicine and education, certain areas commonly come under some type of audit. The time-card print-off example in the previous paragraph is only one such example. These audited areas generally break down into several key functions:

Accounts Receivable and Payable and Bookkeeping: Most organizations today have this area almost entirely automated. Computers tally, invoice, record shipments and receipts, determine taxes due and taxes paid, and perform a host of other activities formerly relegated to the pen and ledger. Where there is a computer, there must be input. The results of this input are always visible on the computer print-out. Thus every error, no matter how small, is permanently documented. Since anyone who continually works with such data can almost automatically tell by the type and degree of error what the level of input was at the source and since most accounting and finance departments are separated into specific areas of functional responsibility, it is fairly easy to establish individual responsibility for most accounting error.

Contracts and Procurement: Here, too, many of the operations fall into the computer- or business-machine-audit cycle; but there are also secondary auditing procedures that automatically back up the former. These include legal-department reviews and changes, customer or vendor reviews, accounting-department audits, and, in many companies, contract and procurement-order checkers making formal inspection of every document produced. In the latter case, these people rarely keep formal defect-data records. They simply return the document to the initiator for rework. Little or no extra effort would be required on their part to record errors by individuals on a weekly report sheet.

General Administrative: It might be said that in any major business or government enterprise there is an auditor behind every post. Years ago, most people tried to avoid the auditor; in today's ZD organization he is welcomed. If the administrative supervisor looks hard enough, he can generally come up with some element of his organization's auditing system that pertains directly to the defect performance of his employees. Though this data may not provide a complete picture of individual accomplishment, it will certainly highlight or bring to the surface any instance of outstanding achievement.

Many of the tasks in these areas also come under machine audit, not only from their own computer runs, but from those of other departments. This is because such areas are usually involved in the data input and output review of many other areas. Also, almost all operational and planning activities are well documented. They are naturally reviewed or audited from time to time. Whether this review is by top management or by the lower levels of management and supervision, any errors or inaccuracies are invariably discovered and brought to the attention of the initiating group. You might say that the business of these functions is "everybody's" business.

OTHER MEASUREMENT CRITERIA

After management has reviewed all existing forms of audit, the use of other existing measurement criteria can be investigated. As with other functions, these areas contain elements that can be readily converted into solid measurement information. Such techniques require a little more effort than a simple review of computer print-outs or an accountant's reports, but they are far less costly than the institution of a completely new measurement/inspection system. Since it would be impractical to review every possible administrative-measurement criterion, they will be considered by administrative-function grouping:

Accounts Receivable and Payable and Bookkeeping: One of the most common criterion used in these areas is the evaluation of complaints and adjustment requests. If a particular clerk has not had any customer or vendor rejections during a given period, it is reasonable to assume that he or she is making a serious attempt at proper documentation and tabulation. This information, although it doesn't indicate that the individual has reached perfection, does show that the effort was above average. From this point on, the supervisor must do a little digging to uncover the complete achievement picture. Another technique that could be used for this purpose is a review of discounts and other adjustments missed during a given period. A regular review of turn-around time on bills and invoices will highlight certain individual's scheduling and planning capabilities—a lost or delayed invoice can bring added losses in discount and special-handling costs.

Contracts and Procurement: A periodic review of materials shipped or received without proper purchase orders will give the supervisor an excellent guideline for determining which buyers are on top of their responsibilities. A review of late or incomplete deliveries can also highlight achievement in other areas; thus, the order clerk or purchaser with a perfect record will probably have other characteristics to back up achievement recognition. (To use this criterion alone would be unfair since many such discrepancies are due to outside influences and are beyond the control of the organization's staff.) Another check would be to provide the requester with a follow-up satisfaction card on which he could note whether or not he received his material on time and in good condition and whether the item purchased answered the requester's need. If no automated review of purchase-order documentation is available, the supervisor should take time to review such documents on a total or sample basis. If sampling is used, it should be regularly scheduled to make sure that the sample covers all individuals in the group.

Finance: Though much of this area comes under standard audit, either within the organization or through the financial institutions with which the organization deals, there remain other elements of documentation that can be used for measurement. Regardless of automated checks and balances, some payroll errors do get out to the employee level. The reports of such error and the fixing of accountability for same can supplement computer information in assuring achievement figures. In any such operation, certain logs and journal entries are common to a large segment of the work force. Periodic checks and reviews will often bring achievements to the surface. Finance is also responsible for discounts and other deductions from payments; so this area can also provide performance information. Secondary audits by the Treasury Department, Social Security Administration, defense-bond and stock-purchase data, and other outside reporting agencies can usually be used to indicate group as well as individual achievement.

Personnel: Since most organizations check their records once a year for changes in family status, addresses, etc., these reviews can be used to highlight personnel-clerk achievement. For instance, the number of changes due to clerical error in name spelling, house numbers, and number of dependents may be reviewed as a measurement criterion as well as being used for corrective action. Insurance-claim processing involves many in-house audit features, and claims are double-checked by the claimant companies and individuals. Travel departments or clerks are usually measured by balancing the number of trips processed against traveler complaints, by examining cost consciousness in making reservations and travel arrangements, and by financial reviews of support documentation. Elements of labor relations can be evaluated through a review and analysis of submitted worker grievances. Wage and salary sections can be evaluated through periodic reviews of workers' wage rates balanced against established standards for specific classifications. Efficiency measurement can determine achievement in the areas of employee-suggestion follow-up, employee participation in company-sponsored activities, training and educational activities, labor turnover, safety, and the provision of adequate food services. All of these items are documented as to time spans, participation, and other factors.

Advertising, Publications, and Public Relations: Many ZD organizations have put these areas under actual quality audit. Such steps will depend on the size of the operation and amount of internally generated material. Such auditing procedures usually consist of a review of the number of type changes due to editorial error; the number of rough layouts and designs prior to final mechanical; print-mechanical checks for art errors; support-documentation accuracy; copy errors found in proofreading; actual inspection and review of final document; in the case of handbooks, the thoroughness in meeting engineering and customer specifications; checks for omissions in approval steps; review of procurement records of vendor and agency documentation; and damage reports on plates, artwork, and mechanicals. Though these areas are considered "creative" in nature (see Chapter 13), the Administrator and supervisors can discover literally hundreds of well-documented activities from which to draw measurement data.

Sales: Though one of the truest methods of measuring sales effectiveness is by the actual sales themselves, there are other criteria that can be easily put to use in these areas. Since most sales people make regular reports of activities, calls, and other customer information, these reports are a very good gauge of sales-personnel performance. For instance, the number of calls versus the number of key customer contacts indicates the amount of planning and preparation behind such activities. The number of both new and active customers balanced against the number of no-order clients during a six-month period can provide similar information. Any other formula in this area would work equally well since a defect to a salesman is the loss of a customer, the loss of a sale, or failure to stay abreast of the customer's needs and activities. Since one of the most useful sales-management tools is information from the field, the completeness of the sales reports themselves can be used as excellent and valuable measurement criteria. Another critical area is expense and travel reports. Achievement in this area should warm the heart of any sales manager. The basic documentation review can be handled by the department secretary, with final evaluation by the supervisor or manager.

Marketing: Since marketing groups deal in data, it should be no trouble to convert some of this information into ZD measurement material. Accuracy of prediction is an excellent criterion in this area. Another would be accuracy of data and data input (both items are usually checked by the data-processing group). Marketing personnel can also be judged on the timeliness of information gathered and its influence on proposal and sales costs. Since marketing groups deal in reports and other written communications, many of their activities may be judged by the same criteria discussed in the advertising and publications section of this chapter. Also, since these reports are reviewed by management, there is usually a certain amount of official and unofficial feedback as to their preparation and effectiveness. Documentation of such information can add to the overall measurement picture.

General Staff: Though these are primarily areas of managerial responsibility, there are certain support functions that will require some type of regular measurement. As mentioned earlier, many of these activities come under audit somewhere within the organization. The supervisor and the Administrator will have to decide just what criteria are the simplest and least expensive to use. Several common criteria that have been used effectively in these areas are effectiveness of controls, timeliness of reports and other documentation, accuracy of data input (computer), effectiveness in reaching planned operational goals, manpower balance and distribution evaluation, effectiveness in manpower and machine loading, and the budget adjustments versus planned expenditures.

Secretarial: Despite the cartoon image of the nail-filing, magazine-reading secretary, she should be one of the most efficient elements in any organization. Most Administrators have run into the situation in which management hesitates to attempt documentation on secretaries or to nominate them for achievement recognition. One common question at Zero Defects workshops is: "How do I measure my secretary?" Experience has proved that secretarial measurement is easy to accomplish if the boss takes a few minutes to think about it. Every secretary has her own personal inspector—her boss. He reads (or should read) everything she types for his signature. If he has any sort of quality awareness about him, he will note erasures, typos, and other common secretarial errors. But typing is only one criterion for secretarial measurement. There are dozens of other criteria of which most bosses are unaware simply because most bosses are unaware of or unconcerned with the dozens of other jobs a secretary performs. Though these activities are usually taken for granted, they do in fact make up a large part of the secretary's total performance. For instance, the secretary usually makes out the boss's expense report—these reports are audited by travel or finance; the secretary usually handles office-supply orders, purchase requisitions, time and payroll documentation, and formalized reports—all of which come under some type of audit; the secretary keeps appointment schedules—the boss certainly knows how often he is caught with two meetings or guests at the same time; and so the activities go on. The reluctance or embarrassment of turning in such documentation on or an achievement recognition of personal secretaries is usually overcome as soon as the first one or two are recognized within an organization. An excellent administrative check on such documentation is to be found in most companies' personnel records. Since secretaries are usually tested for speed and accuracy, all secretarial-measurement input for achievement should be checked against these test records. It is unlikely that a secretary making barely passing grades on such tests would come up with several thousand pages of perfectly typed letters and reports. This is to say that such tests are not absolute in their findings, but they do serve as warnings for the Administrator to review the achievement data.

Summary

Though this review barely scratches the surface of administrative and clerical activities, it does show that there are a host of measurement criteria available if the supervisor and management will only look for them (see Figure 48). In most cases, the defect data is there but it is rarely used for individual-accomplishment documentation. Generally, when a defect appears, it is corrected and that is the end of it. Unless an obvious rash of errors causes the supervisor to speak to a worker about it, administrative personnel rarely hear about their specific errors. That is, existing data is used only to correct defects and reprimand obvious offenders; it is rarely used to praise and recognize achievers. Once the supervisor is convinced that the latter is a far easier and more rewarding chore, this data will take on new importance to both management and the individual worker.

SPECIAL AUDITING PROCEDURES

Where there are no available data sources for ZD measurement, the supervisor or higher management may wish to consider instituting some special form of quality audit. Though these cases are rare, they do come up from time to time in administrative and clerical areas. In reaching such decisions, management must first ask if it is worth it. If the cost of adding an inspector or checker to a section is higher than the cost of the errors or rework, management should take a close look at the situation before instituting such a change. For instance, putting an inspector behind every girl in a typing pool would not only be far too costly, but it would probably drive both inspector and inspected to distraction. Yet, in some areas it may be found that an actual quality audit would provide great savings and be beneficial to both employee and management. In these cases the sections involved should be encouraged to investigate such a possibility. In making such decisions, the ZD program should not be the only requirement factor.

Even where there is no form of recorded defect data, there is always one more avenue of approach—the supervisor. Supervisor observation is one of the best techniques available for ZD achievement measurement since most qualified supervisors are well aware of which worker is doing what and how well. He need only put his observations on paper to provide acceptable measurement criteria for ZD achievement recognition.

NEW TECHNIQUES

As new, automated business equipment is developed and as administrative activities become more and more geared to their use, measurement will become more and more a part of regular business procedure in these areas. Yet, regardless of the degree of automation, there will always be someone who makes input, who operates the machine, and who evaluates or acts on output. As long as this condition exists, management has the responsibility to let the employee

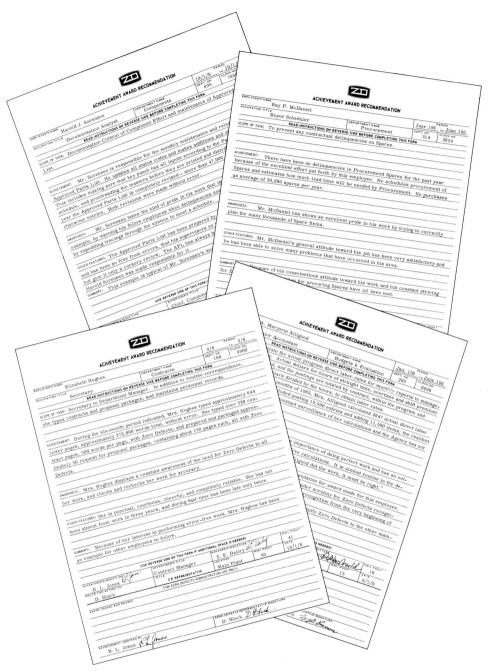

FIG. 48 Individual Achievement Award Recommendations from the administrative and clerical areas. A review of the achievement information will give the reader an indication of some of the basic criteria used in this area.

know where he stands and where his group stands and to recognize achievement wherever it occurs. Though this chapter has dealt primarily with administrative-task measurement, the reader will find certain elements of administrative function in the preceding and following chapters. Since the next chapter covers creative activities, certain administrative supervisors can put much of the material to good use. This is especially true of those in the marketing, advertising, public relations, and planning areas.

The Administrator should always keep the first rule of ZD measurement in his mind when seeking usable criteria: thoroughly investigate every possible existing method of measurement before considering the initiation of new criteria and techniques. Additional measurement techniques should be employed *only* where the estimated value exceeds the cost of such measurement!

13

Measurement of
Scientific/Professional Employees

The measurement of scientific and professional employees seems to give more Administrators more headaches than any other phase connected with the Zero Defects program. There are two prime reasons for the difficulties experienced in measuring scientists and professionals: first, most of these areas have never been under any type of formal quality audit; and second, the individuals within these areas are considered to resist any effort to instill formal inspection or defect audit within their activities.

The reason behind the first condition is that prior to ZD there was little active interest in the documentation of professional error. It was a case of: when you find an error, correct it; if you find too many errors, reprimand the individual; if the errors persist, fire him. Thus, errors resulted in corrective and punitive action alone. Since the *lack* of error was never documented or even highlighted in the mind of the supervisor, this data was rarely used for achievement recognition.

The reason behind the second condition is a natural, built-in defense mechanism. In a design or research project there is a certain amount of trial and error. Scientists and engineers learn from error. This type of error we could call "productive error." But all scientific and professional mistakes can't hide behind this "trial and error" shield. Would the case of a scientist making the same study and taking the same error-elimination steps (simply because he hadn't done his homework) that a fellow had accomplished a year before be considered a worthwhile or productive error? Is an engineering design error-free when the responsible engineer comes up with an element that meets specifications in itself but doesn't marry with the components to the right or left of it? Should an advertising-agency copywriter be praised for coming up with a hard-pulling ad to sell canned soup to business executives when there is marketing data available to show that these people have a direct influence over less than 0.01 percent of the market?

EXISTING DEFECT AUDIT

There is a certain element of activity in any task that comes under some type of formal audit, such as expense-account vouchers, purchase requests, facilities requests, and the other paper work that everyone gets involved in. Yet, here again, we face an attitude problem. Although the finance clerk is chastised for turning in a messy or inaccurate requisition form, this same "defect" is usually shrugged off when traced back to a scientific or creative staff member. "After all, they are professional people, not bookkeepers!" Supervision is reluctant even to bring up the subject unless the problem becomes acute or influences other professional activities within the group.

The Administrator's first task is to bring the *reason* of ZD measurement back into the proper prospective. ZD measures to recognize achievement—not to nag or punish the employee for lack of achievement. The Administrator has a selling job to do, not only to supervision but to the individual scientific/professional employee. Before the individual employee will make an effort in these areas, he must first see the reasoning behind it. The reasoning or quality awareness sell in these audited areas can best be accomplished by hitting the professional where it hurts the most—dead center in his professional ego. The nuclear physicist who tries to argue away a clearly inaccurate facilities request with the statement "I can't be bothered whether or not a form is filled out properly when I have really important scientific problems to solve" is really treading on thin ice. If he can't fill out a simple form, why should he be trusted with part of a million-dollar research program?

Usually management contributes to this attitude problem by taking Dr. X's incomplete and thus unserviceable request and handing it over to a business agent to clean up and resubmit. The result is that Dr. X has wasted his valuable and costly time by improperly initiating the request; the auditor has wasted his time by having to reject and send back the request; the manager has wasted his time by having to settle the controversy; the business agent has wasted his time having to fill out the form the right way; and Dr. X gets his badly needed piece of equipment three weeks late. What is the true cost of the form, even before it gets out of the lab area? In many cases it is more than the cost of the item requested, and all because a man with nine years of graduate, scientific education failed to answer accurately five questions on a 3-cent form.

When the scientific/professional employee is made aware of the additional administrative costs and schedule problems, he will usually try to cooperate. When management recognizes him for this cooperation, he will look upon the task as an achievement rather than a petty nuisance. It will be in these simple, easily audited areas that the Administrator will make his first measurement applications in the scientific/professional element of the organization. With solid measurement (and the auditing figures are usually available) in these fringe areas, coupled with posted reports of declining defect rates, the program will begin to stir up interest for measurement in the other, more creative areas of the work. Since the average professional hates to see money wasted on these support activities, he is usually receptive to this first measurement phase. This is true not only in the areas of specifically scientific endeavor but in any area of professional effort.

ESTABLISHING MEASURING TECHNIQUES

Once the professional's supervisor begins to make use of existing measurement data and the staff under him begins to make an effort toward perfection in these limited areas, he should then turn his attention to the professional tasks themselves. This is where the real problem seems to arise. For several years, ZD Administrators and supervisors in general have been bemoaning the fact that there is no common measurement criterion (thus no common measurement formula) for the measurement of professional endeavor. This is not wholly true. The most common technique for measurement in these areas is supervisor judgment. Reluctance to use such judgment can be overcome in the same manner that it was handled when dealing with production supervision. Just like the manufacturing supervisor who will never admit he doesn't know what his people are doing, the supervisor of scientists and professionals will never say, "Oh, we're just floundering around, and some day we will come up with the answer." Every supervisor has some way of evaluating employee performance. It will be up to the Administrator to help him use this evaluation to recognize individual achievement.

FORMAL MEASUREMENT CRITERIA

While there is no magic formula, there are certain formal criteria common to all scientific/professional activities. There are always standards to measure against, and there is always someone doing the measurement. The only thing lacking in these cases is formal documentation. There are errors made in these areas, and the errors do get detected and corrected; the problem is to find a method of documentation (existing or specially created) to give the supervisor some reference for achievement recognition.

BASIC CRITERIA

There are several basic criteria under which formal measurement can be established in scientific and professional activities: specification groundwork, survey of available facts, skill (careless) error, success of project, and the standard (existing) criteria mentioned earlier in this chapter. The method of error discovery and error documentation may differ from task to task, but the basic criteria generally remain the same.

Specification Groundwork: Any task in engineering design, applied research, industrial design, advertising writing or design—in fact, any professional/creative endeavor—is based on some form of requirement or specification. This specification may be set by a customer, another group within the organization, the supervisor, or even the individual himself. Regardless, there is usually some form of specification calling out the why and the what of a task. If the individual doesn't take the time to know these specifications or simply doesn't work toward them, he will invariably err. If the specifications call for a 5-inch bolt and he designs one 4 inches long, it is an error. If one of the requirements for a metal is that it withstand a temperature of 1000°F and the researcher designs or selects one that will not survive 500°F, then he has made an error (unless, of course, the goal is outside the state of the art). If a copywriter is asked for a 4-inch ad and he comes up with enough copy to fill two pages, he too has failed to meet specifications. Each of these errors is usually caught. Most of them are documented. The design error would be caught in assembly or perhaps earlier by a drawing checker. In either case, there is probably some sort of liaison call slip issued between departments to correct the error. The research error would be found either during testing or earlier in an engineering review of the research findings. The writer would be caught by his art director when it came time to specify type-setting. Regardless, there is usually some sort of paper work in support of these discoveries and the requirement for change.

Survey of Available Facts: Almost every scientific/professional task requires some sort of data or information research (on material other than the specifications themselves) to help the individual do his task right the first time. For an engineer, this activity would include a review of the possibility of an off-the-shelf substitution; looking into the producibility of his design; checking test and evaluation reports on similar items; and a general review of the state of the art in his area. If he fails to do this and designs an item that is impossible to manufacture or spends costly design hours on a part that is already available, then he has made an error. Such errors are usually caught later by manufacturing tooling engineers or at "make or buy" conferences and reviews, and most of them result in some form of formal documentation.

This survey of available facts is almost a way of life with scientists. It is assumed that most researchers spend 90 percent of their time reading and less than 10 percent "doing." Failure to review pertinent facts can easily result in such costly error as duplicating documented experimentation, trying to discover the discovered, and testing the tested. Scientific errors are rarely formally documented at the time and are often discovered only after the individual task is completed. Yet, the fact that they are discovered does make them a part of the criteria of supervisor judgment. When the error is caught during the task—a lab supervisor recognizing a repetitive test or experiment—it will probably involve some sort of documentation, even though it may only be a memo.

Skill (Careless) Error: Like anyone else, the scientific/professional employee may make outright skill or craft errors. For the design engineer these would be a transposed tolerance, a wrong electronic value, or any other careless error. For the scientist it would be misinterpretation of test results, incorrect data input, or faulty information in a report. To a copywriter, it could be a typographical error, a misspelled word, or an error in grammar. In any of these cases, the error usually results in some sort of documentation or change notice.

Success of Project: Since all scientific/professional activity has a goal or end product (regardless of the temporary or transitory nature of such goals), there is always some degree of success and failure to be determined. In a long-term project there may be hundreds of goals or milestones to be met before the final one is reached, but the goals are always there. Though some of these goals may require breaking through the state of the art, there are many goals that do not require such dynamic discovery. Failure to meet them is, in many cases, simply due to individual error.

Though much of this success evaluation depends on supervisor judgment, there are still many elements that come under regular formal documentation. Final test and assembly often disclose blatant engineering-design errors. The same is true for applied-research tasks. And such failures are generally well documented—at times *too* well for the supervisor's comfort. In the case of our advertising writer, his success ratio is documented through readership surveys (Starch, etc.) and sales-inquiry results.

CRITERIA SELECTION

By using the four basic scientific/professional criteria as well as standard criteria (audited forms or reports, etc.), the supervisor can generally come up with a valid measurement technique. To do this, he must review existing, specific inspection or checkpoints that could reveal errors against his basic criteria. For instance, an engineering-design supervisor would ask himself, "Who usually comes up with our specification errors?" He lists them, along with the documentation (if any) that supports the error discovery. He then goes on and does the same with all of the other basic criteria (see Figure 49) until he has a full picture of all available defect-finding elements. Once this is done, he is able to review these elements against each other and against the basic criteria that they support. He may now select the criteria and the form of documentation against which he wishes to evaluate his workers.

Specific Criteria

The supervisor will not want to use every criterion or every available form of inspection or documentation. He will select those that are easiest to use and, if possible, those that are the most important to the success of his operation. In Figure 49, the supervisor has circled Specification Groundwork and Skill or Craft Error. He has rejected the information-survey criterion since he has had few or no problems in this area. He decides not to use the success criterion since his designers rarely work alone on a single component and findings in this area would reflect on a group rather than an individual. (He may wish to use this criterion later as a group-measurement device.) Because of an earlier push on standard criteria, he has all but eliminated error in this area.

Common Documentation

Upon reviewing the two selected criteria, he finds that they both have common documentation and that he will have to go to only two or three sources (checked items) of documentation for the entire picture. That is, by reviewing design-change notices, material-review-board reports, and liaison call actions on a quarterly basis (or daily as this documentation crosses his desk), he can prepare a fairly accurate picture of the accuracy of design within his group (see Figure 50). To these factors he will also add his own supervisory observations. When and if he discovers that a designer is free from error in these documents, he can run a further check with the drafting-checking records to complete the evaluation against the two criteria selected. He uses drafting as a double check on the individuals who show no error under the first three sources since the drafting documentation is generally voluminous and any across-the-board review in this area is time-consuming.

In Figure 50 we see an "open-and-shut case" of outstanding achievement in the case of Mr. Brown. He obviously has no error over the three-month period. According to the criteria set—specification groundwork and skill error—he has been error-free. But what about the other members of the group? Though not perfect, one or more of them may be so close to perfect that they deserve recognition also. The supervisor must add at least one more element—the element of opportunity for error—before he can determine his

	SPECIFICATION GROUNDWORK	SURVEY OF INFORMATION	SKILL OR CRAFT ERROR	SUCCESS OF PROJECT	STANDARD CRITERIA
INSPECTION BY:	Supervisor	Supervisor	Supervisor	Supervisor	Supervisor
DOCUMENTATION BY:	None existing	None existing	None existing	None existing	None existing
REGULARITY & COVERAGE:	All assigned tasks	Key assignment	All assignments	Key assignment	All oversized items
ERROR DISCLOSURE:	Any obvious specification error	Any error showing lack of information survey	Any obvious craft error	Failures due to major design faults	Any documentation error
INSPECTION BY:	Drafting	Procurement	Drafting	Testing	Travel audit
DOCUMENTATION BY:	Checked reports	Review form	Checking reports	Test report MRB action	Reject notice
REGULARITY & COVERAGE:	On all drawings	All production items	All drawings	All production items	All expense vouchers
ERROR DISCLOSURE:	Errors in specification – marriage and tolerances	Failure to use obvious off-the-shelf substitute	Call-out errors. Documentation errors. Basic design errors	Failure on final test due to design error	Return for documentation error
INSPECTION BY:	Manufacturing	Manufacturing	Component Test	Customer final inspection	Timekeeping
DOCUMENTATION BY:	Liaison buffer MRB action on DCN's	Approved callout & design change note	Test reports MRB actions	Customer complaint or public reject	Weekly reports
REGULARITY & COVERAGE:	All production items	All production items	All production items	All purchased items	All tasks
ERROR DISCLOSURE:	Failure to meet marriage speed, balances, material specifications	Design that does not take manufacturability into consideration	Any error traced to craft error	Reject for design error	Excessive over-time, documentation error
INSPECTION BY:	Component test	Value Engineering		Scheduling	
DOCUMENTATION BY:	Test reports and MRB actions	Review forms		Weekly and final reports	
REGULARITY & COVERAGE:	All prod. items	All production items		All major tasks	
ERROR DISCLOSURE:	Test failure due to specification error	Excessive tolerances, ignoring off-the-shelf option, etc.		Failure to meet end date and milestones	

FIG. 49   Criteria-selection work sheet for engineering-design group. The selected criteria are circled, and the documentation to be used in evaluation is checked.

145

NAME	TEST REPTS. OR LIAISON CALL & MRB ACTIONS	SUPERVISORY OBSERVATION	DESIGN CHANGE NOTICES	
L. Jones	///	/	0	
K. Smith	/	0	/	
D. Edwards	//	/	0	
R. F. Brown	0	0	0	
W. Ring	////	//	/	
R. Black	/	0	/	
T. Miles	/	0	0	
N. Miller	0	/	0	
H. Gorman	0	0	/	

FIG. 50   Engineering supervisor's work sheet. By tabulating errors identified by selected documentation (listed at top of columns), the supervisor can quickly identify his leading achievers.

other achievers. For instance, a designer who has two tasks in a three-month period and botches one of them certainly can't be called an outstanding achiever. But a designer working on 100 elements during the same period who also makes one error is 99 percent error-free. He certainly deserves consideration.

ERROR POSSIBILITY

This brings up a fairly valid "formula" for general scientific/professional measurement:

$$\frac{S}{P}\ 100\ =\ \text{percent defective}$$

Where S is the errors discovered under any of the selected criteria (specifications, survey, skill, success, or standard criteria) and P is the possibility for error, or the number of opportunities for error, during a given period.

Where does the supervisor get the possibility figure? He certainly should have some record of assigned tasks during the period. It may be in the form of time charged against task record or a simple list of assignments. A review of the number of actual drawings prepared during the measurement period could also give this information, though this search could prove too time-consuming. In some cases, the supervisor may have to resort to memory or supervisory judgment. In the case of small groups, his judgment would be

NAME	TEST REPORTS OR LIAISON CALLS & MTL. REV. BD. ACTIONS	SUPERVISORY OBSERVATION	DESIGN CHANGE NOTICES	MAY–JUNE–JULY (S) TOT. DESIGN ERROR	(P) ELE-MENTS DESIGNED	PERCENT DEFECT-IVE
L. Jones	///	/	O	4	50	8%
K. Smith	/	O	/	2	73	2.7%
D. Edwards	//	/	O	3	25	12%
R. F. Brown	O	O	O	O	43	0%
W. Ring	////	//	/	7	87	8%
R. Black	/	O	/	2	55	3.6%
T. Miles	/	O	O	/	20	5%
N. Miller	O	/	O	/	48	2.1%
H. Gorman	O	O	/	/	91	1.1%
GROUP TOTAL				21	492	4.3%

FIG. 51 A work sheet with percent defective information added not only gives the supervisor a more complete picture of degree of achievement but also gives him an overall picture of the group's accomplishment (see Group Total).

fairly accurate; with larger groups, the supervisor may need statistical backup. Regardless, there is usually some way to come up with a meaningful possibility figure. As was pointed out earlier, a supervisor will rarely admit that he doesn't know what his workers are doing, what they are working on, and how much they are accomplishing.

In Figure 51, the supervisor has added the possibility figure *P*. In this case it is based on number of elements designed. This particular supervisor obtained the count from his task-time-charge report. When figured against the total design errors for each of his engineers through the formula, the percents defective found in the last column are obtained. A review of these percents show that none of the other engineers are close to Mr. Brown in achievement. The nearest is Mr. Gorman who will probably not be recommended for ZD achievement recognition but who should receive some supervisory recognition for his effort.

GROUP MEASUREMENT

Once the possibility ratio is established for each worker, it is relatively easy to establish group standing. This figure serves three purposes: (1) it can be posted to show the employees just how the group stands; (2) it gives the supervisor a base from which to evaluate his own success with the program; (3) it gives management a guide to evaluate the supervisor's ZD achievement. Since, in the scientific/professional areas, the criteria and measurement methods will vary greatly (as will the possibility factor), the posting of group standings will not stimulate the competition seen on a manufacturing floor or in any other repetitive-task area. Just the same, the professional does like to see where his group stands and will be highly receptive to an improvement trend on a chart. The posting technique would be similar to that of any other group within the organization (see Figure 52) and would be based on the total *P* and *S* factors noted on Figure 51.

The engineering-design supervisor may wish to use an entirely different set of standards and criteria for group measurement. Where he does have test and evaluation records available for most of his group designs, he may wish to use these figures as a measurement of his section's overall achievement. This data would be found checked under the success of project criteria shown in Figure 49. In this way he relieves himself of the time-consuming task of compiling complete statistics on all of his workers (with the exception of his most obvious achievers) and looks to a simpler, more formally documented area for group achievement. And though the documentation is not suitable for individual measurement, it is highly suitable for group and supervisor measurement.

OTHER EXAMPLES

This method of measurement and documentation can be used in almost any area where nonrepetitive, original work is performed. Though the industrial engineer was one of the first to be measured under the Zero Defects

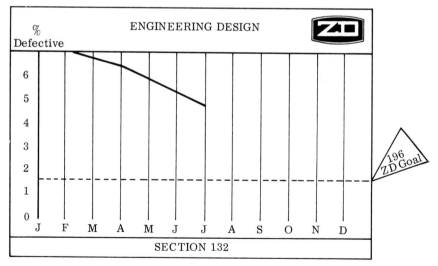

FIG. 52 Posted chart showing percent defective derived from previous figure. This type of posting allows the group to see where it stands without identifying any particular non-achievers.

	SPECIFICATION GROUNDWORK	SURVEY OF INFORMATION	SKILL OR CRAFT ERROR	SUCCESS OF PROJECT (GROUP)	STANDARD CRITERIA
INSPECTION BY:	Supervisor	Supervisor	Supervisor	Supervisor	Supervisor
DOCUMENTATION BY:	Worksheet ✓	Worksheet ✓	Worksheet ✓	None Existing ✓	None Existing
REGULARITY & COVERAGE:	On all tasks	On all tasks	All tasks	All major tasks	all contemplated documentation
ERROR DISCLOSURE:	Total failure to test and study correct requirements	Repetitious effort, experimentation + omissions in test or matl. selection	Any obvious documentation errors and blatant craft errors	Failure to meet scientific goals due to scientific error	Documentation error and omissions
INSPECTION BY:	Engineering Review	Engineering review	Engineering Review	Customer or Management Review	Trade audit
DOCUMENTATION BY:	Review reports ✓	Test report ✓	Review reports	Review Report ✓	Reject notice
REGULARITY & COVERAGE:	on all tasks weekly monthly	on all major tasks	All major tasks	All final reports	All expense reports
ERROR DISCLOSURE:	Failure to follow basic requirement	Repeat of documented test or experiment	Documentation errors, information omissions, Failure to misinterpret test data properly	Failure to meet requirements due to scientific error	Documentation error and omissions
INSPECTION BY:	Test + evaluation	Engineering review		Test + evaluation	Procurement
DOCUMENTATION BY:	Test report ✓	Review reports		Test report ✓	Reject notice
REGULARITY & COVERAGE:	on all required tests	on all major tasks		on all final tests	all reports
ERROR DISCLOSURE:	Failure to test to required levels	Omission of obvious material candidates and test-technique selections		Failure to meet requirement due to scientific error	Documentation error on all facilities and material requests
INSPECTION BY:				Scheduling	
DOCUMENTATION BY:				Weekly report	
REGULARITY & COVERAGE:				All major tasks	
ERROR DISCLOSURE:				Failure to meet dates and milestones	

FIG. 53 Criteria-selection work sheet for research group showing three selected criteria (see text and checked documentation material). Review and Test Reports are also checked under the success of project since these forms of documentation will be used for separate group-measurement criteria.

149

program, several organizations have extended the same techniques to other scientific or professional areas. Two examples from such areas would be the research scientist and the promotional copywriter.

The Research Scientist

This man is perhaps the most difficult single person in the organization to measure effectively. Yet, as shown earlier, he does have certain basic chores that do come under formal audit (standard criteria): facilities requests, expense documentation, budgets, customer documentation, and other basic business activities. He also handles certain documentation under the four other basic criteria. As an example, consider the case of a small research group working on the development of special materials for high-temperature applications. Their work is in the "applied" areas rather than in the realm of "pure" research; that is, they are working toward specific answers to specific problems provided by the engineering staff. Thus, in this case, there are formal specifications or requirements to be met and real measurement techniques for each.

After writing out (see Figure 53) and reviewing all available criteria documentation, the supervisor decides to use the three circled criteria for individual-measurement purposes. He makes this decision because they all have common documentation that is reviewed by him on a regular basis. He enters the three common documentation sources on his work sheet (see Figure 54). The work sheet itself becomes a documentation source for supervisor-discovered errors since he will "tick" them directly on this sheet as he finds them.

Though he has also been having problems with his men on proper initiation of procurement documentation (see standard criteria on Figure 53), he feels that error in this area does not always relate to specific assigned tasks. Thus, he sets aside errors in this area as backup documentation or a final check on Zero Defects excellence. Though he will note these errors on the work sheet, they will not be used for "first round" evaluation.

Since most of the assigned tasks are group efforts in this case, the success criterion will generally reflect on the group as a whole. Thus, the supervisor will reserve this criterion for group measurement and reporting only.

He does not determine a percent defective from his S and P figures on the work sheet since he has no way of calculating the actual number of operations in the individually assigned tasks. Rather, he simply balances the number of noted errors against task load and makes an evaluation by supervisory judgment.

As you can see from the work sheet (Figure 54), both Smith and Brown are defect-free for the period. But two things become evident: (1) Brown has had a heavier load during the period, and (2) Smith has three procurement-documentation errors while Brown has none. Thus, Brown is singled out

NAME	TEST REPORTS	ENGINEERING REVIEW	SUPERVISORY REVIEW	MARCH–APRIL–MAY		
				TOTAL ERRORS	ASSIGNED TASKS	PROCURE-MENT AUDIT
L. Jones	/	//	//	5	10	///
K. Smith	0	0	0	0	5	///
D. Edwards	/	/	0	2	7	//
R. Brown	0	0	0	0	8	0
				GROUP TOTAL		

FIG. 54   Research supervisor's work sheet weighing errors discovered through selected documentation (see Figure 53) against number of assigned tasks. The procurement-form audit was added later as a tie breaker between Smith and Brown since both were clear of errors from the other selected sources. No group totals or percents defective are computed since the supervisor has selected a separate criterion for group accomplishments.

for recognition, and Smith is singled out for a talk on the importance of proper documentation.

For posted group measurement the supervisor simply takes the management reviews from the period and balances the rejected findings or failures to meet requirements against the number of projects reviewed (P), multiplies by 100, and comes up with a percent defective for the group. This is posted in the area (see Figure 55). For this figure to be meaningful as a defect measurement, a failure to breach the state of the art should not be considered a defect.

The Writer

As an example here, let us take a small group of copywriters working on sales brochures and direct-mail pieces. Their product line includes business machines and support equipment. They are required to have some technical knowledge but rely heavily on data inputs from the various product managers within their organization.

The supervisor makes out the standard-criteria-review sheet in an effort to discover the most useful criteria and documentation for individual measure-

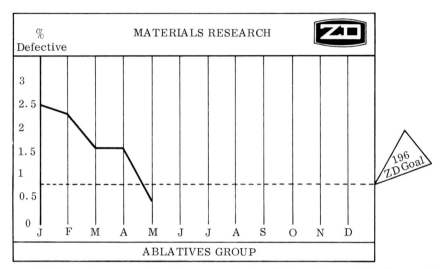

FIG. 55   Research-group-standing chart computed through formula by weighing Success of Project factors noted on this group's criteria-selection sheet.

ment. On the review sheet (see Figure 56), the supervisor has circled all but one of the basic criteria. The success factor was rejected because, in most cases, such review would come six months or more after task completion. The rest are documented on a day-to-day or weekly basis. Since, like most advertising groups, this shop uses the job or traffic ticket to follow any task through to completion, the sign-offs and dates on this document give the supervisor an excellent picture of his employees' accomplishments. And since their work depends so much on product-manager coordination, this man's acceptance or sign-off is of prime importance. The last measurement method, documented in part by purchases of type for writers' changes (to correct spelling errors, punctuation, etc.) and in part from the editorial activities of the supervisor, completes the measurement picture for all of our selected criteria.

When the actual found errors are noted on the work sheet (see Figure 57), the final result looks something like that shown in the two previous examples —except that the supervisor has noted defects per assigned piece in the last column rather than percent defective. In this case, this was done because each piece represents hundreds of words and many data elements. By review, it is found that W. Ring has 0.03 errors per assigned task and is obviously the top achiever for the group. By a little simple mathematics, the supervisor can also note that this man has had one typographical error in approximately 13,000 printed words (his assignments average 500 words each). These facts should certainly be taken favorably into the consideration of the achievement-awards committee.

In this case, the group achievement is simply the sum of the individual achievements with the average defects per piece determined by the formula

	SPECIFICATION GROUNDWORK	SURVEY OF INFORMATION	SKILL OR CRAFT ERROR	SUCCESS OF PROJECT	STANDARD CRITERIA
INSPECTION BY:	Supervisor	Supervisor	Supervisor	Supervisor	Supervisor
DOCUMENTATION BY:	None existing	None existing	Error checklist	None existing	Job Ticket ✓
REGULARITY & COVERAGE:	All tasks	All tasks	All tasks	All tasks	All tasks
ERROR DISCLOSURE:	Any failure to meet basic requirement	Lack of accuracy in support data	Spelling errors, typos, poor art-calcs on final draft	Judgment of effectiveness of piece	Failure to follow proper approval cycles
INSPECTION BY:	Product Manager	Product Manager	Production Chief	Product Manager	Production Chief
DOCUMENTATION BY:	Review memo ✓	Review memo ✓	Job Ticket ✓	Review memo ✓	Type purchase report
REGULARITY & COVERAGE:	All tasks	All tasks	All jobs	All tasks creatively	All tasks
ERROR DISCLOSURE:	Failure to provide Sales aid as requested	Failure to follow data provided.	Errors in production call-outs	Failure to accomplish Sales aim	Writer's change due to written error in final type
INSPECTION BY:	Production Chief			Traffic Chief	
DOCUMENTATION BY:	Job Ticket ✓			Job Ticket	
REGULARITY & COVERAGE:	All jobs			All jobs	
ERROR DISCLOSURE:	Failure to meet Production requirements			Failure to meet final date due to writer error	
INSPECTION BY:	Traffic Chief				
DOCUMENTATION BY:	Job Ticket ✓				
REGULARITY & COVERAGE:	All jobs				
ERROR DISCLOSURE:	Failure to meet pre-determined date				

FIG. 56 Criteria-selection work sheet for advertising group showing four selected criteria (circled) and supporting documentation (checked). The Error Checklist item under Skill or Craft Error is actually supervisor's work sheet shown in Figure 57.

153

NAME	JOB TICKET	SUPERVISORY CHECK LIST	PRODUCT MGR. MEMOS	MARCH-APRIL-MAY		
				NO. OF ERRORS	ASSIGNED TASKS	AVERAGE DEFECTS PER ITEM
L. Jones	//	//	///	7	20	.4
K. Smith	///	//	/	6	22	.3
D. Edwards	/	////	0	5	14	.3
R. F. Brown	/	///	/	5	23	.2
W. Ring	0	/	0	1	26	.03
R. Black	///	##### ///	///	14	16	.9
			GROUP TOTAL	38	121	.3

FIG. 57   Advertising supervisor's work sheet kept on a day-to-day basis. The supervisor also used this sheet as a documentation source by checking personally observed defects in the center column. He has modified the basic formula to give himself an Average Defect per Item figure in the last column since, in this case, this would be more meaningful than a percent defective figure.

P/S = average defect, which is a modification of the percent defective formula 100 S/P. A posting of the group's record is shown in Figure 58.

SUMMARY

Though it is true that no magic formula has evolved for measurement in the scientific and professional areas, the Administrator should never feel stymied. There are always criteria and measurement techniques available if the supervisors and management will only seek them out. It will be up to the Administrator to show the supervisors the way and to provide aid in criteria and technique selection. A positive approach is the only way to answer the excuse that "my work just can't be measured." The success in this area will reflect the determination of the Administrator. The success of many ZD organizations in overcoming this problem proves beyond doubt that it *can* be done.

A word of warning: professional groups tend to set their goals too high. They tend to be harder on themselves than an outside measurement agency would. This is only natural when you ask people to set their own goals. The

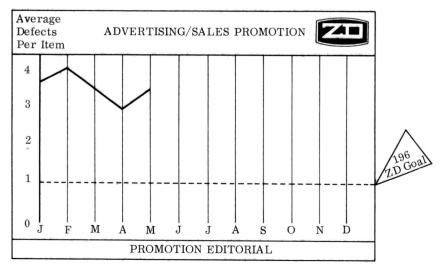

FIG. 58   Advertising-group-standing chart computed by averaging the final column figures in Figure 57 (see Group Total).

Administrator should review all such measurement techniques to assure that goals and criteria are realistic.

One last word on measurement: the Administrator should not be overly concerned about formal measurement procedures. As has been noted before, when all of the other program factors are going well, almost everyone will jump on the measurement bandwagon. And when a supervisor really wants his workers measured and recognized for achievement, he almost always finds a way.

The Zero Defects Program
as a Day-to-Day Management Tool

> *Zero Defects is personal. It makes the employee conscious of
> his role in gaining top product quality.*
> JOSEPH L. MAZEL, *Factory* MAGAZINE, JULY, 1965

14

Employee Recognition

Proper recognition of employee achievement is one of the most important activities in the Zero Defects program. It is, in fact, the very heart of the program. As noted in the last section, recognition is the only reason for the program's concern with measurement. Without recognition, without employee awareness that management knows and cares about outstanding effort, no ZD program can sustain itself for any length of time.

RECOGNITION AS A MANAGEMENT TOOL

The act of recognizing employees for extra effort is certainly not new. Many organizations have suggestion-awards programs, bonus plans, patent-awards plans, overtime premiums, piecework premiums, and other benefits of this sort. Though it may seem incongruous to group a patent award with a piecework premium, they have much in common: they are both given for doing something over and above the actual assigned employee task. In fact, almost all of the awards or recognition systems used by modern management fall into this category. The result of this trend has been that little effort is being made to recognize or reward the man who does his job and does it well, day by day, year in, year out. This consistency of performance may far overshadow the value derived from high productivity or invention.

Management's general attitude toward overall employee achievement of this sort has been, "That's what I pay them to do." The response to management is a mountain of scrap and skyrocketing rework and retest costs. If the employee is being paid to do each and every job right the first time, it appears that almost every employee and every organization in America is shortchanging management. The truth is, management is shortchanging the employee.

This does not mean that every time a worker makes a perfect solder connection, his supervisor should rush onto the manufacturing floor and praise the worker for his accomplishment. But if that solder connection is the worker's one-hundred-thousandth consecutive perfect assembly, management should certainly do something. Zero Defects affords management the opportunity to do just that.

Will this recognition pay off? The answer is a definite yes. Experience has shown that, in every case of Zero Defects recognition, the involved employee has continued to excel at the same rate for extended periods after the original act of recognition. The questions here are: "What type of recognition does the ZD achiever respond to, and why does he react in this positive manner?"

What Type of Recognition?

Perhaps the most surprising thing about ZD recognition is that it need not involve a monetary outlay. If we are to follow the ZD philosophy, it can't. Management hired an employee to do a job and to do it right. It would not make sense to give him a bonus simply for doing what he was hired to do. Such an act would say that, when it hired him, management really didn't expect the worker to do good work. Thus, the man is being paid for mediocre effort. Since employees are keenly aware of management attitude, it is basic to the program that ZD recognition take another approach—one where man-

FIG. 59 Recognition sessions should be kept informal, giving the achiever and top management the opportunity to discuss freely the scope and importance of the individual contribution.

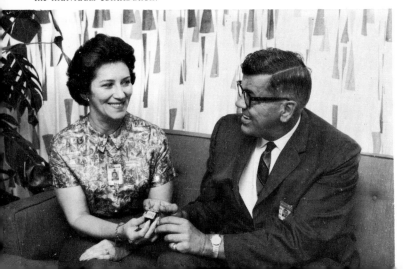

agement openly and honestly demonstrates to the employee that his effort is recognized and appreciated by the organization. To put it in its fundamental state, it is simply management telling the employee it is aware of his achievement. This act is accomplished by face-to-face contact between employee and management.

Why Does It Work?

Much has been said about the management pat-on-the-back approach to employee achievement. Books have been written on the subject. It has been cursed and praised by both management and employee alike. Then why did Zero Defects adopt this controversial technique of recognition? The truth is that, though Zero Defects recognition does contain a certain element of the pat-on-the-back technique, it goes further; it makes sure the worker is hit right between the eyes with the recognition sledgehammer. For example: When a manager calls an employee into his office and, after a brief discussion about job importance, states, "Jones, you have been doing a good job. Keep up the good work," the employee leaves without being sure just what management was trying to tell him. Management could have meant what it said, but, more than likely, " . . . you have been doing a good job. Keep up the good work," meant the discussion was over and the employee should go back to his job.

If, on the other hand, management takes the time and effort to assure the employee that it is aware of his specific accomplishment and that management will be looking for and expecting more of the same in the future, there is no chance of misunderstanding (see Figure 59). The employee leaves the office knowing his every move is important to management and that management cares enough about the individual's task to keep right on caring.

Does this information make the employee happy? Not necessarily. He may even leave a recognition session feeling he has a "monkey on his back." It will, however, make him feel his task is important enough for him to continue performing at an optimum level of craftsmanship. The secret to Zero Defects recognition is in that key program-concept word—"awareness." Zero Defects recognition does not buy the man a new boat or make the down payment on a new house; it buys him a feeling of increased security and makes a management down payment on continued craftsmanship.

Because of these facts, Zero Defects recognition works in spite of any adverse conditions possibly surrounding it. It works every time. It works whether or not the management representative involved is an eloquent, highly motivating speaker. It works even when the employee has won initial recognition simply by chance and does not wish to accept any further responsibility. It works not because it simply involves praise but rather because it assures job-importance awareness.

ZD

ACHIEVEMENT AWARD RECOMMENDATION

EMPLOYEE'S NAME		PERIOD	
Myrtle Anderson		January TO June 196	
OCCUPATION TITLE	DEPARTMENT NAME	DEPT. NO.	CLOCK NO.
Mechanic E&E	Harness Manufacturing	884	3975

READ INSTRUCTIONS ON REVERSE SIDE BEFORE COMPLETING THIS FORM

SCOPE OF TASK: Harness Assembly

ACHIEVEMENT: This employee has completed five months of work without a chargeable defect. She has worked on wire preparation, crimp insertion, plug assembly, soldering, harness boards and all phases of harness manufacturing. She has performed the following tasks without error during this time: 300 plug assemblies; 9,500 wires; 19,000 crimp contacts; and 1,600 solder connections.

AWARENESS: Mrs. Anderson takes great pride in her work; she checks subassemblies to make sure there are no defects before assembly, and inspects the job after she has completed it.

OTHER FEATURES: She has a very good attitude, solves most of her problems and tries to perform to the best of her abilities.

SUMMARY: Mrs. Anderson's work is always excellent, and she instills an attitude of Zero Defects in her fellow workers by her own example.

(USE REVERSE SIDE OF THIS FORM IF ADDITIONAL SPACE IS NEEDED)

SUPERVISOR'S SIGNATURE	SUPERVISOR'S TITLE	MANAGER'S SIGNATURE		MAIL POINT
C. E. Johnson *C. E. Johnson*	Foreman Harness Mfg.	Bill Metter *B. Metter*		18
ROUTE FOR ACTION TO:	TITLE	LOCATION	MAIL POINT	DATE
T. E. King	ZD REPRESENTATIVE	Main Plant	25	9/1-6

FOR ZERO DEFECTS ADMINISTRATION USE ONLY:

AWARD DENIED AND REASON

ACHIEVEMENT VERIFIED BY	ZERO DEFECTS REPRESENTATIVE SIGNATURE
C. E. Johnson *C. E. Johnson*	T. E. King *T. E. King*

FIG. 60 A typical Achievement Award Recommendation, giving complete information for proper evaluation by the awards committee.

RECOGNITION TECHNIQUES

Most Zero Defects organizations follow the same basic recognition pattern of management recognition, public recognition, and personal recognition. The standard recognition technique involves the formal achievement presentation by management; publicizing the achievement to the work force in general; and some form of special, personal touch that brings the importance of the recognition home to the employee and his family.

Achiever Selection

The actual selection of the Zero Defects achiever begins, like everything else in the program, with the first-line supervisor. It is the supervisor who initially recognizes the individual achievement through one of the techniques covered in Part 5 of this book (Performance Measurement). When the supervisor perceives an employee achievement, he initiates an achievement form (see Figure 60 and Appendix B). On this form he outlines the employee's actual achievement and gives support information about the individual's attitude, ZD awareness, and other background information that could be helpful to the recognition-review committee (see Figure 61). The form is then forwarded through the department manager to the Administrator or his department representative. Here it is checked for completeness of information and reliability of support data. The form may be sent back to the supervisor for additional information or forwarded to the industrial relations committee representative for an employee-background check. This step is especially important in large organizations where certain negative factors may exist, unknown to even the employee's immediate supervisor. Once this preliminary check is completed, the achievement is ready for final review.

FIG. 61   This listing includes most of the factors that would go into an individual-achievement evaluation. This type of information should be included on the recommendation form in order that the review committee fully understands the scope of the achievement.

Summary Checklist for Evaluating Zero Defects Achievers

1. Impact of potential error (abort of mission, cost, effect on schedules, etc.).
2. Contribution of the individual or group to the prevention of error.
3. Difficulty of the job and level of skill required.
4. Level of tediousness or boredom of assigned task.
5. Schedule and load impact on error potential.
6. Ability of employee to correct his own errors before being detected by a checker.
7. Attitude of the worker toward work, project and company mission.

ACHIEVEMENT AWARD RECOMMENDATION

EMPLOYEE'S NAME		PERIOD	
W. H. MacIntosh		9/1/6 to 9/1/6	

OCCUPATION TITLE	DEPARTMENT NAME	DEPT. NO.	CLOCK NO.
Support Engineer	Specifications	516	9970

READ INSTRUCTIONS ON REVERSE SIDE BEFORE COMPLETING THIS FORM

SCOPE OF TASK: To carry out design assignments in accordance with specifications set forth by customers and within parameters of final function of finished product, in this case the wheel assembly.

ACHIEVEMENT: Henry MacIntosh's work was 98% accurate during the period under investigation. He checked liaison call sheets and drawings.

AWARENESS: He is interested in doing the complete job right the first time. He tries to avoid making design fixes which usually end up with difficult to solve manufacturing problems later on.

OTHER FEATURES: He continues to try to increase his knowledge of work and to keep up with the state of the art. He is cost-conscious and tries to perform his work within schedules.

SUMMARY: His task leader and the group leader for the wheel assembly both commend his work highly.

(USE REVERSE SIDE OF THIS FORM IF ADDITIONAL SPACE IS NEEDED)

SUPERVISOR'S SIGNATURE	SUPERVISOR'S TITLE	MANAGER'S SIGNATURE	MAIL POINT
N. E. Walton	Chief, Specifications	C. H. Hilton	40

ROUTE FOR ACTION	TITLE	LOCATION	MAIL POINT	DATE
W. F. Stone	ZD REPRESENTATIVE	Main Plant	52	10/1/6

FOR ZERO DEFECTS ADMINISTRATION USE ONLY:

AWARD DENIED AND REASON
Need more specifics: how many call sheets and drawings did he check? How many characteristics per drawing? How many errors per how many thousand characteristics? Has he initiated any cost-reduction methods?

ACHIEVEMENT VERIFIED BY	ZERO DEFECTS REPRESENTATIVE SIGNATURE
N. E. Walton	W. F. Stone

FIG. 62 A rejected recommendation with Administrator's request for additional information (at base of form).

The review is usually conducted by a special-achievement-recognition committee which meets each month. This committee is made up of representatives from employee relations or personnel and a member of each major function within the organization, with the ZD Administrator as chairman. Several days before the meeting, each member is provided with copies of the recognition forms to be discussed, facilitating prompt action during the committee review.

The committee checks each of the achievements against the basic organizational criteria and makes a "go" or "no-go" decision in every case. Where recommendations are rejected, the Administrator conveys the committee findings to each supervisor involved and explains why the achievement was not selected (see Figure 62). In most cases, the reason is that the form did not give enough detailed information regarding the achievement or that the achievement time span did not support the requirement for "constant, conscious desire" to do the task right every time. Experience has shown that many of the committee-rejected recommendations do eventually get accepted. The mere act of rejection drives the supervisor to make an extra effort to document his worker's achievement in a more comprehensive manner.

Administrator Action

Once endorsed by the committee, the achiever is assured of Zero Defects recognition. The next step is for the Administrator to set up the actual recognition activities. He will review all accepted achievement forms for specific achievements having organization-wide promotion possibilities. Though all achievers are acknowledged publicly, some achievements will lend themselves to greater promotional applications than others. For instance, a drill-press operator's achievement of making 120,000 perfect high-tolerance operations over a six-month period will be of interest primarily to people in the manufacturing areas of your organization. On the other hand, a manufacturing secretary's accomplishment of typing 2,000 memos and entering 80,000 pieces of operational data without defect will interest every secretary in the organization. It is a case of getting the most motivational mileage for every dollar spent.

Once advance promotional plans are under way, the Administrator or his departmental representatives see that each member of top management is briefed on the individual-employee achievements in their particular areas of administration (see Figure 63). Specific times are set for the actual recognition sessions and everyone involved is notified of the time and plans.

Recognition by Management

It would be wrong to consider management recognition of achievers in the Zero Defects program a "recognition ceremony." The term "ceremony" brings to mind the stiff, formal award session where an apprehensive employee is ushered into a room full of supervisors and managers, given a few stereotyped words of praise, and handed a check or bond before being sent back to his bench. As with everything else in Zero Defects, the recognition activity is carefully planned and well prepared. There is a specific time and place for every move, and everyone involved knows his responsibilities.

Usually, the employee knows he is going to be recognized for a Zero Defects achievement. In the case of a factory employee (especially a woman), this gives the individual an opportunity to spruce up before going into the

---

INTRA-COMPANY MEMORANDUM

Date November 30, 19

To: .A. Ahlin

cc: N. D. Gray, H. F. Pearson, John L. Bordley

From: R. M. Buck   **Dept.** Zero Defects   , **Mail No.** 331   **Ext.** 2861

Subject: Presentation of Zero Defects Achievement Pin to Mrs. Alice E. Hoffman

---

    Arrangements have been made for you to present a Zero Defects Achievement Pin to Mrs. Alice E. Hoffman, 139-6978, Production Planner. The presentation will be made in your office at 2:30 p.m., on December 3, 1965, with Messrs. Gray, Pearson, and Bordley present. A photographer will record the presentation.

    Mrs. Hoffman's achievement is, briefly, that from July, 1964 to July, 1965, she received, logged and filed more than 80,000 Change Accountability Transmittal Cards and 30,000 drawings, with Zero Defects.

FIG. 63 Top-management information sheet presenting pertinent information about achiever so that management will be fully aware of the worker's specific achievement before the recognition session.

organization's executive suite, thus cutting down to some extent the usual embarrassment that accompanies such a visit. The supervisor and the achiever should both participate in the activities. It is best to keep the session attendance down to these two plus the management spokesman and the ZD Administrator.

The member of top management making the presentation has, as noted earlier, been thoroughly briefed on the employee's achievement. He welcomes the employee and makes sure that everyone is comfortably seated. He then goes into a detailed discussion with the worker and the supervisor on the actual achievement and its contribution to the overall goals of the department and organization. He makes sure that the employee is aware of the fact that management knows everything there is to know about this particular employee's task and his achievement.

The Award Symbol

At this time, a pin or some other form of visible recognition is presented to the worker. Most ZD organizations use a pin because it has more lasting promotional and motivating value than some object that will be removed from the organization and never seen again by the achiever's fellow employees. This pin is usually an adaption of the regular ZD pin, either being made out of a precious metal or utilizing some easily recognizable color differentiation (see Figure 64). If identification badges are worn, the pin should be attached directly to the individual's badge. This will usually make sure that the pin will not be lost and will be worn daily. If badges are not worn, the achievement pin should replace the regular ZD pin on the employee's clothing. It is suggested that the regular pin be actually removed and the achievement pin treated as a replacement to avoid the chance that the employee will take the latter home and save it for special occasions rather than wearing it daily.

At this point, a photographer may enter the office and photograph the actual pinning ceremony. There is nothing more unnerving than the sight of a photographer lounging about the room while the achievement discussion is taking place. He should remain outside until actually needed. A photograph of the event can be of value both promotionally and as a reminder or memento of the occasion for the achiever.

Group Awareness

Upon his return to the work area, the supervisor should call the entire section together to explain the achievement award and relate it to group goals. He should express his hope that every member of the group will soon wear the recognition pin and should suggest ways to accomplish this end. There will naturally be a certain amount of teasing of the awardee by his peers; this should be kept to a minimum, and the seriousness of the group goals be kept paramount.

ACHIEVEMENT FOLLOW-UP ACTIVITIES

The initial management contact will naturally have a strong effect on the individual achiever, but this one act does not complete the ZD recognition cycle. Since the employee has gone out of his way to accept and exhibit the Zero Defects way of life, it is up to management to make an extra effort to recognize this fact.

FIG. 64   ZD achievement pins (lower line) adapted from the original sign-up-pin designs (top line) save the organization money in design and die costs for special pins.

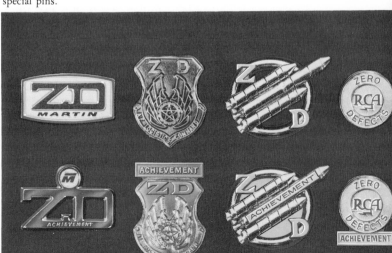

Special Activities

Many Zero Defects organizations follow up the initial achievement recognitions with an event such as an achievers' dinner or a special field trip for the achievers to see the organization's product or service in action (see Figure 65). These activities are designed to make the individual aware of the impact the achievement has had on the organization's end product. The field trip technique is especially useful when the organization deals in a service or produces a component for another organization's end product. It lets the achiever view the fruits of his efforts firsthand. It lets him meet the actual users of his product or service and find out from them just how important a defect-free product is.

Defense-industry ZD organizations have obtained tremendous mileage from this technique. The achiever from an airplane-manufacturing organization who is taken to a navy base to meet the pilots who actually fly his product and see the product in flight cannot help but be impressed by the experience. And, more important, he will surely tell his fellow employees about his experiences and his talks with the user.

It is not necessary to be in defense to use this valuable technique. A drug company could take achievers to a hospital; a paper mill could send them to a large printing establishment; an oil company could make its field trip to a major automobile racetrack. The main point to remember here is that it is important not only that the achiever be impressed by the trip but that all non-achievers get the message as well. Comprehensive follow-up in company papers and on bulletin boards should carry to the rank and file the stories of such excursions.

Personal Involvement

As for achievement dinners and other social occasions: To be effective, there must be some built-in product or task awareness factor. One ZD organization has an achievers' Family Day. Each achiever is invited to bring his entire family to his place of work for a round of activities and a dinner or luncheon. In this way, the achiever's relatives are exposed to his tasks and learn how his efforts contribute to the success of the organization as a whole. This approach is an effort to present the importance of the craftsman's attainment as an object of family pride. Fifty years ago, it was not unusual to hear a woman brag to her neighbors, "My husband is a master mason" or "Albert is senior clerk at Jones and Company." Today she may well say, "He works in construction" or "He's in an office down at Jones and Company."

Direct Family Contact

This family-awareness goal is also accomplished through the simple act of mailing a letter home to the achiever's next of kin (see Figure 66). To be effec-

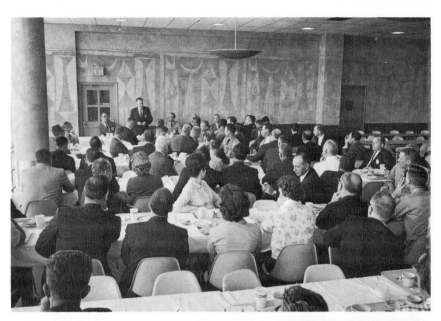

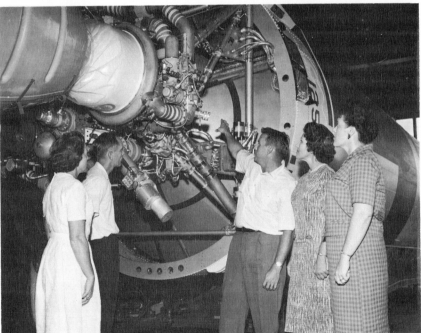

FIG. 65 Special achievers' luncheons (above) and trips to visit the customer to see the product in action (below) help to impress the achiever and the work force in general with management's interest in accomplishment.

MARTIN COMPANY

ORLANDO
DIVISION
Orlando,
Florida
32805

G. T. WILLEY
Vice President and General Manager

September 1, 19

Mrs. Betty Carmean
2800 South Shine Street
Orlando, Florida

Dear Mrs. Carmean:

When Martin-Orlando's Zero Defects Program was inaugurated in July,
1962, each employee was asked to dedicate himself or herself to the
prevention of errors by striving constantly to do every job right the
first time. To this end, every Martin employee signed a pledge card
promising to support the program to the best of his abilities.

So successful has been the program that many companies, all over the
world, as well as agencies of the U. S. Government, have adopted similar
programs and today more than 2,000,000 men and women in this country
are members of Zero Defects teams.

In the past three years, one hundred and seventy-four Martin employees
-- among them your husband -- have received Zero Defects Achievement
Awards in recognition of their exceptional contributions to the success of
the program. Last month, Mr. Carmean was again cited by his supervisors for his outstanding performance, and has again been chosen to
receive the Zero Defects Achievement Award. Only three other individuals
have been so honored. His accomplishment was to develop process plans
and welding tools for 24 crucial NASA signal control units. He performed
this task in a year's time with no welding defects.

On behalf of the Martin Company, I wish to express our continuing
appreciation of your husband's efforts.

Sincerely,

DIVISION OF
**MARTIN
MARIETTA**

FIG. 66 Recognition letter written by the Senior Executive and mailed home to the achiever's next of kin.

tive, this mailing cannot be a form letter or a pre-prepared communication.
The most successful use of this technique has been in organizations whose
management takes the time to send personal letters addressed to husbands,
wives, etc., telling of the specific achievement and asking the recipient to share
the organization's pride in the individual's accomplishment. This letter usually
comes from the desk of the Senior Executive and carries his personal signature. In large organizations, it would be impractical for the Senior Executive
to dictate every letter. The actual letter preparation can be handled by the

department representative or the department manager—in fact, by anyone who is close to the achievement and has all the facts at hand. Special care should be taken by the Administrator to assure that the correct person receives the document. Employee records should be double-checked for addresses, names, and current marital status. For instance, it could prove embarrassing to the achiever and/or the recipient if such a letter were to be sent to an ex-wife (divorced) or to a husband who had recently passed away.

Another technique is to bring the consumer to the organization for a special achievers' gathering. He can address achievers at a special luncheon, or talk to them individually; a combination of both will prove quite effective. If the individual talks take place in the achiever's work area, the rest of the work force will profit from exposure to the user too. For example, Jack Jones, a machinist achiever, meets Mr. Benson, president of a large automotive concern (and the organization's chief customer), at a special luncheon. Later in the day, Mr. Benson is brought to Jack's work area and Jack gets to show the guest just what his group does with the product. He also introduces Mr. Benson to the rest of his group. The impact is obvious. The entire group discovers that (1) the customer is aware of and vitally interested in their operation, and (2) the customer has a high regard for achievement in their area of activity.

Promotional Follow-up

Most Zero Defects organizations time their achievement-recognition activities to coincide with other program-sustaining efforts. For instance, when ZD impact weeks are held on a quarterly basis, the achievement activities can be held during these periods. This high-impact type of promotion cycle, discussed in the next chapter, has proven the most successful sustaining technique for the Zero Defects program.

Publication Tie-in

Since impact week is timed to coincide with publication of the company paper, most organizations feature individual achievement as the theme of the issue. If a large number of achievements are being recognized, it is recommended that a special recognition insert be added to the regular publication (see Figure 67). Since, according to the ZD philosophy, any one achievement is as important as any other, *all* should be covered in the special edition. To keep the issue interesting, the write-up should not feature one pin-presentation picture after another. Photographs of the workers on the job for which they are being recognized are more interesting and usually offer more to the reader.

Posting Achievements

As discussed previously, a poster series on these achievements should be used at this time (see Figure 68). Since the achievement itself offers potential

Employees Perform Outstanding Zero Defects Tasks

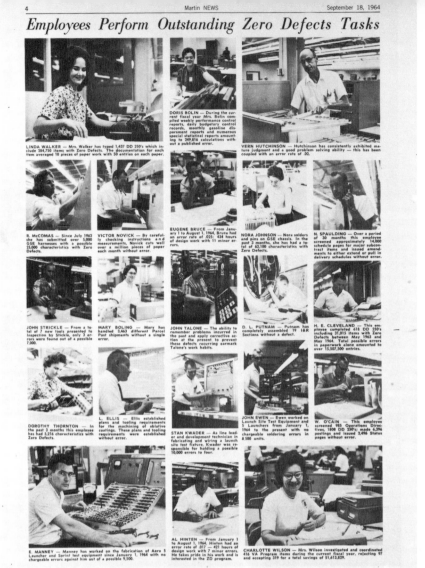

FIG. 67 A special achiever insert in a company paper highlights the accomplishments of award winners for a specific period.

problems of worker association and interest, these posters should be prepared on a limited-run basis. One method is to preprint a poster format leaving space for inserting a photograph and some copy. Then, when one or two of a type are needed, the Administrator's staff can simply paste the worker's photo into the space provided, with some enlarged typewriter type telling of the achievement. In cases where the achievement has application throughout the organization (secretarial, etc.) the Administrator may wish to go to a longer print run. Since it doesn't make much sense to heavily promote a paint-shop achievement in a typing-pool area, poster placement should be carefully studied and formal plans made for each presentation.

Extra Mileage

Many ZD organizations have discovered a great deal of sales and public relations potential in these achievements. For instance, the photo of a worker standing next to "his" 200,000 perfect parts may be picked up by local press and even national news services. Each achievement is, in itself, a human-interest story (see Figure 69). Publication of such information not only draws attention to the individual's achievement, but it also goes far to convey the image that the organization is actively pursuing a program to provide defect-free goods and services.

Many times, ZD organizations feature these achievements in company advertising. There is certainly no better method of getting the quality-of-product story across. Regardless of the technique, the payoff is twofold: (1) the customer is made aware of the organization's extra effort, and (2) the employee sees that his company thinks enough of the achievement to feature it in an ad.

REVIEW

Zero Defects achievement recognition is more than just a lollipop given to the worker for being a good boy. It not only rewards, but it motivates and directs. It is never an end in itself; it always features a driving force for more and better achievement in the future. When properly tied to realistic goals

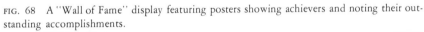

FIG. 68   A "Wall of Fame" display featuring posters showing achievers and noting their outstanding accomplishments.

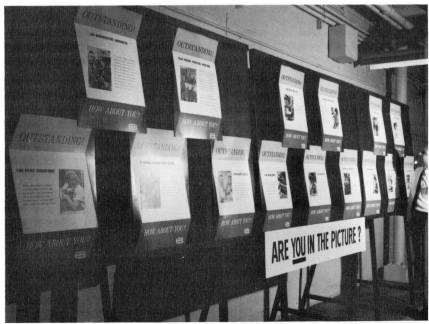

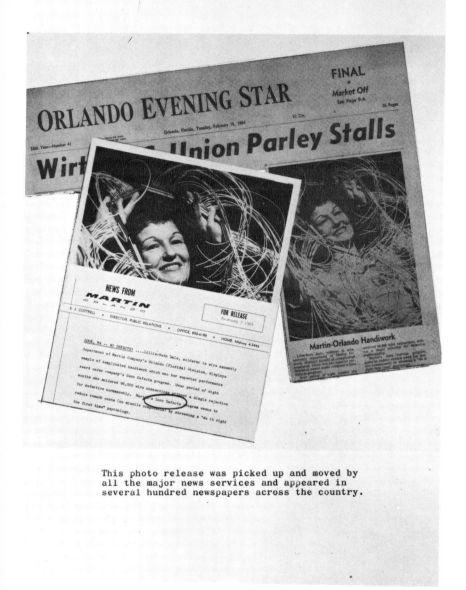

This photo release was picked up and moved by
all the major news services and appeared in
several hundred newspapers across the country.

FIG. 69 Achievement press release.

and product or service awareness, Zero Defects recognition can provide management with one of its most effective employee relations tools.

The key to effective recognition—the key to the entire program—is active management participation. Without this involvement, the recognition phase becomes no more than a rubber-stamp affair. With complete management and supervisor support, the recognition phase will carry more than half the Administrator's program-sustaining load.

I don't have a Zero Defects program for 20,000 people—my program is directed towards one person (the individual).
A. G. STRICKLAND,
ZD ADMINISTRATOR, LOCKHEED GEORGIA COMPANY

15

Directing a
Continuing Program

Sooner or later every ZD organization is faced with the problem: "What can we do or say about the program that we haven't tried before?" This problem is not peculiar to Zero Defects: every motivational effort from United Appeal to the annual safe-driving campaign meets this question. The big advantage in Zero Defects is that it has built-in sustaining factors inherent to the basic program itself. The recognition phase, discussed in the previous chapter, is one of these self-perpetuating factors. If properly implemented, it will keep interest alive in even the most inaccessible areas. Measurement and recognition will help the Administrator to win new friends for Zero Defects and to solidify support from those elements on the fringes of the program. Though there is no formal, set procedure for this phase (as there is for the indoctrination, recognition, and ECR phases), there are several proven approaches that can be applied to any ZD organization.

SUSTAINING THEORY

Review of Indoctrination Techniques

One factor is common to almost all early program promotion: it is the effort to get a general message (the ZD philosophy and concept) to a specific audience (the individual employee). The recognition-phase promotion gets specific information (individual achievement) to a general audience (everyone in the work force who can associate with the achievement and be motivated by it). The next step is to get a specific message to a specific audience. This technique opens many new motivation and promotion avenues to the Administrator who thinks himself stymied.

The Law of Diminishing Returns

Aside from the fact that the *specific*-promotion/motivation technique offers "something new" to the Administrator, it also has some very solid reasoning behind it. Experience has shown that serious, well-coordinated ZD programs usually result in substantial drops in rework and scrap costs during the first year. For instance, a particular production-line section may drop its defect rate from 3½ percent to 1½ percent over the initial twelve-month period. This type of result is not unusual, nor is it unreasonable to expect such a result. The impact of the kickoff and other early activities will carry the employees this far. But is it reasonable to expect them to halve the rate again in the second year? Or will the rate of decline level off as we near zero? The answer should be obvious: the closer they move to zero, the more difficult is their task. Each additional 0.1 percent may require just as much and more employee effort as did the initial 1½ percent.

The employees have to, in fact, "grind away" at every possible defect cause as they near their goal. Little things become important as this process develops. Where a general task awareness may have been all that was needed to motivate the employee to remove sloppy workmanship from his day-to-day activities, he will now need more specific help to remove the minute differences that stand between a good effort and near-perfect results.

The Specific-defect Attack

As noted earlier, recognition promotion contains some element of attacking a specific defect with a specific remedy. A secretary seeing that another has built up a performance record which has qualified her for ZD achievement, will direct her own activities accordingly. If she decides to work toward an exceptional standard, she will need help. Zero Defects must provide this help either through additional management motivational effort or through specific tools and training. Much of this aid can be provided by the first-line supervisor, but the Administrator will have to supply some additional backup.

We are not suggesting that a management representative be assigned to hold each employee's hand. In the first place, management doesn't have the time or manpower, and secondly, the employee wouldn't like it. What is suggested is that both management and the ZD administration be ready and willing to help when the supervisor discovers that the rank and file need it.

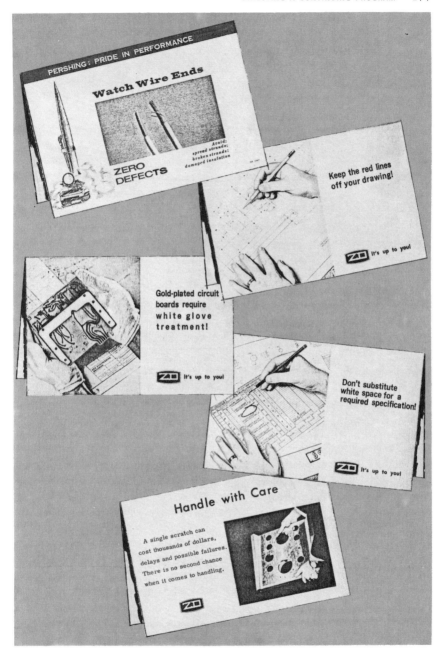

FIG. 70   Simple, cheap, and to the point, small table tents produced in limited runs highlight problem areas specific to interested groups.

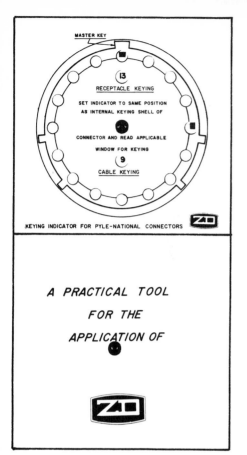

FIG. 71 A low-cost circular rule for identification of connector plugs and sockets was prepared as the result of a supervisor Error Cause Identification.

SPECIALIZED TECHNIQUES

At first glance, specialized support may seem to have a high-cost potential. Actual experience has proven the opposite. This type of sustaining promotion is much less expensive than that of the indoctrination phase. Specific support may include anything from a brief management talk to a simple table tent identifying a common defect or defect cause (see Figure 70). It seldom involves complex training gear, brochures, or even posters.

Supervisor Support

One common method used in this type of support is for the supervisors to point out problem areas to the ZD Administrator or his representatives. The Administrator must make the first move to let the supervisors know that assistance *is* available. Requests for specific-problem-area assistance may come through the ECR channels as a supervisor Error Cause Identification or they may simply be oral or written requests.

An example of such action would be a production-line supervisor who discovers an increase in surface scratches due to careless or improper handling.

He naturally speaks to his workers about the problem and asks them to be more careful. Though some improvement is seen, the scratches continue to occur. At this point, the supervisor takes his problem to the Administrator, who reviews the actual effect such scratches have on the end product. It is discovered that a scratch or burr on this particular surface can cause the product's electric system to short out and can actually ruin the entire finished item. The Administrator and one of the electronic engineers visit the area and show the employees the harm this type of defect can cause. They bring along a unit that failed the final test because of such an error. Usually, workers respond to this sort of explanation and try to avoid any further defects. All the Administrator has done is to use a technique derived from the earlier product/quality awareness phase.

Another situation would be the case of workers having trouble identifying the correct part for assembly. This happens often where color coding is impractical and hundreds of thousands of similar parts are available in supply bins. One ZD organization had a problem with matching connectors. It was discovered that parts-matching information was available in specification manuals located some distance away from the work area. It would have been too expensive to supply each line or worker with a set; even if this information were supplied, the line worker would have to waste valuable time searching through it. The answer was to have a draftsman draw up two circular scales showing the parts match. These were reproduced on card stock, cut out, and grommeted together (see Figure 71). All the worker had to do was match the outer circle with the inner circle to discover which plug matched what socket. All it cost was about two hours of drafting time, a few dollars in printing costs, and about thirty minutes in assembly. The result was that twenty-five employees didn't make errors in matching connectors. Rework on such errors had cost the organization anywhere from $25 to $50 per error.

This sort of specific aid does not pertain to manufacturing activities alone. Take the case of damaged and messy page frames found in one organization's production typing pool. The supervisor was aware that the typists' desks were cluttered, contributing to the problem, but he could not identify any direct cause. None of his workers had come up with the error cause either. The Administrator, being somewhat removed from their activities, was invited in to take a fresh look at the problem. After reviewing the fact that the typists' desks were cluttered with everything from finished manuscripts to handwritten input copy, he inquired why it was necessary to have all that material on the desk tops. The fact that the typists needed to refer to the material constantly brought about his second question: why didn't they use the sorting shelves and files in their desk pedestals to keep the finished pages protected, yet handy? A look into one desk gave him the answer. The girls were using the file drawer to hold their purses and shoe bags. Further checking disclosed there was no room available in the area for personal-effects lockers; so he

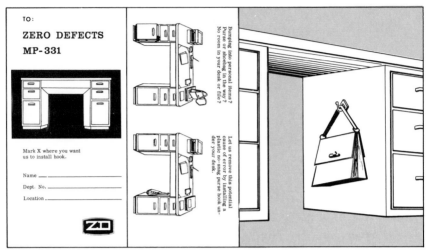

<small>TO:

ZERO DEFECTS
MP-331

Mark X where you want
us to install hook.

Name ____

Dept. No. ____

Location ____

Bumping into personal items?
Purse or shoebag in the way?
No room in your desk or file?

Let us remove this potential
cause of error by installing a
plastic no-snag purse hook under your desk.</small>

FIG. 72   Extended ECR application. This purse-hook offer was the result of an Error Cause Identification request for a technique for keeping a desk free of personal effects.

looked for a less obvious answer. The solution turned out to be simple: small plastic hooks were attached to the inside of each desk wall on which the girls could hang their purses and shoe bags (see Figure 72). Freed of the problem of where to put their personal effects, they put the desk files to correct use, and the defect rate took a downward curve. The hooks cost 12 cents each—a single typed page frame is valued at $1.75.

The point here is that both the supervisor and the individual employee will encounter problems that normal procedures or even ECR can't seem to solve. It is the Administrator's function to provide an answer or, at least, to provide a probable avenue of corrective action. What if the Administrator is deluged with this type of request? If this point is ever reached, he should be the happiest Administrator in the country. He then would have proof positive that his program was a complete success; for he no longer would need to go out and ask the individual to support the program—it would be a case of the individual coming to the program for help.

Administrator Action

The Administrator may also initiate specific-problem-area support action of his own. Such action is usually the result of problem identification through some other program phase. For instance, he could offer a specific solution to other areas having a likelihood of similar problems. The purse-hook solution was in fact offered to every secretary in the organization involved and over 90 percent of the girls requested this device. As mentioned earlier, this particular technique is a natural extension of the ECR program. The Administrator should review all such actions for possible wider application. The recognition phase offers similar possibilities. When the Administrator discovers a new and effective measurement criterion used in a hard-to-measure area, he should forward this information to supervisors having measurement problems with similar tasks.

Recognition promotion can also be directed to specific areas and individuals. If the Administrator learns that a certain area has not produced any achievers and, through follow-up, discovers the reason is lack of achievement, he may wish to take positive promotional action. He can go back through his achievers and select those having tasks similar to those in the low-achievement area. These achievements may be posted or distributed on information sheets to all the employees in that area. The message here is that "it can be done," and real examples of effort by fellow employees back up the Administrator's story.

Awareness of Specific Support

Though the primary reason for getting down to specifics is to counteract the law of diminishing returns, there is another strong sustaining factor in such activity. Such action, whether on the supervisor level or with the individual employee, presents proof positive that management will back up its policies with action. It helps to assure every employee that his problems are management's problems. It brings new importance to the individual task. It returns us to the basic program concept—a strong reason for every employee to have a constant, conscious desire to do every job right the first time (see Figure 73).

OTHER SUSTAINING TECHNIQUES

One of the primary rules for efficient program administration is to use what you have. Do not use new media or techniques simply because they haven't been used before. If the Administrator keeps his eyes open, he will continually discover new program vehicles existing within his own organization.

Special-events Tie-in

A visit by an important customer or government official always provides possibilities for the alert Administrator. Though these people may not have been specifically invited to support the program, their presence can be turned into a ZD plus. A few minutes spent talking to employees in a specific problem area or a short meeting with a group of supervisors may be all that the man's schedule will allow. Yet, even such brief exposure will pay off when the effects of several such visits are tallied up.

In cases where organization-wide vacation shutdown is the policy, the Administrator should always reemphasize ZD upon the employees' return. A back-to-work theme has almost unlimited promotional possibilities, such as a rededication week, a reemphasis of ECR, a back-to-work rally, a new product awareness drive, and others.

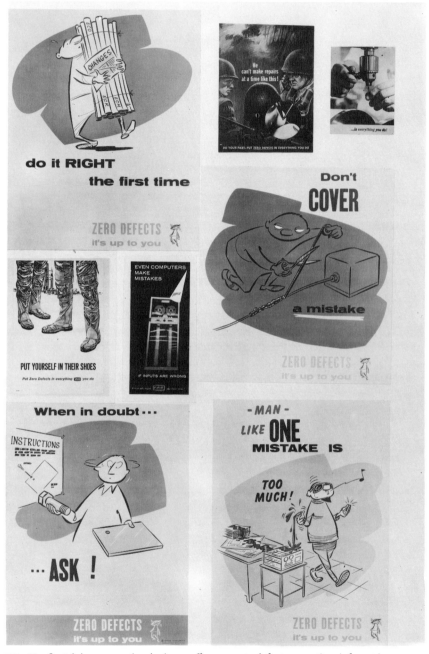

FIG. 73 Sustaining promotional pieces offer concrete defect-prevention information or are directed toward specific areas of interest.

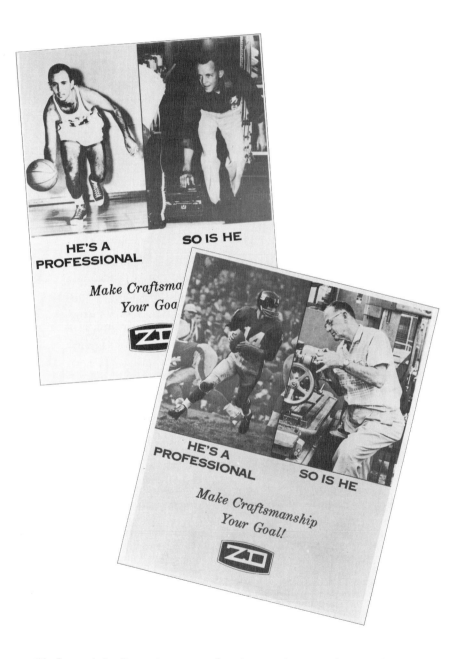

FIG. 74   Sports tie-in. Comparison posters featuring popular sports figures and achievers.

Several organizations have successfully tied their programs to seasonal activities and sports. One organization compares its achiever "pros" with famous professionals making sports headlines (see Figure 74). Another relates excellence in seasonal recreational activities to tasks within the plant. This treatment goes back to the basic philosophy, in accordance with which an employee is shown that he seeks perfection in his bowling game but does not set such high standards on the job.

A new-product introduction is always the signal for a new Zero Defects drive. All workers need to be made aware of the product, its importance to the company, its service to the customer, and the need for quality effort in every step of the production process. With new products usually come new management, new organizations, and new production lines. All the management and supervisors involved should be brought into the program and the importance of ZD to the new product put across.

New Employees

Like new projects, new employees who have not been exposed to the program must be watched for by the Administrator. The employee relations committee representative can be asked to help out in this area. The Administrator should receive the names and assignments of all new hires; he can then mail a simple reminder to the new employee's supervisor or manager, recalling their obligation to present the program to the new hire. This reminder could also

FIG. 75   If at all possible, a special Zero Defects section should be included in any general, new-employee material.

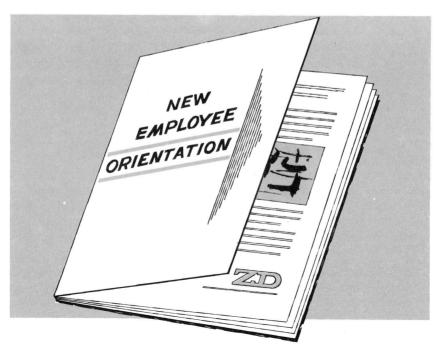

include a pledge card and a pin to stimulate action. If the organization has formal new-employee indoctrination sessions, ZD can simply be inserted as part of the program (see Figure 75).

The Administrator should also be made aware of all promotions. A person previously indoctrinated as a supervisor who is promoted to a higher management position assumes a new role in the Zero Defects program. If possible, the Administrator should handle these upgraded briefings personally. This special attention will add to the man's new stature and make him a stauncher supporter of the program and its goals.

Timing

Too much of anything wears thin. If sustaining promotion is improperly timed, ZD attitudes can become like those of the pit band in a burlesque house: the program's most active supporters can become immune to the message. A steady stream of ZD promotion and publicity causes the same reaction as no promotion or publicity at all. The impact technique, mentioned in Chapter 10, prevents oversaturation with ZD promotional material. A well-timed program featuring four to six impact weeks through the year will keep the program message before the employees. By tying recognition activities and other special events to impact dates, the program will always have something new to say and will never become dull routine (see Figure 76).

The schedule of impact periods should remain flexible enough to take advantage of special or unplanned events. The Administrator should be organized well enough to implement one of these program-impact sessions with one or two weeks notice. Thus, he will always be able to keep his program current and in the mainstream with the rest of the organization's activities.

FIG. 76 Internal promotion should be scheduled so that specific messages reach the audience at specified times. A schedule plan such as this will help to avoid a confused haze of promotional material and will allow each internal program its own emphasis period. The open dates are retained for special events and extra-emphasis promotions for the existing programs.

PROMOTION SCHEDULE						
	Jan	Feb	Mar	Apr	May	June
1–15	Bonds	Open	Safety	ZD Anniversary	Value Engineering	Open
16	ZD	Value Engineering	Security	Safety	Security	Vacation Notice

PROMOTION SCHEDULE						
	July	Aug	Sept	Oct	Nov	Dec
1–15	Vacation	ZD	Education Courses	Value Engineering	ZD	Security
16	Open	Security	Safety	United Appeal	Open	Safety

Sharing

At this printing there are over 1,000 ZD organizations in the United States. Almost without exception, each of these groups has produced some unique or different type of promotion to meet a specific need. If the Administrator keeps in contact with his opposites in industry in his immediate area, he will have access to dozens of new ideas each year. In many cases the applications may be so similar that poster art work and other promotional material may be borrowed and used as is at little additional expense. Other Administrators will welcome such exchanges since all parties gain under such circumstances.

SUMMING UP

Sustaining an organization's Zero Defects-program impact depends on the Administrator's imagination and perseverance. All the tools are at his disposal. Almost all of the earlier steps provide natural avenues of promotional and motivational carry-on. If the Administrator stays with his program and makes sure that all the basic work is accomplished, the program will largely sustain itself. As long as the Administrator continues to grind away at the defect problem, with the realization that any defect, no matter how small, is one defect too many, the program will continue to show the outstanding accomplishments almost always associated with first-year effort.

As the Zero Defects concept spreads—and all indications are that it will—industry and government Administrator workshops will spring up with regularity on the business scene. Defense industry Administrators have already organized to facilitate sharing ideas and techniques. As more commercial organizations join the ranks, this exchange should increase in scope and value. Like any other professional, it behooves the Administrator to keep abreast of his field. He should try to attend seminars, workshops, and other activities as a contributor to this new and exciting quality awareness method. Last year alone, over 100 articles about ZD appeared in trade magazines, professional journals, and consumer media. Most of this material was well presented, and almost all provided new and fresh ideas about many facets of the ZD program.

Thus, the Administrator who actively participates in his profession and keeps his own interest alive can't help but communicate his enthusiasm and determination to the rest of the program organization.

16

The Future of Zero Defects

So far we have covered the philosophy, the history, the implementation, the recognition, and the sustaining factors of the Zero Defects program. These are all things of the past or present. As to the future, the challenge of the program is even greater because of the rapidly changing influences in our business and industrial community—automation, high specialization, and mounting pressure on management as well as on the individual worker. During these challenging times, programs like Zero Defects can and will keep these spiraling activities in their proper perspective. ZD is needed to add continuity to the overall picture.

Just how does Zero Defects fit into the overall picture? What role will it play in the lives of Americans thirty years from now? In these days of rapidly changing technologies, no one has the complete answer to the question, but some general conclusions can be drawn from what we have seen so far.

First of all, both government and industry have one common major goal: the best possible product or service, at the lowest possible price, delivered to the customer when he wants it. Any organization that meets these criteria is well on its way to success. The prime elements are quality, cost, and schedule. ZD directly supports all three. The quality element is obvious. The program's record of scrap and rework savings supports the cost element. The reduction of lost time through elimination of rework and reinspection hours takes one of the basic burdens off the scheduling element. Thus, Zero Defects can and will assure management a strong market position in the years to come.

Keeping Ahead of Competition

ZD is not a panacea for the world's business ills. It creates the proper environment or attitude necessary for other, more mechanical, business remedies to take effect. For example, as competition becomes keener, companies must come up with new and better products or services if they are to maintain their market position. This accelerated push into research and development can't be done on a hit-or-miss basis. The old argument that research can't be rushed was washed down the drain in World War II. Yet, this attitude prevails in many of our labs and design studios today. Prior to ZD, management rarely had the tools needed to measure and evaluate personal performance in these areas. With the advent of ZD, the very people who had resisted measurement and other sound business practices began looking for these techniques themselves, not so that management could play "watchdog," but so that the individual could see where he stood and thus plan his future efforts in a way that past mistakes would not be repeated. This was not a case of the ZD Administrator *doing* something. It was a case of the program setting the stage and creating the environment so that others could take action. The result is that many ZD organizations now have every area of their operations under some sort of sound, businesslike evaluation system. Top management's reins have been tightened—not by the "driver"—but by individuals down at the other end doing the "pulling."

The Challenge of Automation

What becomes of Zero Defects as automation sets in? Automation is becoming a fact of business life; automation is drastically changing the social and economic picture. Since it is a real factor, what can management do to make the transition easier and more rewarding all the way around? ZD provides a natural answer. When we reflect on the influences that brought about the need for Zero Defects, we find that these same factors are even more evident in the automated operation. The dial-reading, button-pushing worker has an even more drastic problem of product or purpose identification. If he makes an error, he can usually blame it on the machine and get away with it. After all, the machine makes the product or provides the service. As tasks become more technical and less physical, they become, in fact, easier. Today's automated systems warn the operator of impending error, take their own corrective action, or simply stop and wait for the operator to find the problem and to start the activity down the correct trail once more. Yet when an error does creep in, it is usually a big one. The worker who previously made fifty operations in a day now makes ten times that many in an hour. A single defect can multiply itself into a tremendously costly mess in a few minutes under such circumstances. Unless constant, conscious awareness can be pumped into what may seem like a simple, automatic job, scrapping costs can skyrocket.

Automated inspection and rejection methods do not completely protect the producer. When a human inspector misses an error, it is usually because of a momentary breakdown of his defect-awareness facilities. In the case of a machine, the breakdown becomes repetitive and can continue until some other device further down the line (perhaps days later) calls it to the operator's attention. Thus, one input error by the operator of the inspection device is compounded. Whereas the human inspector had to be alert eight hours a day, the automated-inspection-machine operator faces this problem only at the time of data input and during periodic checks. Alertness is no longer a way of life but rather something to be turned off and on like an automobile engine. ZD can give the operator purpose of action and provide sound reason for a constant, conscious attitude of defect awareness.

To sum up: As human mass-production techniques give way to automation, management must not make the mistake of reducing the importance of the individual again. As new machines and new tasks are created, ZD must be right there assuring the employee that management still relies on individual accomplishment.

Change

As industry, commerce, government, and social order change, so do policies and techniques governing these activities. ZD fifty years from now will probably no more resemble today's program than ZD today resembles the quality-assurance programs of ten years ago. This change is inevitable and natural. What will remain the same will be the basic individual needs that created the program in the first place.

As long as there are people, there will always be challenges. Management, unions, government, and the individual can meet these challenges as long as there are avenues of common interest for all to walk upon. By keeping the ZD program alive, by constantly adding to and building upon the program's sound foundation, these avenues can be kept open indefinitely.

At the start, there was only an idea and a name—Zero Defects. A few people took it to heart and made a program out of it. Another group came along and added Error Cause Removal. Dozens more contributed to the implementation techniques behind the program. Later, thousands of individuals contributed methods of measurement, extending the program into almost every task and endeavor in business and industry. Some of these changes took place so rapidly and automatically that the reasons for the changes and advances often weren't discovered until long after they had been accepted. ZD was and *is* changing to meet the needs of the millions of people who have adopted it. It is alive, and as a living program, it is bound to stay in a state of flux.

Change for the sake of change is generally wasteful; but progressive, purposeful change is a symbol of the organization that means to stay in business and continue growth regardless of the economic picture or competitive influences. So it is with ZD. The Administrator should not grab at everything that comes to mind in an effort to come up with "something different." He should take what he has, apply it to everything in his path, and come up with the new only where the old won't serve his purposes. This, in fact, is the story of ZD. ZD is nothing new: it is a case of sound business practices being put to use on a carefully organized basis.

A NEW PHASE FOR ZD

In an effort to follow this philosophy of change, the author is offering a new phase to the basic program procedure. And like many of the other program phases, it is really not new but is, rather, a reemphasis of another sound business practice. What is important is that it fills a gap by taking another look at one of the things management generally takes for granted.

To comprehend fully the importance of this phase, we must first go back to the very beginning of the ZD program. The program was needed because management took it for granted that a worker would normally try to do a good job on every task and that defects were the result of momentary slips due to human frailty—"nobody's perfect."

The program pioneers put that old saw to bed by using the following line of reasoning: a worker does some things with a reasonable degree of perfection; he expects perfection in certain instances and turns his back on it in others; why can't he be made to see that he can attain this same reasonable degree of perfection in everything? Then, to set the stage, our pioneers provided the worker with the best possible tools, the best possible education, and went to work on the remaining worker-attitude problem with outstanding success.

Now, along came some other people who said these program pioneers were assuming too much. Their success would be greater if they would go back to that tool or facility and take another look. They suggested that since Zero Defects was beamed at the individual, the individual should participate in the question of defect-free tools, facilities, and procedures. In that way he would be calling his own shots and would not be able to say "I made an error because I didn't have the proper resources." Thus, the successful ECR phase was born.

What assumption is left? *Education!* Can it be that we assumed too much in this aspect also? Whether we did or did not, the subject is worth looking into.

THE NATURE OF EMPLOYEE EDUCATION

In order to make a decision, we must first inspect some other assumptions that surround the worker "knowledge" question. How are employees trained?

There are many answers to this question, but the most common are experience, college and technical schools, and company-sponsored training sessions. An organization can gain the benefit of the first two by selective hiring. The last comes with management initiative and investment. In this day and age, the "unskilled" worker has all but disappeared from the business scene. Almost everyone has some sort of formal training behind his task or general work requirement. Thus, if anything is lacking, it is to be found in the very nature of this training.

Is it enough to show a man how to do a task, let him practice until he feels he can do it reasonably well, give him a test to check out, and then put him to work? This is how most companies and schools handle the problem. But perhaps we are not giving the individual everything he needs to do the job and do it well. Is it enough to show a man how to make a good solder connection on a certain type of plug assembly when that will be his only task for the next six months to a year? At first glance it does not seem that he needs anything else.

The truth is that this is where management should make its basic ZD wishes known. Obvious management action at this primary phase of the learning cycle can, and will, do much to make the rest of the program phases fall into line in the eyes of the individual. Through ECR we have shown him that management cares about his individual needs as far as facilities and procedures are concerned. Through the basic program activities, we have shown him that management cares about each and every task in the organization. Through recognition, we have shown him that management is aware of achievement (or lack of the same) and expects top performance from everyone involved. Why does management usually take a back seat when it comes to the education that prepares the individual to meet its goals?

A PLAN OF ACTION

This phase, in which management can insert its presence and needs into employee education, is perhaps the least complicated and least costly portion of the ZD program. Any thinking Administrator should be able to come up with dozens of ways the ZD philosophy and concept can be interjected into in-house training programs. Regularly scheduled management visits to training sessions is one method. Another would be to include a management presentation into every lesson plan—whether the course is welding, marketing, high-speed typing, sales techniques, or any other course the organization sponsors. And by a presentation, we do not mean a brief appearance by management on graduation day. The individual is being trained to do something more than simply weld, type, or sell and this should be built into the basic framework of the course.

What about the employee who receives his training outside the organization?

Does management have less responsibility to this individual? Management that sits back and says it has no control over this element is no different from the worker who says, "I know I can't do it perfect every time," when he hasn't even tried.

How long has it been since your top management ventured into the academic world to explain industry's and government's needs and desires to the student? Of course, the Senior Executive appears at a graduation ceremony once or twice a year to receive a degree and to tell the class that there is a world of opportunity outside the ivy-covered walls. But where were business and government management when the student was looking for solid facts, when he was in class trying to learn? The school can only present skill or knowledge. The true importance of the knowledge becomes evident only when the student leaves school and enters the outside world of business and industry.

How long has it been since one of the key members of your management spoke before an audience of students? How long since your director of manufacturing visited the classes in your community's trade schools? How many times has your administrative executive spoken to the freshman class of the nearest business school? Have you ever thought of sending the Senior Executive's secretary on a field trip to the local secretarial schools?

If the answers are no or never, it is certainly not because the schools do not welcome such visits and talks. It is doubtful that there is a school or instructor in the country who would not welcome a qualified expert from business or government with open arms. What better way to put our passing-grade complex into proper perspective for the student?

The possible objection to such activities, that they are a "buckshot" approach and do not reach a specific employee audience, does not stand up. For years, business, industry, and government organizations have been making grants and offering scholarships to schools and universities. This is done with the full knowledge that most of the people affected will never work for the grant-giving organization. It is done with the hope that those who do will be well prepared for the task ahead and of service to the sponsoring organization. It is done with the knowledge that general improvement in the standards of the profession involved results in gains for everyone in the field.

THE ROLE OF ZD IN OUR NATION'S FUTURE

By constantly being aware of change and by adjusting the program to meet each new challenge, management can keep the Zero Defects contribution to our local and national economy alive for many years to come. By reviewing what has passed and by looking for new adaptions for the future, every organizational program can maintain the same impact and vitality seen on kickoff day. As the individual succeeds, so does the industry and the nation. The key force in the whole structure is the individual—the individual worker, supervisor, manager, and executive. Zero Defects must never be thought of as a thousand-man program or even a ten-man program; to guarantee continued success, it must always be a one-man or individual program.

To consider the true role of ZD in our nation's future economy, study our national goals and desires. If ZD helps to meet those goals, it has a place in the plans of our government. These goals can best be seen through the eyes of the individuals who make up our country. Take the housewife, for example.

Have Shoppers Stopped Looking?

Not long ago, a housewife wandering down the aisle of a department store would invariably turn an object over to see what country's stamp the item carried. She did it out of habit, born of a need for reassurance that the item in question was not a flimsy product imported from country X. Nowadays, country X has managed to remove this concern from the minds of shoppers. Quality and fine workmanship have replaced an image of papier-mâché and plaster.

Meantime, what has happened to the formerly reassuring image of our own stamp? Has it lost its value because it is no longer necessary to be wary of the products of others? Or have the items carrying "Made in USA" actually dropped in quality over the past thirty years? Regardless of the reason, "Made in USA" is not the seal it once was. While others have improved, we have either regressed or stood still.

How do you improve a country's product image? We only have to look to country X for the answer. Rapid as the improvement was, its reputation for quality of product was not accomplished overnight or as the result of efforts in one product or product line. It was the direct result of thousands of companies and millions of workers striving for a bigger share of domestic and world markets. Names like Nikon, Sony, Honda, and Datsun are now not only accepted but are respected throughout the world.

What can our government do to meet this challenge? Nothing. Special tax relief and protective tariffs do not contribute to the quality of the national product. If anything, they may appear to reflect a government attitude that our products can't compete quality- and cost-wise on the open market. The government can only offer advice and encouragement. This it has done by

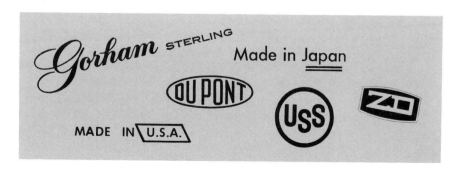

endorsing programs such as Zero Defects to American industry. From this point on it is really up to the individual. If "Made in USA" is ever to regain its place as the hallmark of world quality, it will be through the efforts of millions of Americans doing their day-to-day tasks with the firm conviction that craftsmanship still has a place in modern-day United States of America. No matter how you cut it, pride in performance is a personal thing.

Zero Defects—*it's up to you!*

APPENDIX A

APPENDIX A   Zero Defects pledge card.

The Zero Defects Program is aimed at providing a conscious effort, on the part of each of us, to get every job done right the first time.

Its goal is personal excellence which will eliminate defects by prevention.

It will assist our Company in its campaign to provide "more defense per dollar."

It will enable our Employees to give the nation a company product of which each of us can be proud.

ZERO
DEFECTS

Front

I freely pledge myself to constantly strive for improved quality of workmanship and will be ever conscious that I am an important part in each of our successes.

signed...........................

Prevention Not Detection

Back

APPENDIX **B**

APPENDIX B-1   Typical Achievement Award Recommendation form (front).

ZD

ACHIEVEMENT AWARD RECOMMENDATION

EMPLOYEE'S NAME		PERIOD
		TO

OCCUPATION TITLE   DEPARTMENT NAME   DEPT. NO.   CLOCK NO.

READ INSTRUCTIONS ON REVERSE SIDE BEFORE COMPLETING THIS FORM

SCOPE OF TASK:

ACHIEVEMENT:

AWARENESS:

OTHER FEATURES:

SUMMARY:

(USE REVERSE SIDE OF THIS FORM IF ADDITIONAL SPACE IS NEEDED)

SUPERVISOR'S SIGNATURE   SUPERVISOR'S TITLE   MANAGER'S SIGNATURE   MAIL POINT

ROUTE FOR ACTION TO: TITLE   LOCATION   MAIL POINT   DATE
     Z D REPRESENTATIVE

FOR ZERO DEFECTS ADMINISTRATION USE ONLY:

AWARD DENIED AND REASON

ACHIEVEMENT VERIFIED BY   ZERO DEFECTS REPRESENTATIVE SIGNATURE

APPENDIX B-2   Typical Achievement Award Recommendation form (back).

INSTRUCTIONS

THIS FORM IS TO BE COMPLETED BY A SUPERVISOR WHO BELIEVES THAT ONE OF HIS SUBORDINATES DESERVES OUTSTANDING RECOGNITION FOR HIS CONTRIBUTION TO THE ZERO DEFECTS PROGRAM. COMPLETE THE ENTIRE FORM EXCEPT FOR THE AREA LEFT FOR ZERO DEFECTS ADMINISTRATION. BE BRIEF, BUT BE SURE TO GIVE ENOUGH INFORMATION SO THAT A PERSON NOT FAMILIAR WITH YOUR GROUP'S ACTIVITIES CAN THOROUGHLY UNDERSTAND THE BASIS OF YOUR RECOMMENDATION.

SCOPE OF TASK: DESCRIBE THE TASK THE EMPLOYEE WAS ASSIGNED WHICH LED TO THE ZERO DEFECTS ACHIEVEMENT.

ACHIEVEMENT: DESCRIBE HOW THE EMPLOYEE HAS CONTRIBUTED TO THE ZERO DEFECTS PROGRAM. GIVE SPECIFIC DETAILS AND PERTINENT FACTS AND FIGURES.

AWARENESS: DESCRIBE THE EMPLOYEE'S INTEREST AND EFFORTS IN OTHER ASPECTS OF THE ZERO DEFECTS PROGRAM, SUCH AS PRIDE IN HIS WORK, REDUCING ERRORS, SUGGESTIONS FOR IMPROVEMENTS, PREVENTION OF OTHERS' ERRORS AS WELL AS OWN, ETC.

OTHER FEATURES: DESCRIBE OTHER FEATURES OF THE EMPLOYEE'S WORK, SUCH AS GENERAL ATTITUDE, JUDGMENT, PROBLEM SOLVING ABILITY, IMPROVEMENT IN JOB PERFORMANCE, ETC.

SUMMARY: DESCRIBE ANY ADDITIONAL FACTORS NOT COVERED PREVIOUSLY THAT YOU CONSIDER IMPORTANT TO THIS RECOMMENDATION.

ONCE YOU HAVE COMPLETED THIS FORM, SECURE THE APPROVAL OF YOUR DEPARTMENTAL MANAGER AND FORWARD THE FORM TO THE DEPARTMENT ZERO DEFECTS REPRESENTATIVE.

THE REPRESENTATIVE WILL REVIEW THE RECOMMENDATION AND EITHER: 1. APPROVE IT AND SEND IT TO THE ZERO DEFECTS AWARDS COMMITTEE, OR 2. DISAPPROVE IT AND RETURN IT TO THE DEPARTMENT MANAGER. THE AWARDS COMMITTEE WILL NOTIFY THE REPRESENTATIVE AS TO WHEN AND HOW THE EMPLOYEE IS TO RECEIVE RECOGNITION.

APPENDIX C

APPENDIX C-1   Typical ECR form (snap outs shown on next three figures).

APPENDIX C-2   Front of first and second sheets of ECR form.

ZERO **ZD** **DEFECTS**   QAN - 07159

ERROR CAUSE IDENTIFICATION

NAME		LOCATION	MAIL POINT

OCCUPATION TITLE		DEPT.	CLOCK NO.	☐ HOURLY / ☐ SALARY

IN ORDER THAT A BETTER JOB BE PERFORMED TOWARD THE GOAL OF ERROR-FREE PERFORMANCE, I AM IDENTIFYING THE FOLLOWING CAUSE OR POTENTIAL
CAUSE OF ERROR:

_____

_____

_____

_____

_____

_____

_____

_____

_____

_____

_____

_____

_____

_____

_____

_____

IMPORTANT INFORMATION

IF, IN ADDITION TO IDENTIFYING ERROR CAUSE, YOU FEEL THAT YOU HAVE A WAY TO SOLVE IT, PLACE THIS SOLUTION IN THE ABOVE AREA.
IF ADDITIONAL SPACE IS REQUIRED, USE A SEPARATE SHEET, ATTACH IT TO THIS FORM AND PLACE A CHECK IN THE FOLLOWING BLOCK.   ☐

THE ERROR CAUSE IDENTIFICATION PORTION OF THE ZERO DEFECTS PROGRAM IS NOT A SUBSTITUTE FOR THE SUGGESTIONS AWARDS PROGRAM.

IF YOUR SOLUTION IS ADOPTED, AS A COST REDUCTION TECHNIQUE, YOU MAY ALSO BE ELIGIBLE FOR A SUGGESTION AWARD.   REMEMBER, YOU MUST FILL OUT
AN ADDITIONAL FORM TO BE ELIGIBLE FOR THE SUGGESTION AWARDS PROGRAM.

ERROR CAUSE IDENTIFICATION IS NOT NECESSARILY RESTRICTED TO YOUR OWN WORK AREA - THE SITUATION MAY EXIST ANYWHERE IN THE PLANT.

IN ALL CASES, THE DECISION OF THE COMPANY WILL BE FINAL.   ALL IDEAS SUBMITTED BECOME THE PROPERTY OF THE COMPANY.

APPENDIX C-3   Back of first and second sheets of ECR form.

SUPERVISOR'S COMMENTS

SUPERVISOR'S NAME	ROUTE FOR ACTION TO: (NAME)	DATE TO BE RETURNED

ANSWER AND PLAN OF ACTION

EMPLOYEE RESPONSIBLE FOR ANSWER AND ACTION	DEPARTMENT NUMBER	CLOCK NUMBER

EMPLOYEE REVIEW		ADMINISTRATIVE REVIEW	
SATISFIED WITH FINDINGS: ☐ YES ☐ NO		ACTION BY: ☐ SUPERVISOR ☐ COMMITTEE	
SATISFIED WITH DECISION: ☐ YES ☐ NO		☐ OTHER DEPT. ☐ ADMIN.	
EMPLOYEE'S SIGNATURE	DATE	ADOPTED: ☐ YES ☐ NO	IN EFFECT: ☐ YES ☐ NO
		PROPOSED ACTION DATE:	SUSPENSE FILE: ☐ YES ☐ NO

APPENDIX C-4 Last sheet of ECR form.

ZERO **DEFECTS**   QAN - 07159

ERROR CAUSE IDENTIFICATION

NAME	LOCATION	MAIL POINT

Your ECI has been received and recorded, and we take this opportunity to thank you.

If any additional information is needed during the investigation of your ECI, you will be contacted. Your ECI will be forwarded immediately to the activity involved for a possible solution.

If you have any question regarding the disposition of your suggestion, kindly refer to the above ECI number.

Z D ADMINISTRATOR

APPENDIX **D**

Management Guide to Zero Defects

Supervisor's Handbook; For Management Use Only

ZERO DEFECTS—WHY?

The Zero Defects program offers timely support for the objectives of our determined effort to eliminate waste wherever it occurs in the programs of the Federal Government. I regard producing defect-free materiel—doing the job right the first time—as one of the finest means of getting the most for every dollar we must spend. LYNDON B. JOHNSON, PRESIDENT OF THE UNITED STATES

There is a very practical reason for contractors to give serious thought to the implementation of a workmanship motivation program such as Zero Defects. We of the Defense Department make every effort to spend our money where we can get the best deal—considering quality, performance, schedule, and cost. All of these factors are elements in evaluating the performance of our contractors. Thus, anything—anything at all—to improve your performance will enhance your own competitive posture and position. GEORGE E. FOUCH, DEPUTY ASSISTANT SECRETARY OF DEFENSE

This, in the words of the President and the Department of Defense, is why Zero Defects was conceived and why it must become a way of life. It is essential to our survival.

A Way of Life

July, 1962, saw the kickoff of the first Zero Defects program in American industry. Results surpassed the highest expectations: 54 percent reduction in the defect rate of manufactured hardware in the first year and an additional 25 percent the second year —approximately 2 million dollars saved in two years.

Obviously, Zero Defects is worthwhile. This fact has become apparent to the Department of Defense and to hundreds of other defense and commercial companies who have accepted the Zero Defects challenge.

Achieving such a Zero Defects record was no small undertaking in a large organization. It took the combined efforts of all employees with heavy emphasis by management. And it will take an even harder effort to continue and to surpass this record.

To reach our ultimate goal—to really motivate the individual to perform beyond the level usually demanded—requires a carefully planned and enthusiastically executed sustaining program. Zero Defects must continue to be a way of life for each individual.

The Supervisor's Role

Success of the Zero Defects program, particularly in sustaining the program, depends on you—the supervisor. Personal contact is absolutely necessary because Zero Defects must become a personal challenge to each employee, and only you have this daily personal contact. The employee is much more likely to accept the challenge if it is presented to him on a personal basis by you, his supervisor. Remember, in this action you have the complete support of top management.

You have a major share of the responsibility for (1) measuring your employee's Zero Defects achievements, (2) indoctrinating employees new to the company and your group, (3) motivating your people to strive constantly to raise their personal standards, and (4) identifying problem areas and instituting corrective action.

In these tasks, you will be supported by management and by a continuing promotional communication program of the Zero Defects administration. Do not hesitate to ask the help of your manager, Zero Defects representative, or Zero Defects Administrator. Management is behind you and the program 100 percent.

The Zero Defects administration, headed by the Administrator, is charged with running the Zero Defects program. The Administrator and his division representatives are the link between director-level management and the supervisory staff. Your primary contact is with the division Zero Defects representative. When you need assistance or information, see your representative. Furthermore, if you feel you have a unique approach to any part of the Zero Defects program, by all means inform the Zero Defects representative.

Remember two things about Zero Defects. First, you, as well as the employee and the company, benefit from the Zero Defects achievement. Your reputation, position, and future depend on the performance of your people. Second, Zero Defects may work without your 100 percent effort, but with it, Zero Defects will be an outstanding success for our customers, your people, and you.

Measuring and Recognizing Your People

The Zero Defects program, as any other motivational program, must offer some form of reward. Just what forms of reward are best? You know from your own experience that a personal "pat on the back" by the boss and the personal self-satisfaction of a job well done are what counts. Given these, most people will keep on doing a good job and will even strive to do a better job.

Measurement by the Supervisor. Measurement of Zero Defects effort within his own organization or department is almost exclusively the supervisor's responsibility. No one else can do it as well because no one else has the personal day-to-day contact with the employee. Supervisory judgment—your judgment—is the basis of all Zero Defects measurement.

Obviously, the object of the measurement of individual achievement is improvement in the performance of a task. Total Zero Defects may not be possible immediately. Thus, Zero Defects recognition must be given for the constant effort and desire to produce defect-free work, even though the result is not yet 100 percent.

On the basis of 100 percent performance, there may well be a number of employees in your group who qualify for recognition. Striving toward no mistakes is the goal of the program and the primary basis of measurement, but it is not enough upon which to base recognition. Other factors must be considered in your evaluation, including:

- Impact of potential errors (abort of mission, cost, effect on schedule, etc.)
- Difficulty of the job and the level of skill required
- Level of tediousness or boredom of the task
- Ability to prevent errors and correct errors before detection
- Experience on the job
- Attitude toward work, project, and company mission
- Degree of improvement in performance

Although these secondary measurement criteria have been successfully used in a variety of situations, they are not necessarily the only valid criteria. A particular situation in your area may call for others. If other criteria work for your group, use them. It is recommended, though, that you discuss such criteria with your manager and your Zero Defects representative.

How Do You Measure? Just how does a supervisor measure Zero Defects achievement? Through the normal supervisory duties of directing your people. Daily, constant observation of your people will give you a good indication of the performance standing of each. This supervisory observation, however, is only part of your measurement. When you recommend a person, you will be required to back up your recommendation with facts and figures. Thus, you must have specific data on which to base your recommendations. This means data on quantities of work done without defects in such terms as hours (1,800 hours machining defect-free), percent (0.05 percent typing errors), and functions (382 engineering functions defect-free).

You have available three common sources for such data: existing quality records, existing data not ordinarily used for quality rating, and special measurement techniques used to measure specific situations. Whatever data you use, do not base a recommendation on the dollars saved by avoidance of potential errors. The Zero Defects program aims to eliminate defects of all kinds and costs. Any defect is bad, regardless of its cost.

In each of the following areas of measurement (production, creative and professional, administrative, and service), an example of a recommendation is shown on an Achievement Award Recommendation form.* On each of these forms, you will note

---

*The implementing organization should fill out samples of the first sheet of the recognition form (see Appendix B) with appropriate information on a typical achiever for each area mentioned. One each for Production, Creative and Professional, Administrative, and Service.

that specific facts and figures are given in describing the achievement. Such information is very important since the Zero Defects recognition must be based on specific and verifiable achievements. Inclusion of complete information on the form will save both you and the Zero Defects representative time.

Production: In areas such as production, the work is often repetitive and results in definite end items. Here measurement is relatively easy because numerous types of quality records are readily available. Supervisory judgment can be substantiated by quality records of defects per unit of work or period of time.

Creative and Professional: Measurement of Zero Defects achievement in this area is usually considered difficult and often, impossible. But Zero Defects achievements in creating designs, concepts, and theories can be measured, and the criteria and data for such measurements do exist. In almost every case, this data is currently documented but is not recognized or used for ZD measurement. For example, when specifications call for a black box to mate with adjacent components and it does not, a measurable defect has been made. Whether correction is instigated by verbal orders or through a design change notice, the supervisor is usually aware of the defect. More often than not this defect data goes unused except for an occasional reprimand. Why not use the data to recognize those whose work is defect-free?

In general, five criteria apply to nearly all creative and professional tasks. Individual recognition through application of the criteria to a specific task, however, requires of the supervisor a comprehensive knowledge of his people and the details of their tasks.

- SPECIFICATION-REQUIREMENT ERROR: These errors, resulting from careless analysis of a specification, show up in DCN's, liaison call notices, material review board reports, test-result reports, and RT&E reports.
- INFORMATION-REVIEW ERROR: These errors are caused by lack of, or a careless, review of previous work and lead to duplication and misdirection of effort. Defects such as designing a unit that is readily available as an off-the-shelf item often are documented in value engineering and value or buy reports. The defect of designing a unit which cannot be manufactured usually shows up in liaison call reports. Other such errors are documented in the sources listed previously.
- CRAFT ERROR: Defects due to simple professional mistakes—such as slipping a decimal point, transposing a formula symbol, or misspelling—are usually noted in daily observations by the supervisor. However, they are documented in almost all of the previously mentioned sources.
- TASK SUCCESS: The degree of success or failure of a task should be measured at each task milestone rather than waiting for the conclusion of the task. This factor is one of the best yardsticks with which to measure group effort and thus, the achievement of a supervisor or manager. Customer acceptance is obviously the source of this data.
- ADMINISTRATIVE ERROR: Mistakes in procurement forms, job cards, expense and trip reports, and schedules are almost always covered by normal documentation.

If additional criteria are needed for specific situations, you can let your people set their own criteria. You must, however, examine these criteria to see if they are realistic and then submit them to the Zero Defects Administrator for review. Only in this way can the Administrator ensure that Zero Defects recognition is based on a relatively uniform standard of measurement.

Administrative: If you supervise an Administrative group, many forms of checking and periodic reporting are already available which are evaluated by the government for quality the same as a piece of hardware. In areas where no standard procedures exist, it is not too difficult to establish criteria. For instance, the following administrative factors can be used:

- NUMBERED FORMS: Such forms as purchase orders are normally audited; thus, a record can be kept of errors.
- TABULATION CARDS: Key-punch machines automatically keep a record of errors.
- TYPING: Make use of the normal review of typed material, but have a record made of the number of errors.

Service: If you supervise a service group, you probably will have to adapt some of your existing records not now used for quality measurement. Supervisory judgment is very important since maintenance men, painters, forklift operators, and other service personnel do not ordinarily work directly on a product. Most of their operations are not normally covered by quality-reporting systems. However, most do have characteristics that can be easily used as measurement standards. For example, transportation workers usually move objects only through a dispatching and trip-ticket system. Also, there is usually some system for accident reporting and accounting for damaged goods. This information can be used to record such factors as how many trips were completed without accident and how many items were handled without damage.

All Areas: However you measure achievement, remember four things:

- Your basic tool is your judgment as the employee's supervisor, backed up by data which give concrete facts and figures.
- Recognition is of prime importance in motivating your people to do outstanding work, and measurement is the basis of recognition.
- Only outstanding achievement should be recognized.
- Measurement must be on a completely unbiased and impartial basis.

When Do You Measure? Since measurement is based on supervisory judgment and observation, you will be informally evaluating your people on a daily basis. Once you have spotted a potential Zero Defects achievement, you should compare that person's performance against the quality records you use to verify your judgment. After verification, you should evaluate the worker on the secondary criteria suggested in the previous section.

The employee's achievement for recognition must be recorded on the Zero Defects program Achievement Award Recommendation form. Follow the instructions shown on the back of the form. (A complete form is shown in Appendix B.) The completed form should be submitted to your department manager for approval and then forwarded to the division Zero Defects representative.

It is a good idea to evaluate each employee's Zero Defects efforts on a periodic basis. This way no one is overlooked. When you make the evaluation is up to you, but a natural time is when you make an employee's performance evaluation. Regardless of your timing, turn in recommendation forms on the first of the month.

The question occasionally arises: "What do I do when an employee already has received Zero Defects recognition but is still doing Zero Defects work?" The answer is, recommend that employee for recognition again on the basis of continued or new achievement.

Small-group Measurement

There may be times when you feel that a Zero Defects achievement is due to the efforts of a team of employees and that the team effort deserves recognition. This form of recognition is valid under certain conditions, but it should be avoided if possible. The primary purpose of the Zero Defects program is to motivate the individual person; thus recognition of groups loses much of the motivational effect on the individual. Perhaps the best rule to follow is to recognize a group for superior team performance only if each individual in the group deserves an award for his own individual achievement. If all members of the group do not deserve recognition, do not recognize the group but only the outstanding individuals. Other factors important to group recognition are:

- The team should not be larger than two or three members.
- Small-group achievement must be measured against the same standards as those used for the individual worker.
- If in doubt, call the Zero Defects representative or Administrator.

Recognition of Achievement

Your Zero Defects achievement recommendations will be reviewed by the Zero Defects award council. If the council approves your recommendation, you will be notified about when and where the recognition will be given. If at all possible, you should personally attend the ceremony with the employee. When an employee in your group receives recognition, you deserve to share in this recognition.

The recognition pin will be awarded by top management, but you will award the employee his certificate of Zero Defects recognition. This should be done before your assembled group to get the most motivational value from the award. You should also personally congratulate the person on his or her achievement. As was said previously, one of the greatest motivating forces for any employee is a pat on the back from management.

Maintaining Interest

The Zero Defects administration has a carefully planned program to sustain the interest of your people toward the goal of Zero Defects. This program is designed to show the employee (1) how his job is related to the products and (2) how his efforts are paying off for him personally as well as for the company and the customer. Banners, posters, table tents, signs, news articles, special assemblies, talks by management, and local news and television stories will be used to keep employee interest in Zero Defects high. To help keep you up to date in these and other aspects of the Zero Defects program, special seminars and workshops will be scheduled for supervisors. In these sessions, you will have the chance to learn new techniques of motivation and measurement as well as how the program is working in other parts of the company.

Your part in the sustaining activities is to maintain the personal relationship you established with your people. As in other phases of the Zero Defects program, personal contact is an absolute must. You are the only one who can provide this on a daily basis. There are a number of actions you can take:

- Use your group meetings to promote the concept and practice of Zero Defects.

- Promote Zero Defects in your daily contact with individuals.
- Establish the feeling that each of your people is an important member of the Zero Defects team in your group and the company.
- Call on your department manager, Zero Defects representative, or Administrator to talk to your people.
- Keep in touch with other groups to benefit from their experiences.
- Call your people's attention to accomplishments that they have made possible, such as a successful missile firing.
- Keep your people aware of their daily performance and achievements as well as of their chances of receiving recognition.
- Call attention to failures to show what happens when Zero Defects work is not done. But never publicly tie a failure to an individual. Zero Defects rewards achievement; it does not punish failure.
- Call on the Zero Defects Administrator for assistance with any specific problems.

Along with lending the "personal touch" to the sustaining program, you can judge by their Zero Defects achievement the amount of sustaining effort that is required in your group. If you find numerous errors and few achievements, both you and the Zero Defects administration need to work harder to motivate your people.

Above all, *get to know your people, gain their respect,* and boost Zero Defects at every opportunity.

Indoctrinating New Employees. When a new employee joins your group, especially if he is new to the company, discuss the concept and practice of Zero Defects with him or her at the earliest possible opportunity. Employees new to the company will be briefly introduced to the Zero Defects program during the initial indoctrination. However, it really is up to you as the new employee's supervisor to explain the personal aspect of Zero Defects. The new employee may well sign the Zero Defects pledge card when he "hires in," but he probably will not really understand or believe the personal commitment required of him unless you explain it to him personally. Just like all your other people, the new employee must believe that Zero Defects is important to his supervisor, his manager, and himself.

Pinpointing Problem Areas. If a sudden rise in the number of defects is noted in an area, investigate and determine the cause immediately. If necessary, call in the Zero Defects representative or Administrator and tailor a motivational program to counteract your specific problem.

You can hold special meetings with your group to explain the problem and how it can be corrected. Various promotion techniques also can be used. They should be inexpensive and yet easy to see and understand. In a maintenance area where dirty fuel filters are a problem, a Zero Defects reminder card can be placed inside the top lid of each worker's tool box. In a plating department where workers are carelessly handling gold-plated circuits, Zero Defects table tents with a reminder phrase on them can be placed on the work tables. Displaying the results and cost of an error, particularly if a damaged product can be obtained, is also very effective.

Where do you get such visual aids? See your Zero Defects representative. He will help you determine what is needed and then get them produced. This can be handled in forty eight hours if necessary. Also, he may already have some visual aids prepared for another application which will match your needs. In any case, the visual aids will be supplied at no cost to your group.

Along with pinpointing problem areas, you should periodically check your group's work functions for new ways to apply Zero Defects. Also, encourage your people to watch for new applications.

Error Cause Removal. Error Cause Removal is a tool to help the employee identify facilities or procedures which cause or could cause errors. With Error Cause Removal the employee can improve the chances of doing outstanding work. As a supervisor, you have two functions in Error Cause Removal: (1) inform the employee of the concept and practice of Error Cause Removal, and (2) investigate and then initiate action to correct problems identified by the employee.

Error Cause Removal is a definite part of the sustaining phase of the Zero Defects program. The concept and procedures for both employee and supervisor are explained in detail in the Zero Defects Error Cause Removal supervisor's handbook.

Key Points to Remember

To sum up the supervisor's role in sustaining the Zero Defects program, these are the important points to remember:

- Success of the Zero Defects program sustaining phase depends primarily on the supervisor.
- Only the supervisor has the daily personal contact with the people necessary to keep motivation high.
- The Zero Defects program will be a success only when the individual accepts as a personal challenge the concept of doing the job right the first time.
- Recognition of Zero Defects achievement is a prime factor in motivating the employee, and measurement of achievement is the basis of recognition.
- Recognition must be on a personal level since Zero Defects must be accepted by the individual as a personal challenge.
- Supervisory judgment, backed up by records and measuring techniques, is the basis of recognition.
- Measurement and recognition must be completely unbiased and impartial.
- Small groups of two or three employees can be recognized for superior team effort, but only under certain conditions.
- New employees must be indoctrinated with the concept and practice of Zero Defects, particularly the personal aspect, as soon as they join the organization.
- Error Cause Removal will help the employee identify facilities or procedures which cause or could cause errors.
- Sustaining interest in the Zero Defects program requires a constant effort to show the employee how Zero Defects benefits him or her personally.
- The supervisor must show a personal interest in the employee's Zero Defects efforts.
- Existing records should be used as sources of measurement data whenever possible.
- New measurement techniques should be devised when none of the existing ones suffice. (Check these out with the Zero Defects representative or Administrator before using them.)
- People will work to the performance level set by management.

APPENDIX E

Error Cause Removal

Zero Defects Supervisor's Handbook; For Supervisory Use Only

> *Directed at motivating people to prevent mistakes by developing a constant, conscious desire to do their job right the first time, the program uses every available management communications technique to achieve this end.* JAMES F. HALPIN, DIRECTOR, QUALITY, MARTIN COMPANY, ORLANDO DIVISION

Error Cause Removal: the Concept

Error Cause Removal is one of the important ways and means of keeping the Zero Defects program alive. A distinct part of the program, Error Cause Removal is most of all a tool to assist the employee to do each job right the first time! With it, the employee can identify facilities, processes, or procedures which cause or could cause mistakes and which make it difficult to perform defect-free work. Management can then use this information to eliminate these causes of error.

Regardless of the care with which an industrial complex is designed or equipped, some of the employees will face individual problems caused by the facilities. A left-handed employee operating a facility designed for the average right-handed employee may daily face small problems—each one of them a potential error causer. These problems are vitally important to the individual employee, yet may not be noticed by supervision.

At this point, a thought often occurs to the supervisor: Won't the employees take advantage of Error Cause Removal to alibi their mistakes and suggest costly and impractical facility changes? No! Experience has shown that employees use Error Cause Removal to improve their work. When combined with proper knowledge of the job,

215

Error Cause Removal frees the employee to concentrate on doing his job right the first time. The same experience also has shown that the Error Cause Removal phase of Zero Defects does not result in massive changes. Actual surveys and pilot studies indicate that changes are minimal from the company-cost standpoint. Typically:

- Ninety percent of the problems were corrected on the spot by the employee's immediate supervisor.
- Less than 10 percent required changes in procedures or minor facilities alterations which were handled by such departments as plant engineering.
- Less than 1 percent required costly and immediate facility or procedure modification.

Error Cause Removal gives the employee the opportunity to identify actual or potential causes of error, therefore improving his chances to do Zero Defects work.

Error Cause Removal: the Supervisor's Role

As a supervisor, you have two important functions in Error Cause Removal: (1) to inform the employee of the concept and practice of Error Cause Removal and (2) to investigate and take corrective action immediately after an employee identifies a problem.

You as a supervisor are the key to success of Error Cause Removal. You have the direct daily contact with the employee. Only *you* can explain Error Cause Removal to the employee on a personal basis and make or initiate corrections to problems caused by inadequate or improper facilities. Remember, more than 90 percent of these corrections can be handled by the supervisor using normal operating procedures.

Employee Indoctrination

The entire purpose of Error Cause Removal is to help the employee remove facilities or procedures problems which interfere with achieving Zero Defects. In your indoctrination, this is a philosophy that you must sell to the employee. Once he is wholeheartedly convinced that Error Cause Removal is designed to help him, he will enthusiastically participate, improving his defect record and that of your group. The degree of benefit received from Error Cause Removal is directly proportional to both the employees' and your intelligent use of the Error Cause Removal concept.

Personal contact with your employees, either individually or in small groups, is the most satisfactory method of presenting this phase of the Zero Defects program. If indoctrination must be done in large meetings, the employees should be given the opportunity to ask questions. If possible, discuss Error Cause Removal with your employees personally in the days following such a meeting.

You will be backed up by your department Zero Defects representative and the Zero Defects Administrator. Promotional material such as posters, table tents, brochures, and articles in company publications will provide support. Also, do not hesitate to call on your manager to help in the indoctrination. Management is behind you, and you as a supervisor must convey this to the employees. Before he does anything, the employee must feel that management cares.

Problems and Solutions

Error Cause Removal must not be confused with such programs as value engineering and suggestion awards. You must make it very clear to the employee that Error

Cause Removal is designed to identify and correct only those problems which cause or could cause errors. Thus, suggestions such as "How we can save money by cutting down paper consumption" have no place in Error Cause Removal. Such suggestions properly belong in the suggestion program.

The employee should not be limited to identifying problems with which he is personally involved, although this is the primary purpose of Error Cause Removal. He should be encouraged to identify any potential problem he sees. If the employee has a possible solution to the problem he identifies, he should submit both problem and solution on the Error Cause Identification form. Moreover, if the problem and solution meet the criteria for the employee suggestion program, they should also be submitted on the suggestion form. This will enable the employee to be rewarded for his suggestion while avoiding confusion between Error Cause Removal and existing suggestion programs. Error Cause Removal is not a substitute for the suggestion program.

Reporting Procedure

To identify existing or potential error-causing facilities or procedures, the employee must fill out an Error Cause Identification (ECI) form. (A small-size example of the ECI form is shown in Appendix C.) Actually your employees will probably come to you first to discuss the problem. But be sure they fill out an ECI form each time. The Zero Defects Administrator needs a form for each Error Cause Removal occurrence to direct the program. More importantly, a problem and the corrective action taken in your group may have application in another group. The ECI form is the only sure method of correlation. Any significant correction made in your group will be publicized for possible use in other groups.

On the form itself: The employee fills in the front. When you check it, be sure the problem is explained clearly and completely and that the employee's job information and location are complete. Tear off the third sheet and give it to the employee. This is his receipt and acknowledgment for having identified a problem.

The back of the ECI form is for your use, as well as that of the Zero Defects representative and the Administrator. The Comments section is for your evaluation of the problem. The Answer and Plan of Action section is for a summary of the corrective action. If you make or initiate the correction, you should fill in this data. If someone else makes the correction he should fill in the information. If the problem is not really a problem or if it is and cannot be corrected for some reason, this should be explained here. Whoever fills in this section should sign his name, department, and badge number in the appropriate place.

The Employee Review section is for the employee to indicate his satisfaction with the action taken on his ECI submittal. The Administrative Review section is for the use of the Zero Defects Administrator.

Correction Procedures

Problems with facilities fall into three general categories:
1. Those which the immediate supervisor can solve on his own, using normal procedures
2. Those which require action by department-level management
3. Those which require action by director-level management

Ninety percent of the problems fall into category 1—the ones *you* have to correct. About 10 percent involve category 2 and less than 1 percent category 3.

Whatever the category, you, as the supervisor, have the primary responsibility for correcting the problem or seeing that is brought to the attention of your superiors, if you cannot correct it. Your first action is to verify that a problem exists and to determine what must be done to correct it.

If the problem can be corrected on the spot, do so. Once the problem is corrected, have the employee complete the Employee Review section on the back of the ECI form. When you have completed the reverse side of the form, with the exception of the Administrative Review section, give the original to the employee and send the carbon copy to the Zero Defects representative or Administrator.

If the problem cannot be solved on the spot, there are several courses of action. A category 1 problem which requires help from another department, such as plant engineering, should be solved with the normal procedure for such cases. A category 2 problem which you feel is beyond your authority should be taken to your manager. He can then take the necessary action to correct the problem. With any category of problem, remember to keep your manager advised and seek his help whenever you need it.

When a problem falls in category 3 and cannot be corrected through normal company channels, you should indicate the results of your investigation on the ECI form. Besides stating the problem, you should define any possible corrections. Depending on your particular departmental procedures, this may be done with your manager or with only his approval. Whichever is the case, the form must be forwarded to the Zero Defects representative or Administrator. The Administrator will take the necessary action to correct the problem or bring it to the attention of the appropriate director. When the problem is corrected, it will again be up to you, as the employee's supervisor, to have him complete the Employee Review section of the ECI form.

Again, both you and the employee must complete the appropriate sections of the ECI form and send the carbon copy to the ZD Administrator at (location) _____

Immediate Action

Immediate action on an ECI form is imperative. No more than two weeks should elapse between submission of an ECI form by an employee and correction of the problem or, at least, notification of the problem status. Rapid follow-up convinces the employee that management is interested in his individual problems and that everything possible is being done to make his work potentially error-free.

Negative Replies

Undoubtedly, there will be occasions when an employee identifies something which is not truly a problem. There will also be problems which cannot be solved for financial or policy reasons and others which can be solved, but not immediately. If the problem is not realistic, you must tactfully convince the employee that the problem does not exist or, at least, that it is not caused by the facility. (Often the problem may really be caused by some unconscious action of the employee himself.)

Do not just write "No action required" in the Answer and Plan of Action section of the ECI form and leave it at that. Fully explain the reasons in writing on the form and verbally to the employee. Also, be sure to have the employee fill in the Employee Review section.

When the problem cannot be solved because the solution is too costly or company policy does not permit solution, this must be carefully explained to the employee. When the problem is real but for some reason cannot be corrected immediately, the reasons must again be explained to the employee and a date for future correction should be established.

A negative reply properly presented will provide a positive example of management's concern for the employee's problem. If the employee is convinced that management has seriously considered his problem, he will accept such a reply more readily.

Typical Cases

What kind of problem falls under the Error Cause Removal program? Almost anything that interferes with an employee's doing his job. The three cases described in the following paragraphs are typical of the kinds of problems that your employees will bring to your attention through the ECI form. The first one involves a simple matter and is typical of 90 percent of the cases.

A secretary found that she had to put her handbag either on the floor under her desk where it got dirty and was in the way of her feet or on top of her desk where it was in the way of her work. In either place it bothered her, both physically and psychologically. When the potential error-causing problem was brought to the attention of her supervisor through an ECI form, he secured a self-sticking plastic hook. By fastening it to the side wall of the center opening under the desk, the secretary was provided with a place to hang her handbag.

The following case is typical of the less than 10 percent of the ECIs that require help from another group.

A lamp-service man whose job was to replace burned-out fluorescent tubes used a cart to carry the fluorescent tubes and a ladder. The ECI form he submitted stated he had no place to put his ladder when it was not in use except on top of the cart where the fluorescent tubes were kept. This occasionally resulted in a broken tube. The employee suggested a pair of hooks be attached to the side of the cart from which the ladder could hang. He also submitted a design for the hooks. Agreeing with this solution, the supervisor contacted the metal shop and filled out the necessary service request to have the hooks fabricated and installed. Since the employee suggested a solution to the problem, he was also eligible for an award under the suggestion program.

The third case is typical of the less than 1 percent that require action by higher management.

A sheet-metal worker submitted an ECI form stating he had insufficient room to manipulate large sheets of metal into his sheet-metal break. The problem was that he had a working area of less than 4 feet between the machine and the wall of an adjacent production area. Investigation by the supervisor showed that the problem was real and even that some element of danger was involved when large, sharp-edged sheets had to be handled in such a confined space. At least 2 additional feet of space were needed for adequate and safe working room. Investigation also showed that the wall was semipermanent and that any move would interfere with the adjoining production area.

After discussing the problem with his manager and concluding that corrective action could not be taken, the problem was brought to the attention of the Zero Defects representative. On reviewing the supervisor's findings and ascertaining that a relatively major correction was required, the representative sent the form to the Zero Defects Administrator. Discussing the problem with the plant engineering department, the Zero Defects Administrator found that the production line was scheduled to be modified in three months to compensate for a projected model change. The decision was made to design the modified production line so that the wall could be moved back a minimum of 2 feet, giving the required working space on the sheet-metal break. Until the change could be made, to avoid both accidents and defects, no large pieces of metal were handled on the machines.

Error Cause Removal: Key Points

These key points should be remembered when the Error Cause Removal technique is used:

- Error Cause Removal is a tool to help the employee to do a better job.
- Error Cause Removal is a distinct part of the Zero Defects program.
- Error Cause Removal improves the employee's, as well as the group's, Zero Defects record.
- The more intelligently an employee uses Error Cause Removal, the more it will help him do Zero Defects work.
- Employees are irritated by things that are inconsequential to the organization but large to the individual.
- Error Cause Removal removes the excuse of not having proper facilities to do Zero Defects work.
- The employee must thoroughly understand the Error Cause Removal concept.
- The supervisor is essential to Error Cause Removal because he has the personal contact with the employees.
- Ninety percent of the problems highlighted by Error Cause Removal can be corrected by the employee's supervisor.
- Corrective action and replies to the employee must be fast, preferably within two weeks.
- Negative replies must be carefully explained.
- Error Cause Removal must be differentiated from the suggestion program and other in-house programs.

Index